Roshan Lall Gupta's
Recent Advances in
SURGERY

Roshan Lall Gupta's
Recent Advances in SURGERY

Volume 18

Editor

Puneet MS DNB (Surgery) MNAMS FACS
Professor
Department of Surgery
Institute of Medical Sciences
Banaras Hindu University
Varanasi, Uttar Pradesh, India

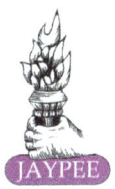

JAYPEE BROTHERS MEDICAL PUBLISHERS
The Health Sciences Publisher
New Delhi | London

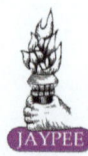 **Jaypee Brothers Medical Publishers (P) Ltd**

Headquarters
Jaypee Brothers Medical Publishers (P) Ltd
EMCA House, 23/23-B
Ansari Road, Daryaganj
New Delhi 110 002, India
Landline: +91-11-23272143, +91-11-23272703
+91-11-23282021, +91-11-23245672
Email: jaypee@jaypeebrothers.com

Corporate Office
Jaypee Brothers Medical Publishers (P) Ltd
4838/24, Ansari Road, Daryaganj
New Delhi 110 002, India
Phone: +91-11-43574357
Fax: +91-11-43574314
Email: jaypee@jaypeebrothers.com

Overseas Office
JP Medical Ltd
83 Victoria Street, London
SW1H 0HW (UK)
Phone: +44 20 3170 8910
Fax: +44 (0)20 3008 6180
Email: info@jpmedpub.com

EU GPSR Authorised Representative
LOGOS EUROPE, 9 rue Nicolas Poussin
17000, LA ROCHELLE, France
Phone: +33 (0) 6 67 93 73 78
Email: Contact@logos europe.eu

Website: www.jaypeebrothers.com
Website: www.jaypeedigital.com

© 2024, Jaypee Brothers Medical Publishers

The views and opinions expressed in this book are solely those of the original contributor(s)/author(s) and do not necessarily represent those of editor(s) or publisher of the book.

All rights reserved. No part of this publication may be reproduced, stored or transmitted in any form or by any means, electronic, mechanical, photocopying, recording or otherwise, without the prior permission in writing of the publishers.

All brand names and product names used in this book are trade names, service marks, trademarks or registered trademarks of their respective owners. The publisher is not associated with any product or vendor mentioned in this book.

Medical knowledge and practice change constantly. This book is designed to provide accurate, authoritative information about the subject matter in question. However, readers are advised to check the most current information available on procedures included and check information from the manufacturer of each product to be administered, to verify the recommended dose, formula, method and duration of administration, adverse effects and contraindications. It is the responsibility of the practitioner to take all appropriate safety precautions. Neither the publisher nor the author(s)/editor(s) assume any liability for any injury and/or damage to persons or property arising from or related to use of material in this book.

This book is sold on the understanding that the publisher is not engaged in providing professional medical services. If such advice or services are required, the services of a competent medical professional should be sought.

Every effort has been made where necessary to contact holders of copyright to obtain permission to reproduce copyright material. If any have been inadvertently overlooked, the publisher will be pleased to make the necessary arrangements at the first opportunity.

Inquiries for bulk sales may be solicited at: jaypee@jaypeebrothers.com

Roshan Lall Gupta's Recent Advances in Surgery (Volume 18)

First Edition: **2024**

ISBN: 978-93-5696-555-3

Dedicated to

My wife, Ritu Ragini
Son, Akshat and daughter, Aanya

CONTRIBUTORS

Aditya Baksi
Assistant Professor
Department of Surgical Disciplines
All India Institute of Medical Sciences
New Delhi, India

Ajay K Khanna
Professor
Department of Surgery
Institute of Medical Sciences
Banaras Hindu University
Varanasi, Uttar Pradesh, India

Arunima Verma
Professor
Department of Surgery
Tata Motors Hospital
Jamshedpur, Jharkhand, India

Arvind Kumar
Chairman
Institute of Chest Surgery
Chest Oncosurgery and Lung
Transplantation
Medanta—The Medicity
Multi-Specialty Hospital
Gurugram, Haryana, India

Ashish Singh
Associate Professor
Department of Surgical
Gastroenterology
Sanjay Gandhi Postgraduate Institute
of Medical Sciences
Lucknow, Uttar Pradesh, India

Asuri Krishna
Additional Professor
Department of Surgical Disciplines
All India Institute of Medical Sciences
New Delhi, India

Basila Ameer Ali
Associate Consultant
Punyashlok Ahilyadevi Holkar
Head & Neck Cancer Institute of India
Mumbai, Maharashtra, India

Belal Bin Asaf
Associate Director
Institute of Chest Surgery
Chest Oncosurgery and Lung
Transplantation
Medanta—The Medicity
Multi-Specialty Hospital
Gurugram, Haryana, India

Bhavika Kothari
Assistant Professor
Breast Surgical Oncology
Tata Memorial Centre
Homi Bhabha National Institute
Mumbai, Maharashtra, India

Gaurav Agarwal
Professor
Department of Endocrine and
Breast Surgery
Sanjay Gandhi Postgraduate Institute
of Medical Sciences
Lucknow, Uttar Pradesh, India

Gurudutt P Varty
Fellow
Gastrointestinal and HPB Surgical
Oncology
Department of Surgical Oncology
Tata Memorial Centre
Mumbai, Maharashtra, India

Gurushankari Balakrishnan
Senior Resident
Department of Surgical Oncology
Cancer Institute
Chennai, Tamil Nadu, India

Koti Sridhar Reddy
Senior Resident
Department of Urology
Institute of Medical Sciences
Banaras Hindu University
Varanasi, Uttar Pradesh, India

Kumar Prabhash
Professor
Department of Medical Oncology
Tata Memorial Hospital
Mumbai, Maharashtra, India

Kush Parikh
Senior Resident
Department of Surgical Gastroenterology
Sanjay Gandhi Postgraduate Institute of Medical Sciences
Lucknow, Uttar Pradesh, India

Likhita Subhash Singh
Senior Resident
Department of Surgery
Jawaharlal Institute of Postgraduate Medical Education and Research
Puducherry, India

Magnus Jayaraj Mansard
Senior Consultant
SIMS Hospital
Chennai, Tamil Nadu, India

Mahesh Thombare
Associate Professor
Department of Surgical Gastroenterology
DY Patil Medical College, Hospital and Research Centre
Pune, Maharashtra, India

Manish S Bhandare
Professor
Gastrointestinal and HPB Surgical Oncology
Department of Surgical Oncology
Tata Memorial Centre
Mumbai, Maharashtra, India

Mohan V Pulle
Senior Consultant
Institute of Chest Surgery
Chest Oncosurgery and Lung Transplantation
Medanta—The Medicity Multi-Specialty Hospital
Gurugram, Haryana, India

N Ananthakrishnan
Professor
Department of Surgery
Mahatma Gandhi Medical College and Research Institute
Sri Balaji Vidyapeeth
Puducherry, India

Probal Neogi
Professor
Department of Surgery
Moti Lal Nehru Medical College
Prayagraj, Uttar Pradesh, India

Puneet
Professor
Department of Surgery
Institute of Medical Sciences
Banaras Hindu University
Varanasi, Uttar Pradesh, India

R Kalayarasan
Associate Professor
Department of Surgical Gastroenterology
Jawaharlal Institute of Postgraduate Medical Education and Research
Puducherry, India

RA Sastry
Professor
Department of Surgical Gastroenterology
Krishna Institute of Medical Sciences
Hyderabad, Telangana, India

Rahul
Associate Professor
Department of Surgical Gastroenterology
Sanjay Gandhi Postgraduate Institute of Medical Sciences
Lucknow, Uttar Pradesh, India

Contributors

Rinelle Mascarenhas
Senior Resident
Department of Endocrine and
Breast Surgery
Sanjay Gandhi Postgraduate Institute
of Medical Sciences
Lucknow, Uttar Pradesh, India

Rohit Kumar Singh
Senior Resident
Department of Surgery
Institute of Medical Sciences
Banaras Hindu University
Varanasi, Uttar Pradesh, India

S Suresh Kumar
Additional Professor
Department of Surgery
Jawaharlal Institute of Postgraduate
Medical Education and Research
Puducherry, India

Sameer Trivedi
Professor
Department of Urology
Institute of Medical Sciences
Banaras Hindu University
Varanasi, Uttar Pradesh, India

Sanjeet Kumar Rai
Assistant Professor
Department of Surgical Disciplines
All India Institute of Medical Sciences
New Delhi, India

Saurabh Bokade
Senior Resident
Department of Surgical Oncology
Tata Medical Centre
Kolkata, West Bengal, India

Shailesh V Shrikhande
Deputy Director
Tata Memorial Hospital, Mumbai
Professor and Head, Cancer Surgery
Chief, Gastrointestinal and HPB Service
Tata Memorial Centre
Mumbai, Maharashtra, India

Shaleen Agarwal
Director
Liver Transplant and HPB Surgery
Center for Liver and Biliary Sciences
Max Super Specialty Hospital
New Delhi, India

Sikhar Kumar
Consultant Medical Oncology
Yashoda Hospital
Hyderabad, Telangana, India

Sunil Kumar
Senior Consultant
Department of Surgery
Tata Main Hospital
Manipal Tata Medical College
Jamshedpur, Jharkhand, India

Vani Parmar
Chief
Breast Surgical Oncology
Punyashlok Ahilyadevi Holkar
Head & Neck Cancer Institute of India
Mumbai, Maharashtra, India

Vanita Noronha
Professor
Department of Medical Oncology
Tata Memorial Hospital
Mumbai, Maharashtra, India

Vikram A Chaudhari
Professor
Gastrointestinal and HPB Surgical
Oncology
Department of Surgical Oncology
Tata Memorial Centre
Mumbai, Maharashtra, India

Vikram Kate
Professor
Department of Gastrointestinal Surgery
Jawaharlal Institute of Postgraduate
Medical Education and Research
Puducherry, India

Virinder Kumar Bansal
Professor
Department of Surgical Disciplines
All India Institute of Medical Sciences
New Delhi, India

VK Kapoor
Professor
Department of Surgical Gastroenterology
Mahatma Gandhi Medical College and Hospital
Jaipur, Rajasthan, India

PREFACE

The 18th edition of *Roshan Lall Gupta's Recent Advances in Surgery* is the key book covering advances in the field of surgery. It covers the latest topics in surgery like artificial intelligence, third space endoscopy, indocyanine green use in surgical practice and many others. This book deals with recent changes in the evaluation and management of patients. It will help postgraduate students to enhance 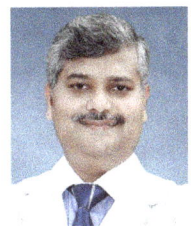 their knowledge about the subject, and also young surgeons to keep abreast with the recent developments, finally benefiting the patients.

The content of the book has been prepared by the eminent surgeons and academicians who are masters in their field and edited by me. The current guidelines and evidences are collectively presented in the chapters in an extremely simplified manner for better understanding of the readers. This book will help postgraduate students in their MS/DNB Exit Examination and enhance knowledge of surgeons, improving their surgical practice and patient care. I hope this book will serve as a benchmark in adding knowledge related to recent developments in the field of surgery.

Puneet

ACKNOWLEDGMENTS

I thank all the authors for their contribution to this edition. The text is in simple language and student-friendly for easy understanding, and appropriate for young surgeons to adapt in clinical practice. I am quite hopeful that this edition will be informative. I am thankful to M/s Jaypee Brothers Medical Publishers (P) Ltd, New Delhi, India, for publishing this book.

CONTENTS

1. Artificial Intelligence in Surgery 1
   Puneet, Shaleen Agarwal, Probal Neogi

2. Indocyanine Green in Surgical Practice 17
   Kush Parikh, Rahul, Ashish Singh, Puneet

3. Third-space Endoscopy 41
   Arunima Verma, Rahul, Saurabh Bokade, Sunil Kumar

4. Acute Appendicitis: Recent Concepts 53
   R Kalayarasan, S Suresh Kumar, Vikram Kate, N Ananthakrishnan

5. Neuroendocrine Tumors of the
   Gastroenteropancreatic System 74
   Gurudutt P Varty, Vikram A Chaudhari, Manish S Bhandare, Shailesh V Shrikhande

6. Newer Terminology in Ventral Hernia Repair 100
   Sanjeet Kumar Rai, Aditya Baksi, Asuri Krishna, Virinder Kumar Bansal

7. Management of Benign Biliary Stricture 113
   Mahesh Thombare, Magnus Jayaraj Mansard, VK Kapoor

8. Obscure Gastrointestinal Bleed 136
   RA Sastry

9. Management of Adrenal Incidentaloma 151
   Rinelle Mascarenhas, Gaurav Agarwal

10. Enhanced Recovery After Surgery for
    Gastrointestinal Surgery 173
    Vikram Kate, Likhita Subhash Singh, Gurushankari Balakrishnan, N Ananthakrishnan

11. Recent Trends in Thoracic Surgery 194
    Belal Bin Asaf, Mohan V Pulle, Arvind Kumar

12. Immune Profiling and Therapies in Cancer 211
    Sikhar Kumar, Vanita Noronha, Kumar Prabhash

13. Venous Ulcer 223
    Rohit Kumar Singh, Ajay K Khanna

14. Paget's Disease of Breast 249
    Vani Parmar, Bhavika Kothari, Basila Ameer Ali

15. Management of Testicular Tumors 258
    Sameer Trivedi, Koti Sridhar Reddy

Index *281*

CHAPTER 1

Artificial Intelligence in Surgery

Puneet, Shaleen Agarwal, Probal Neogi

■ INTRODUCTION

Intelligence is the ability to acquire, understand, and apply the knowledge to achieve the goals. However, artificial intelligence (AI) means designing intelligence in an artificial device. In simple words, in the era of computer science, intelligent machines are created which work and react like human brain. It may perform tasks that require human intelligence such as visual perception, recognizing speech, and decision-making.[1] Thus, AI may be described as an attempt to build a machine that can think like human, able to learn, and also utilize its own knowledge to solve the problem/issue.[2,3] The term AI was coined by John McCarthy in 1956.

The concept of intelligent machines is not new, and such machines have been a part of human imagination for millennia. In fact, the earliest description of such a machine can be found in Greek literature in the form of a mechanical servant named "Talos." Leonardo da Vinci described the design for a mechanical computer; however, it was in 1623 that Wilhelm Schickard built the first calculating machine called the "calculating clock" that could add or subtract six-digit numbers. Kurt Gödel, one of the leading logicians of the twentieth century, published his "incompleteness theorems" in 1931 that laid the foundation for the development of first programming language. The first operational computer was designed by Alan Turing in 1945. Alan Turing is widely considered to be the father of theoretical computer science and AI.

Artificial intelligence is a relatively new discipline of science that is an amalgamation of various other fields such as mathematics, computer science, philosophy, and biological sciences. The interaction and cross integration of these subjects promoted growth, provided vision, and simulated creation, leading to the development of AI.[2,4] In the present era, theoretical understanding of neuron is increasing in biology, and computer scientists have also started preparing the prototype of the functional neurons on chip. Frank Rosenblatt (1958) first made a computational model of neurons called "Perceptron." AI was first used by Gunn in 1976 for the evaluation of abdominal pain.[1]

TERMINOLOGIES AND SUBFIELDS IN ARTIFICIAL INTELLIGENCE

The various AI technologies used in healthcare services include: Machine learning (ML), natural language processing (NLP), artificial neural networks (ANNs), computer vision (CV), reinforcement learning (RL), robotics, and cybernetics.[2,3]

Machine learning: It is a subset of AI. It enables machines to learn and provide predictions based on recognized patterns. ML may be supervised or unsupervised; in supervised, computer utilizes partial labeled data, while in unsupervised, structure is detected in the data without explicit programming to make predictions. Thus, supervised learning uses algorithms to predict a known outcome, and unsupervised learning searches for patterns within data. ML enables to utilize multiple algorithms to calculate predictions with high level of accuracy that may be unattainable with present conventional statistics.[3,5] Next is RL, in which a program learns from its own success and mistake to complete the task.[6]

Natural language processing: It is a subfield in AI. It enables the computer to understand human language; it not only recognizes simple words but also semantics and syntax in analyzing the data. NLP is utilized in the analysis of large database of electronic medical record and detect whether any adverse events or any complications have developed in the postoperative period. NLP can comb the electronic record to identify specific word and phrases that suggest complications such as anastomotic leak following colorectal surgery.[3,7]

Artificial neural networks: They are a subset of ML, an important component in many AI applications, and are inspired by the biological nervous system. Each of these neural networks works as a computational unit, and they are connected to each other. Deep learning networks comprised many layers of neural networks and can perform complex task.[3,8]

Computer vision: Machine is trained to recognize images and videos. It is now used in the image acquisition and interpretation with its applications in diagnosis, image-guided surgery, and virtual colonoscopy. With ML and CV, image and video-based analysis of longitudinal studies and decision-making in surgery are made. The laparoscopic video of sleeve gastrectomy can accurately (92.8%) note the missing or unexpected steps.[3,9]

ARTIFICIAL INTELLIGENCE IN HEALTH CARE

Applications of AI in health care have increased rapidly, and AI is now being utilized in almost all aspects of health care right from laboratory research to various facets of patient management. AI is being utilized for drug discovery, clinical trials, medical risk prediction, medical data security, and detection of fraud. Its application extends from diagnosing the disease using medical image analysis and improving genetic interpretation to treating the disease and monitoring. Algorithms have been laid down for interpreting radiographs, mammograms, and cancers on computed tomography (CT) scans. AI also finds application in pathology for objective evaluation of microscopic findings in various pathological conditions, especially oncopathology.

With the shift to digital medical record keeping and most healthcare facilities now becoming paperless, humongous volumes of medically relevant data have accumulated. Analysis of electronic health records (EHRs) offers promise in extracting clinically relevant information and making diagnostic evaluations as well as in providing real-time risk scores for transfer to intensive care, predicting outcomes such as in-hospital mortality, readmission risk, prolonged length of stay, and improving decision-making strategies. Proof-of-concept studies have aimed to improve the clinical workflow, including automatic extraction of semantic information from transcripts, recognizing speech in doctor–patient conversations, and even summarizing doctor–patient consultations.[2]

Artificial intelligence has the potential to bring about uniformity in clinical practice, improve efficiency, and prevent avoidable medical errors that will affect almost every patient during their lifetime. By providing novel tools to support patients and augment healthcare staff, AI could enable better care delivered closer to the patient in the community. AI tools could assist patients in playing a greater role in managing their own health; primary care physicians by allowing them to confidently manage a greater range of complex diseases, and specialists by offering superhuman diagnostic performance and disease management. Finally, through the detection of novel signals of disease that clinicians are unable to perceive, AI can extract novel insights from existing data.[2,3]

■ APPLICATIONS OF ARTIFICIAL INTELLIGENCE IN SURGERY

In recent years, the progressive use of AI in clinical practice has helped surgeons in clinical decision-making, diagnosis, predicting preoperative risk, intraoperative monitoring, and postoperative care. It also limits human errors, particularly in difficult and critical situations.[10] AI is being used in the diagnosis of cancer and real-time monitoring of the intensive care patients.[11,12] The use of AI in surgery is at much slow pace than in medicine and radiology; it is because of the high stakes in surgery and also complex decision-making involved. The use of AI in surgery involves algorithms and developing semiautonomous device that can perform various interventions/surgical procedures in interaction with the surgeons. The enthusiasm toward the use of AI in surgical practice is growing, and with all technological innovations in recent years, it will increase over time.

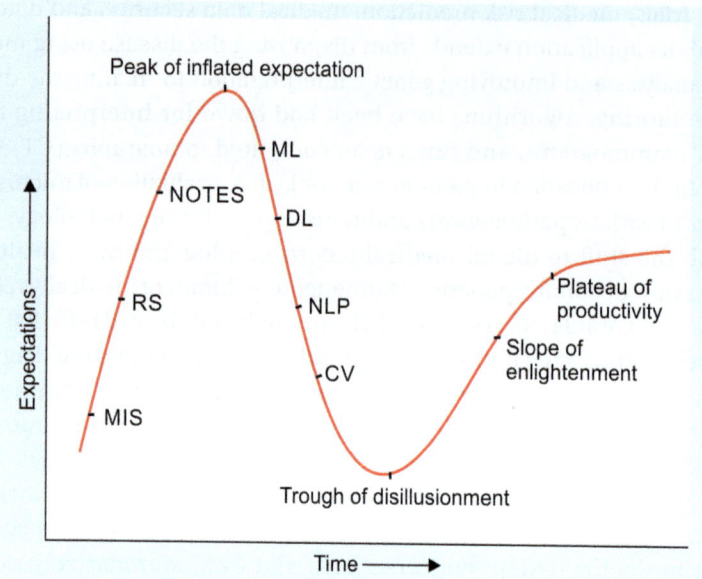

Fig. 1: Gartner hype cycle for artificial intelligence tools in surgery. (CV: computer vision; DL: deep learning; MIS: minimal invasive surgery; ML: machine learning; NLP: natural language processing; NOTES: natural orifice transluminal endoscopic surgery; RS: robotic surgery)

Artificial intelligence in surgery follows the Gartner hype cycle, according to Roger's diffusion of innovation theory, which is a classic S-shaped curve and has several phases before true innovation. The phases include: (1) Peak of inflated expectations, (2) ML, deep learning, NLP, CV, (3) trough of disillusionment, and (4) slope of enlightenment, followed by a long plateau phase. In this phase, real work occurs and is known as plateau of productivity **(Fig. 1)**.[10,13]

The application of AI in surgery ranges from evaluating a patient, making a diagnosis, counseling and preparing for surgery, performing the surgery, anticipating complications, to managing them, and providing postoperative care. Thus, the role of AI in surgery can be described as **(Fig. 2)**:

- *Preoperative:* It includes imaging, endoscopy, tissue diagnosis, surgical decision-making, and risk assessment.
- *Intraoperative:* It includes anesthesia, CV and context-aware assistance, surgical phase recognition and avoiding near misses, augmented reality (AR) and navigation surgery, and AI-assisted robotic surgery.
- *Postoperative:* It includes postoperative monitoring, possible procedures to reduce complications, early diagnosis of complications, and postoperative pain management.

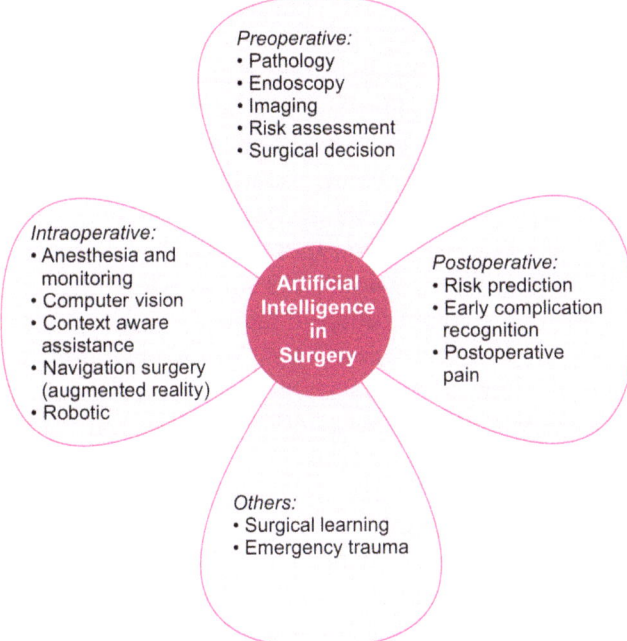

Fig. 2: Use of artificial intelligence in surgery.

ROLE OF ARTIFICIAL INTELLIGENCE IN PREOPERATIVE PHASE

Artificial Intelligence and Gastrointestinal Endoscopy

Artificial intelligence is currently being used to increase the diagnostic yield of endoscopy for detection of polyps as well as to differentiate hyperplastic from adenomatous polyps based on endoscopic images. It can also be used to differentiate malignant versus nonmalignant tissue and identify the depth of invasion and margins of endoscopic resection. An important feat achieved through AI is the evaluation of huge numbers of endoscopic images obtained by wireless capsule endoscopy as well as an integrated ultrasound system in the capsule for evaluation.[14]

Artificial Intelligence and Radiology

3D Visualization and Virtual Simulation

The preoperative assessment of the lesion is traditionally evaluated on two-dimensional (2D) images of CT and/or magnetic resonance imaging (MRI). The three-dimensional (3D) visualization of the liver lesion accurately interprets the lesion and also provides its relation to the surrounding structure.[15]

The first use of 3D visualization of liver lesion was performed by Marescaux in 1998.[16] 3D reconstruction of 2D images of CT scan and MRI for liver lesion improves the preoperative planning and visualization of spatial relationship of the tumor and surrounding intrahepatic structures, identifying the normal vascular and biliary anatomy and its variations. It can assess the resectability of the liver lesions (hepatocellular carcinoma and colorectal metastasis) by performing virtual hepatectomy and also provide the information on future liver remnant.[17] Studies have demonstrated that patients operated following 3D planning have less hepatic inflow occlusion time, less operative time, and reduced postoperative complications.[18] Similarly, reduced intraoperative bleeding is reported with preoperative 3D reconstruction planning.[19] 3D reconstruction in hilar cholangiocarcinoma can predict tumor invasion into hilar vessels, variant hilar anatomy, and future liver volumes. These informations are vital in planning major radical resection, which has high morbidity as well as mortality. Similarly, 3D planning exclude peripancreatic vessel involvement in pancreatic cancer, resulting in significantly reduced blood loss, operative time, and hospital stay.[20]

3D Printed Models

Artificial intelligence converts the 3D reconstructed images with 3D printing technology into real physical models. The 3D printing was first used by Zein et al. in 2013.[21] The 3D images and reconstruction as described above are useful, but the display remains on a 2D screen. Thus, this limitation is overcome by 3D printing, which is useful in liver lesions and transplantation. 3D printed model in operating room can precisely locate the site of lesion and its relations to its surrounding structures, useful in planning exact line of transaction. 3D printing is extremely helpful in planning liver resection in large and complex lesions of liver to avoid posthepatectomy decompensation. 3D printed liver models also be used in assessing size discrepancies between recipient and graft in living donor liver transplantation, particularly in small infants and neonates.[22] Low-cost 3D printed models of liver can also be used for medical education, for better understanding of liver anatomy, and practice hepatectomy. Recently, 3D bioprinted models of liver are used in tissue engineering and in artificial liver.[23]

Artificial Intelligence and Surgical Decision-making

The surgical decision is a shared decision of patient in respect to treatment, compliance, and satisfaction. However, sometimes decisions are complex and involve high stakes that may affect the patient outcome. Surgical decision-making is sometimes dominated by hypothetical/deductive reasoning and individual judgment. These factors can lead to bias, error, and can potentially harm the patient. Traditional predictive analytics and clinical decision-support systems are intended to augment surgical decision-making, but their clinical utility is compromised by time-consuming manual data management and suboptimal accuracy. AI can help the surgeons to improve the accuracy and efficiency in diagnosis. ML identifies the complex relationships between various variables, analyzes large data from patient history, laboratory findings, and images to predict the most probable diagnosis. Similarly, AI may assist and support the diagnosis, also recommend further investigation required, and suggest the best treatment modality based on current evidence. In future, integration of AI with surgical decision-making will augment the decision for intervention, informed consent, identification of risk factors, and postoperative complications.[2,10] AI tool extract data from large EHRs in the form of knowledge, which improves the decision-making of surgeons.

Artificial Intelligence and Risk Assessment

IBM Watson Oncology has been developed for the oncologists to provide current evidence and also to guide them in decision-making; however, it was not able to do so.[24] The various cardiac risk assessment models (such as revised cardiac risk index and Gupta perioperative risk for myocardial infarction)[25,26] and American Society of Anesthesiologists (ASA) classification fail to predict the risk accurately. AI-based platform containing vast data can identify and predict the risk accurately. My Surgery Risk platform, which uses EHR data, has shown to predict perioperative risk accurately. ML-based platform develops as Predictive OpTimization Trees in Emergency Surgery Risk (POTTER) calculator, based on the American College of Surgeons National Surgical Quality Improvement Program (ACS-NSQIP) database. It accurately calculates the perioperative risk involved and associated mortality.[27] POTTER integrated with EHR data can also identify the risk of surgical site infection (SSI), pneumonia, sepsis, cardiac complications, and postoperative intensive care unit stay.[28]

ROLE OF ARTIFICIAL INTELLIGENCE IN INTRAOPERATIVE PHASE

Artificial Intelligence in Anesthesia and Monitoring

Artificial intelligence has found application during the induction and maintenance phase of anesthesia. Monitoring the depth of anesthesia (DOA) requires the assessment of a multitude of parameters and is a complex task. AI utilizes the bispectral index (BIS), which is derived from electroencephalogram data, to maintain tight feedback and control of DOA. McSleepy automated intravenous infusion machines use the BIS along with vital signs to maintain DOA by administering propofol, narcotics, and muscle relaxants. However, the maintenance of DOA is a critical balance between infusion and assessment of parameters, and underdosing or excessive DOA may be caused by equipment imbalance; therefore, automated anesthesia is still in its infancy and not ready to be adopted in general practice.[29,30]

Apart from induction and maintenance, automated regional anesthetic blockade has been performed by the da Vinci® system, and the Magellan robot has been used to place peripheral nerve blocks. Intraoperative intelligence can help to predict return of consciousness after general anesthesia, and neural networks can predict postinduction hypotension as well as the rate of recovery from neuromuscular blockade. In an unblinded randomized clinical trial (HYPE trial), the use of a ML-derived early warning system compared resulted in less intraoperative hypotension with standard care. In supra major abdominal surgeries such as cytoreductive surgeries or hyperthermic intraperitoneal chemotherapy, it is recommended to use cardiac output monitoring.[29,30]

Computer Vision and Context-aware Assistance in Surgery

Artificial intelligence based CV may be used to standardize, automate, and scale the surgical performance. It gives an opportunity for the computer-based performance assessment of the surgical skills such as suturing and knotting. It also includes assessment of tissue handling and fluidity of motion. Now, the operation theater utilizes anesthesia and surgical machines that regularly provide status report. Such heterogeneous sensors stalled in operation rooms are known as context-aware assistance.[31] AI-based system is used, which identifies the various phases of surgery. Thus, any deviation or delay in any surgical step is identified and informed to the surgeon. OR black box system (similar to aircraft) captures various data (such as audio, video, and physiological parameters from the monitor) during surgical procedure. Recently, studies are evaluating this analytical data of black box with the patient outcome.[32]

Navigated Surgery

Three-dimensional reconstruction and printing as well as 3D reconstructed images do not synchronize with actual surgery.[15,33] This limitation can be overcome with the help of computer software that combines the preoperatively acquired 3D reconstructed images and intraoperative real-time information. It is possible with augmented virtuality (AV) (virtual environment that is controlled by real information) or AR (virtual information based on real images of patient). Thus, AV, AR, or mixed reality (MR) is a reliable surgical navigation that avoids the chance of misinterpretation and improves oncological safety with maximal functional preservation.[34] During AR-based navigation, reconstructed images are superimposed on the real organs on monitor display during surgery which may be utilized for pancreatectomy, small neuroendocrine tumor of pancreas, and liver lesion.[35]

Artificial Intelligence and Minimally Invasive Surgery

Artificial intelligence has significant potential to improve the effectiveness and safety in minimally invasive surgery. AI can develop advanced navigation and guidance systems to improve the precision surgery. AI-based image analysis tools provide real-time guidance to operating surgeon, which can assist to diagnose unexpected complications and event.[4,15] With the help of ML algorithms, various patterns are identified from data of past surgeries, helping surgeons in executing best surgical approach. Bile duct injury during laparoscopic cholecystectomy is well known and associated with high morbidity and also invites medico-legal litigation. AI-based models developed for laparoscopic cholecystectomy using four anatomical landmarks (the common bile duct, cystic duct, lower edge of the left medial liver segment, Rouviere's sulcus) can be easily identified intraoperatively,[36] resulting in much reduced risk of bile duct injury. AR technology can be used where 3D reconstructed images of CT/MRI of the liver, superimposed with virtual image of the liver in 1:1 ratio, can help surgeon in hepatectomy.[37] AR has vital role in education of the trainees in laparoscopy. AR-based models will improve skills of the trainee for laparoscopic surgical procedure and also decrease learning curve significantly.[15]

Artificial Intelligence and Robotic Surgery

"Robot" is defined as "a mechanical device that is capable of performing a variety of complex human tasks on command or after being programmed in advance."

Medical robot can be divided into two types:
1. Remote controlled
2. Automated or semiautomated

In the remote controlled or synergistic type, the surgeon has direct real-time control of the robotic instruments from a console placed away from the patient and robotic arms. Da Vinci® Surgical System by Intuitive and Versius® system by CMR are examples of remote-controlled robotic systems. In the automated type of robots, the physician does not have to continuously control the motion of the robot; instead, the physician defines its task and monitors its execution, for example, the AcuBot robot used for CT-guided interventions.

Currently available surgical robotic platforms such as the da Vinci™ (Intuitive Surgical, Inc., Sunnyvale, CA) or the Versius system by CMR are real-time tele-manipulators in a "master-slave" configuration. These systems

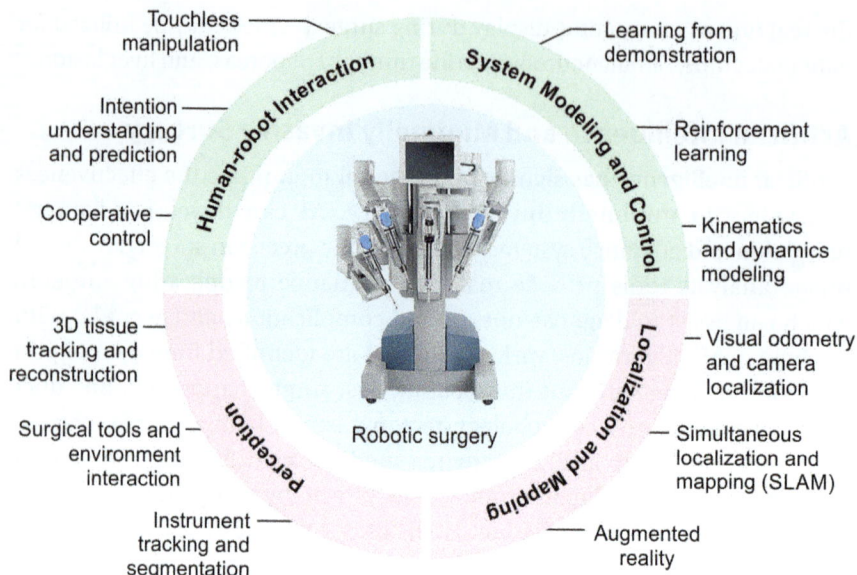

Fig. 3: How artificial intelligence (AI) can enhance utility of robotic surgery? (3D: three dimensional)

consist of a patient-site platform with four robotic operating arms and a video-laparoscopic cart (slave). There is also a surgeon-site console (master) equipped with a stereoscopic 3D camera offering an immersive environment to the surgeon with a sound depth perception and ergonomic handles, which command the robotic effectors replicating human hand movements into a precise and downscaled fashion. The limitation of depth perception of laparoscopic procedure can be overcome by 3D intraoperative views in robotic surgery, which is also 10-fold magnified **(Fig. 3)**. This helps surgeons in dissection of delicate tissue, increased dexterity, and intracorporeal suturing even in narrow space.[38] The sense of touch is missing in both in laparoscopy and robotic surgery; this limitation is also been overcome with use of AR.[39] The see-through visualization technology in AR helps surgeon with port placement as per patient anatomical variation and lesions. AR allows identification of intrahepatic vascular structures with high accuracy, and its benefit has been reported in hepatic resection. The augmented endoscopic view provides the information of resection margin around tumor with high accuracy. With recent advancement, robots are enabled to automatically do simple surgical activities in vitro as suturing and knot tying.[40] However, complete autonomy to robots in surgery is still far ahead to attain, and surgeons continue to control them because of complex decision-making and safety of the patients. The major intraoperative limitations while using 3D overlays arise when an unexpected object appears suddenly in field view of surgeon, causing inattentional blindness.[41]

ROLE OF ARTIFICIAL INTELLIGENCE IN POSTOPERATIVE PHASE

Machine learning algorithms use EHR data to predict the outcomes in terms of SSI, sepsis, and bleeding following various surgical procedures. They provide more accurate prediction than ASA and ACS-surgical risk calculator. The most dreadful complication following bowel suturing or anastomosis is the leak. AI-based analysis can accurately predict anastomotic leak following bariatric and colorectal surgery.[28] Similarly, AI can also predict risk of postoperative pancreatic fistula (POPF) following pancreaticoduodenectomy.[42] AI-based nociception level (NOL) index has been developed to minimize postoperative pain.

Artificial Intelligence in Surgical Learning

Artificial intelligence has potential to change the present-day training of the surgeon. In recent years, training of surgeons is changing with the introduction of simulators and specific task allocations in the same. The creation of AI-based simulation surgical training allows the trainees to acquire skill in managing complex surgical task in a controlled environment. This method has been seen to improve the confidence of the trainee as well as his/her performance. Simulation-based training has an advantage that it provides real-time feedback to improve surgical skill, can also assess the performance, and cause no harm to the actual patient. The personalized training program may be developed as per the need of the trainee based on feedback.[4,43] AI has ability to improve all components of surgical training, including knowledge, surgical skill, and decreasing learning curve of complex surgical procedure.[44] AI enhances attitude training through virtual patient cases and also helps trainees in developing attitudes and behavior required for successful surgeons.

Artificial intelligence in Emergency and Trauma Surgery

The video-consulting emergency (VCE) protocol is developed, which improves the decision-making between the emergency physician present onsite and remote surgeon. The devices used are usually smartphone, FaceTime, and Acute Abdominal Decision Making (AADM*) model.[10,45] The Artificial Intelligence in Emergency and Trauma Surgery (ARIES) project was formulated following an international web survey that was endorsed by the World Society of Emergency Surgery for the use of AI in emergency and trauma surgery.[46] The use of AI in emergency and trauma surgery may be utilized in monitoring and decision-making and prevent errors.

LIMITATIONS OF ARTIFICIAL INTELLIGENCE

The media hype about AI has created unrealistic expectations that lead to disappointment and disillusionment. AI is not a "magic bullet" that can yield answers to all questions. There are instances where traditional analytical methods can outperform ML or where the addition of ML does not improve its results. AI is as good as the data that is used to generate the various management algorithms. The results will depend on the questions asked and the datasets that are available. Any glitches in these components will result in an incorrect algorithm. The following are important limitations of AI that are needed to be addressed in future:[3]

- *Challenges related to machine-learning science:* Artificial intelligence algorithms have the potential to suffer from multiple shortcomings, including inapplicability outside the training domain, bias, and brittleness (tendency to be easily fooled). Important factors for consideration include dataset shift, accidentally fitting confounders rather than true signal, propagating unintentional biases in clinical practice, and the challenge of generalization to different populations.
- *Logistical difficulties in implementing AI systems:* Many of the current challenges in translating AI algorithms to clinical practice are related to the fact that most healthcare data are not readily available for ML. Data are often soiled in a multitude of medical imaging archival systems, pathology systems, EHRs, electronic prescribing tools, and insurance databases, which are very difficult to bring together. Even if we understand the underlying mathematical principles of such models, it is difficult to interrogate the inner workings of models to understand how and why it made a certain decision. This is potentially problematic for medical applications, where it is essential to have approaches that are not only well-performing but also trustworthy, transparent, interpretable, and explainable.
- *Achieving robust regulation and rigorous quality control:* A fundamental component of achieving safe and effective deployment of AI algorithms is the development of the necessary regulatory frameworks. This poses a unique challenge given the current pace of innovation, significant risks involved, and the potentially fluid nature of ML models. The comparison of algorithms across studies in an objective manner is challenging due to each study's performance being reported using variable methodologies on different populations with different sample distributions and characteristics. To make fair comparisons, algorithms need to be subjected to comparison on the same independent test set that is representative of the target population, using the same performance metrics. Without this, clinicians will have difficulty in determining which algorithm is likely to perform best for their patients.
- *Ethical and medicolegal aspects of AI:* The ethical and legal implications of AI are heavily debated. It has already been explained that if the algorithm is flawed, AI will generate inaccurate results. Those errors are different

from ones that occur because of network loss or computer malfunction. AI was initially used only to augment clinical decision-making, but with its current development and autonomy, flaws in the device that harm patients, resulting in medical negligence, require that responsibility needs to be predetermined. The allocation of responsibility was traditionally to the surgeon, but with the self-learning capability of AI, it may not be possible for the surgeon to override certain procedures.

Till date, no consensus has been reached with regards to legal implications of integration of advanced AI systems in surgery and healthcare practices in general. The responsibility of AI and autonomous robotic surgery is classified as (1) accountability; (2) liability; and (3) culpability. Accountability means the capacity of a system to explain its actions, liability is subject to action by the legal system, and culpability relates to punishment. Accountability can be determined by recording the actions, but the issues of liability and culpability require a consensus to adapt to the scenario of AI and robotics.

The medical records also carry sensitive personal information which may cause legal issues and concerns about the breach in personal privacy. There are many countries in the world that have formed legal systems for protecting personal information. Like in US, Health Insurance Portability and Accountability Act (HIPAA) established in 1996, similarly, in Europe, General Data Protection Regulation established in 2016.[47] The International Medical Device Regulators Forum classified the software used in AI for medical use as "Software as a Medical Device (SaMD)."[48] The policies need to be established which can regulate the devices used for medical purpose although such policies have been implemented in the US, Japan, Korea, and few other countries.

■ CONCLUSION

Artificial intelligence is expected to be widely used in healthcare system. Various research centers and governments are keen on building robust AI technologies. AI will augment patient care and can be used in preoperative evaluation, planning, and assessment of postoperative complications. Intraoperatively, automated anesthesia, AR, VR, and robotic surgery with AI technology would improve the safety, comfort, and outcome of the patient. AI in OR will not replace the surgeon; however, it will expand the capacity and capability of the surgeon with enhanced vision and dexterity. AI-based simulation surgical training allows the trainees to acquire skills in managing complex surgical tasks in a controlled environment. The use of AI in surgical learning will enhance the training quality and surgical competence, which will further improve patient care. AI is a powerful tool that is emerging fast; however, legal and ethical issues associated with AI still need to be addressed.

REFERENCES

1. Köse E, Öztürk NN, Karahan SR. Artificial intelligence in surgery. Eur Arch Med Res. 2018;34(Suppl. 1):S4-6.
2. Malhotra K, Wong BNX, Lee S, Franco H, Singh C, Cabrera Silva LA, et al. Role of artificial intelligence in global surgery: a review of opportunities and challenges. Cureus. 2023;15(8):e43192.
3. Park CW, Seo SW, Kang N, Ko BS, Choi BW, Park CM, et al. Artificial intelligence in health care: current applications and issues. J Korean Med Sci. 2020;35(42):e379.
4. Hashimoto DA, Rosman G, Rus D, Meireles OR. Artificial intelligence in surgery: promises and perils. Ann Surg. 2018;268(1):70-6.
5. Deo RC. Machine learning in medicine. Circulation. 2015;132(20):1920-30.
6. Sutton RS, Barto AG. Reinforcement Learning: An Introduction. Vol. 1. Cambridge: MIT Press; 1998.
7. Melton GB, Hripcsak G. Automated detection of adverse events using natural language processing of discharge summaries. J Am Med Inform Assoc. 2005;12(4):448-57.
8. Hinton GE, Osindero S, Teh YW. A fast learning algorithm for deep belief nets. Neural Comput. 2006;18(7):1527-54.
9. Volkov M, Hashimoto DA, Rosman G, Meireles OR, Rus D. Machine learning and coresets for automated real-time video segmentation of laparoscopic and robot-assisted surgery. 2017 IEEE International Conference on Robotics and Automation (ICRA), Singapore. IEEE; 2017. pp. 754-9.
10. Pakkasjärvi N, Luthra T, Anand S. Artificial intelligence in surgical learning. Surgeries. 2023;4:86-97.
11. Hunter B, Hindocha S, Lee RW. The role of artificial intelligence in early cancer diagnosis. Cancers. 2022;14(6):1524.
12. Filho IMB, Aquino G, Malaquias RS, Girao G, Melo SRM. An IoT-based healthcare platform for patients in ICU beds during the COVID-19 outbreak. IEEE Access. 2021;9:27262-77.
13. Zhou XY, Guo Y, Shen M, Yang GZ. Application of artificial intelligence in surgery. Front Med. 2020;14(4):417-30.
14. Okagawa Y, Abe S, Yamada M, Oda I, Saito Y. Artificial intelligence in endoscopy. Dig Dis Sci. 2022;67(5):1553-72.
15. Loftus TJ, Tighe PJ, Filiberto AC, Efron PA, Brakenridge SC, Mohr AM, et al. Artificial intelligence and surgical decision-making. JAMA Surg. 2020;155(2):148-58.
16. Marescaux J, Clément JM, Tassetti V, Koehl C, Cotin S, Russier Y, et al. Virtual reality applied to hepatic surgery simulation: the next revolution. Ann Surg. 1998;228:627-34.
17. Mise Y, Hasegawa K, Satou S, Shindoh J, Miki K, Akamatsu N, et al. How has virtual hepatectomy changed the practice of liver surgery? Ann Surg. 2018;268:127-33.
18. Fang CH, Tao HS, Yang J, Fang ZS, Cai W, Liu J, et al. Impact of three-dimensional reconstruction technique in the operation planning of centrally located hepatocellular carcinoma. J Am Coll Surg. 2015;220:28-37.
19. Cai W, Fan Y, Hu H, Xiang N, Fang C, Jia F. Postoperative liver volume was accurately predicted by a medical image three-dimensional visualization system in hepatectomy for liver cancer. Surg Oncol. 2017;26:188-94.

20. Miyamoto R, Oshiro Y, Nakayama K, Kohno K, Hashimoto S, Fukunaga K, et al. Three-dimensional simulation of pancreatic surgery showing the size and location of the main pancreatic duct. Surg Today. 2017;47:357-64.
21. Zein NN, Hanouneh IA, Bishop PD, Samaan M, Eghtesad B, Quintini C, et al. Three-dimensional print of a liver for preoperative planning in living donor liver transplantation. Liver Transpl. 2013;19:1304-10.
22. Soejima Y, Taguchi T, Sugimoto M, Hayashida M, Yoshizumi T, Ikegami T, et al. Three-dimensional printing and biotexture modeling for preoperative simulation in living donor liver transplantation for small infants. Liver Transpl. 2016;22:1610-4.
23. Faulkner-Jones A, Fyfe C, Cornelissen DJ, Gardner J, King J, Courtney A, et al. Bioprinting of human pluripotent stem cells and their directed differentiation into hepatocyte-like cells for the generation of mini-livers in 3D. Biofabrication. 2015;7:044102.
24. Somashekhar S, Sepúlveda M, Norden AD, Rauthan A, Arun K, Patil P, et al. Early experience with IBM Watson for Oncology (WFO) cognitive computing system for lung and colorectal cancer treatment. J Clin Oncol. 2017;35:8527.
25. Lee TH, Marcantonio ER, Mangione CM, Thomas EJ, Polanczyk CA, Cook EF, et al. Derivation and prospective validation of a simple index for prediction of cardiac risk of major noncardiac surgery. Circulation. 1999;100:1043-9.
26. Gupta PK, Gupta H, Sundaram A, Kaushik M, Fang X, Miller WJ, et al. Development and validation of a risk calculator for prediction of cardiac risk after surgery. Circulation. 2011;124:381-7.
27. Bertsimas D, Dunn J, Velmahos GC, Kaafarani HMA. Surgical risk is not linear: derivation and validation of a novel, user-friendly, and machine-learning-based Predictive OpTimal Trees in Emergency Surgery Risk (POTTER) calculator. Ann Surg. 2018;268:574-83.
28. Bari H, Wadhwani S, Dasari BVM. Role of artificial intelligence in hepatobiliary and pancreatic surgery. World J Gastrointest Surg. 2021;27;13(1):7-18.
29. Hashimoto DA, Witkowski, Gao L, Meireles O, Rosman G. Artificial intelligence in anesthesiology: current techniques, clinical applications, and limitations. Anesthesiology. 2020;132(2):379-94.
30. Singh M, Nath G. Artificial intelligence and anesthesia: a narrative review. Saudi J Anaesth. 2022;16(1):86-93.
31. Vercauteren T, Unberath M, Padoy N, Navab N. CAI4CAI: the rise of contextual artificial intelligence in computer-assisted interventions. Proc IEEE Inst Electr Electron Eng. 2020;108:198-214.
32. Goldenberg MG, Jung J, Grantcharov TP. Using data to enhance performance and improve quality and safety in surgery. JAMA Surg. 2017;152(10):972-3.
33. Sauer IM, Queisner M, Tang P, Moosburner S, Hoepfner O, Horner R, et al. Mixed reality in visceral surgery: development of a suitable workflow and evaluation of intraoperative use-cases. Ann Surg. 2017;266:706-12.
34. Okamoto T, Onda S, Matsumoto M, Gocho T, Futagawa Y, Fujioka S, et al. Utility of augmented reality system in hepatobiliary surgery. J Hepatobiliary Pancreat Sci. 2013;20:249-53.
35. Okamoto T, Onda S, Yasuda J, Yanaga K, Suzuki N, Hattori A. Navigation surgery using an augmented reality for pancreatectomy. Dig Surg. 2015;32:117-23.

36. Tokuyasu T, Iwashita Y, Matsunobu Y, Kamiyama T, Ishikake M, Sakaguchi S, et al. Development of an artificial intelligence system using deep learning to indicate anatomical landmarks during laparoscopic cholecystectomy. Surg Endosc. 2021;35(4):1651-8.
37. Li L, Yu F, Shi D, Shi J, Tian Z, Yang J, et al. Application of virtual reality technology in clinical medicine. Am J Transl Res. 2017;9:3867-80.
38. Giulianotti PC, Sbrana F, Bianco FM, Elli EF, Shah G, Addeo P, et al. Robot-assisted laparoscopic pancreatic surgery: single-surgeon experience. Surg Endosc. 2010;24:1646-57.
39. De Paolis LT, De Luca V. Augmented visualization with depth perception cues to improve the surgeon's performance in minimally invasive surgery. Med Biol Eng Comput. 2019;57:995-1013.
40. Hu Y, Zhang L, Li W, Yang GZ. Robotic sewing and knot tying for personalized stent graft manufacturing. In: 2018 IEEE/RSJ International Conference on Intelligent Robots and Systems (IROS), October 1, 2018, Madrid, Spain. Singapore: IEEE; 2019. pp. 754-60.
41. Marcus HJ, Pratt P, Hughes-Hallett A, Cundy TP, Marcus AP, Yang GZ, et al. Comparative effectiveness and safety of image guidance systems in neuro-surgery: a preclinical randomized study. J Neurosurg. 2015;123:307-13.
42. Han IW, Cho K, Ryu Y, Shin SH, Heo JS, Choi DW, et al. Risk prediction platform for pancreatic fistula after pancreatoduodenectomy using artificial intelligence. World J Gastroenterol. 2020;26:4453-64.
43. Winkler-Schwartz A, Bissonnette V, Mirchi N, Ponnudurai N, Yilmaz R, Ledwos N, et al. Artificial intelligence in medical education: best practices using machine learning to assess surgical expertise in virtual reality simulation. J Surg Educ. 2019;76:1681-90.
44. Dedy NJ, Bonrath EM, Zevin B, Grantcharov TP. Teaching nontechnical skills in surgical residency: a systematic review of current approaches and outcomes. Surgery. 2013;154:1000-8.
45. De Simone B, Ansaloni L, Sartelli M, Coccolini F, Paolillo C, Valentino M, et al. The acute abdomen decision making course for the initial management of non traumatic acute abdomen: a proposition of the World Society of Emergency Surgeons. Emerg Care J. 2019;15(1).
46. De Simone B, Abu-Zidan FM, Gumbs AA, Chouillard E, Di Saverio S, Sartelli M, et al. Knowledge, attitude, and practice of artificial intelligence in emergency and trauma surgery, the ARIES project: an international web-based survey. World J Emerg Surg. 2022;17(1):10.
47. Solanki SL, Pandrowala S, Nayak A, Bhandare M, Ambulkar RP, Shrikhande SV. Artificial intelligence in perioperative management of major gastrointestinal surgeries. World J Gastroenterol. 2021;27(21):2758-70.
48. Pelayo S, Bras Da Costa S, Leroy N, Loiseau S, Beuscart-Zephir MC. Software as a medical device: regulatory critical issues. Stud Health Technol Inform. 2013;183:337-42.

CHAPTER 2

Indocyanine Green in Surgical Practice

Kush Parikh, Rahul, Ashish Singh, Puneet

■ INTRODUCTION

Medical imaging utilizes wavelengths across the entire electromagnetic spectrum through various techniques to visualize the human anatomy for clinical benefit. It can be used for diagnosis, treatment, and monitoring of various medical conditions. Fluorescence-guided surgery (FGS) is an imaging technique that enables real-time visualization of a desired anatomical structure distinct from the surrounding tissues during a surgical procedure that may not be apparent under white light conditions.

The basic configuration of an FGS system comprises a light source with accompanying excitation filters for the fluorescence contrast agent, often administered prior to surgery. The emitted fluorescence signal from the probe is then received by a fluorescence detector. Unwanted signals (excitation light and autofluorescence) are eliminated by initial passage of the light through appropriate emission filters in the probe, followed by passage through collection optics to focus the desired signal on the detector. Subsequently, it is transferred to an attached monitor for visualization. The final image quality is influenced by multiple factors. Hence, careful selection of components of the imaging system is required for the desired output.[1]

Fluorescence-guided surgery scores over traditional imaging techniques on various grounds. It has a better resolution, high sensitivity, reproducibility, and is easy to operate. Ongoing research to improve the probes and surgical system has helped to expand its potential clinical applications.[2] Fluorescein sodium, methylene blue, and indocyanine green (ICG) are the few fluorescent dyes approved by the Food and Drug Administration (FDA) for clinical practice. Out of these, ICG has gained widespread acceptance for intraoperative FGS in numerous surgical procedures, and advances in FGS imaging systems have expanded the horizons of its application.[1]

■ PROPERTIES

Indocyanine Green Molecule

The Kodak Research Laboratories developed ICG in 1955 for near-infrared (NIR) photography. In 1959, it was approved by the FDA for clinical use.[2,3] Since its inception in the 1950s, its use was largely restricted to cardiac output measurement, delineating the anatomy of the retinal vessels and measuring the functional capacity of liver prior to major hepatic resection in cirrhotic patients for more than two decades. After 1980, the development and advancements in imaging systems and the discovery of new photometric measuring units resolved many technical difficulties and widened the scope of application of ICG for real-time intraoperative assistance.[4]

It is a sterile, anionic, water-soluble but relatively hydrophobic, tricarbocyanine molecule with a molecular mass of 776 Da. It is available in a lyophilized powder form and remains stable at room temperature. It is reconstituted prior to use. ICG is not readily soluble in normal saline but is soluble in distilled water (1 mg/mL). After reconstitution with distilled water, it can be mixed with saline or other crystalloid solutions. ICG usually contains sodium iodide as an additive agent and the native molecule is unstable when exposed to ultraviolet (UV) light. Hence, it is packed in an amber-colored glass bottle.[2]

Optical and Fluorescence Properties

The absorption and fluorescence spectrum of ICG is in the NIR region.[5] The basic principle of ICG fluorescence is that once the molecule is excited on stimulation with NIR spectrum light, it emits fluorescence. It largely depends on the solvent and the concentration of the drug used. ICG absorbs light with wavelengths between 600 and 900 nm and emits fluorescence between 750 and 950 nm.[5] On excitation, using either a laser beam or by NIR, the absorption peak ranges from 750 to 800 nm, and the emission peak is around 800–850 nm **(Fig. 1)**. The fluorescence emitted by ICG can be detected using specifically designated scopes and camera.[1,2,5,6]

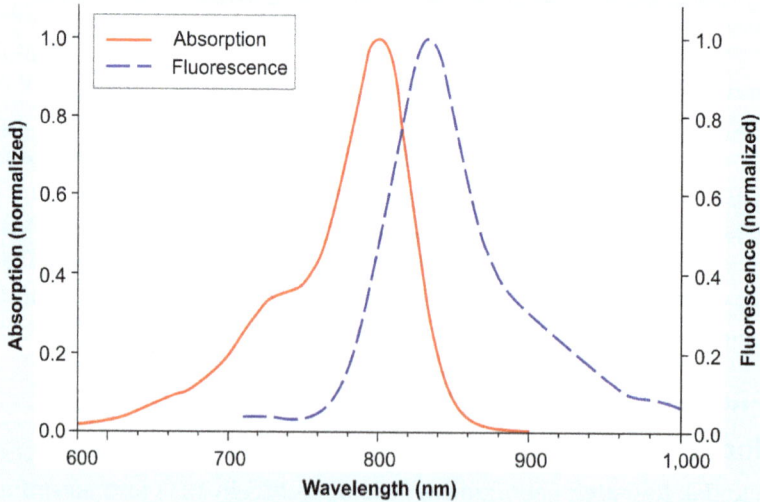

Fig. 1: Absorption and emission wavelength spectrum of fluorescence shown by indocyanine green (ICG) dye.[6]

PHARMACOKINETICS

After intravenous/intralesional administration, the ICG molecule rapidly binds to plasma proteins in the circulation and interstitial fluid: Albumin and β-lipoprotein (particularly to the lipid portion of the lipoprotein complex). The intravascular half-life of ICG is 180–250 seconds. It is taken up by the hepatocytes and excreted in an unconjugated form in the bile with the help of glutathione S-transferase transporter protein without any modification, about 8 minutes after injection. Excretion depends on liver function and vascularity.[2,5]

DOSAGE AND SAFETY PROFILE

The commonly used commercial preparation of ICG is available as a 25-mg dry lyophilized powder per vial (trade name "Aurogreen" by Aurolab) with a sterile syringe filter (0.2 μm) and 5 mL of sterile distilled water for reconstitution. After reconstitution, the solution must be used within 10 hours. In standard clinical practice, the usual dose of ICG administered is 0.2–0.5 mg/mL/kg, which is well tolerated and well below the toxicity level (5 mg/kg or more). Few reports have documented adverse allergic reactions to the drug, although deaths have not been reported.[7]

It is advised to use the dye with caution in pregnancy. Its use is contraindicated in neonates and premature infants undergoing exchange transfusion for hyperbilirubinemia, patients with uremia and chronic kidney disease, and patients allergic to iodine (due to the presence of sodium iodide). Exposure to UV light should be avoided as ICG becomes unstable and has a tendency to form metabolites on exposure to UV light.[2,3,5]

EQUIPMENT AND TECHNIQUE

Equipment

Indocyanine green fluorescence imaging and angiography can be performed intraoperatively during both open and minimally invasive procedures (laparoscopy/robotic). The operating room needs to be equipped with special equipment and surgical system for fluorescence imaging and angiography. The list of necessary equipment is as follows (**Figs. 2 and 3**):
- Light source—white light and NIR spectrum light
- Camera system—capable of vision both in white light and in NIR spectrum.

Note: For fluorescence imaging in open surgery, a charge-coupled device (CCD) camera with a light-emitting diode (wavelength 760 nm) as the light source and a cut filter to filter out light with wavelengths below 820 nm as the detector is required. During minimally invasive surgery, fluorescence and imaging are achieved through a laparoscopy system consisting of a small

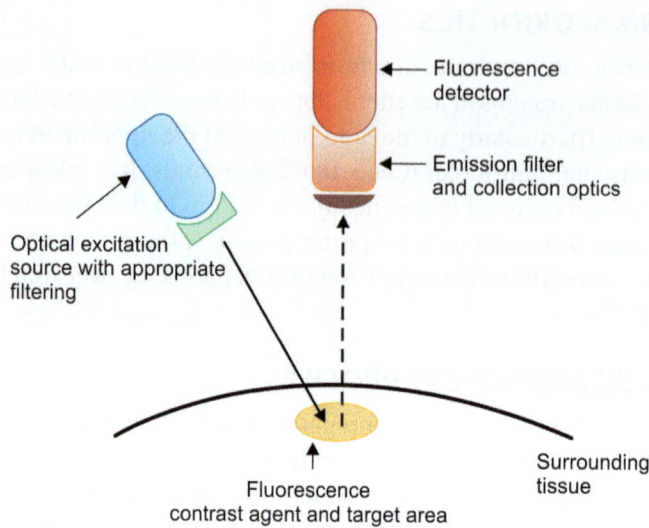

Fig. 2: Basic configuration of fluorescence imaging system: Consists of an excitation source, appropriate excitation, and emission filters depending on the choice of contrast agent, followed by collection optics and a fluorescence detector.[1]

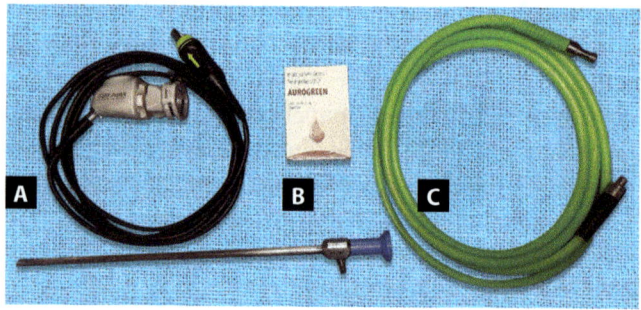

Figs. 3A to C: (A) Near-infrared (NIR) imaging + white light imaging enabled camera with cable and 30° laparoscope; (B) Indocyanine green (ICG) drug kit; (C) Light source cable.

control unit, a CCD camera, a xenon light source, and a 10-mm laparoscope containing specially coated lenses that transmit NIR light.
- Image acquisition unit and recorder
- Monitor screen
- ICG drug

Example:
The Stryker AIM 1588 + SPY-PHI technology system for open and laparoscopic surgery.

Firefly imaging system integrated in the da Vinci Xi Robotic Surgical System by Intuitive Surgical **(Figs. 4 and 5)**.

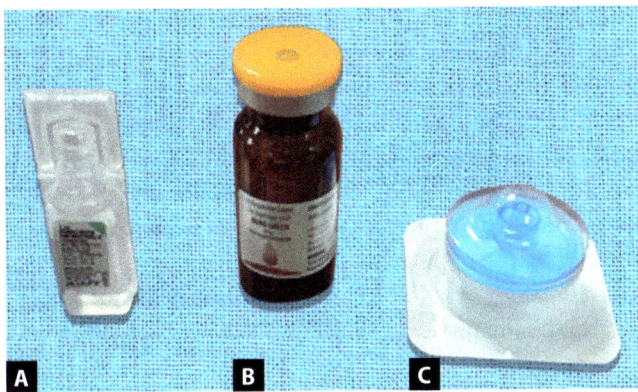

Figs. 4A to C: Indocyanine green (ICG) drug kit components (Aurogreen by Aurolab Ltd). (A) Sterile water for reconstitution; (B) Amber-colored drug vial; (C) Sterile drug filter.

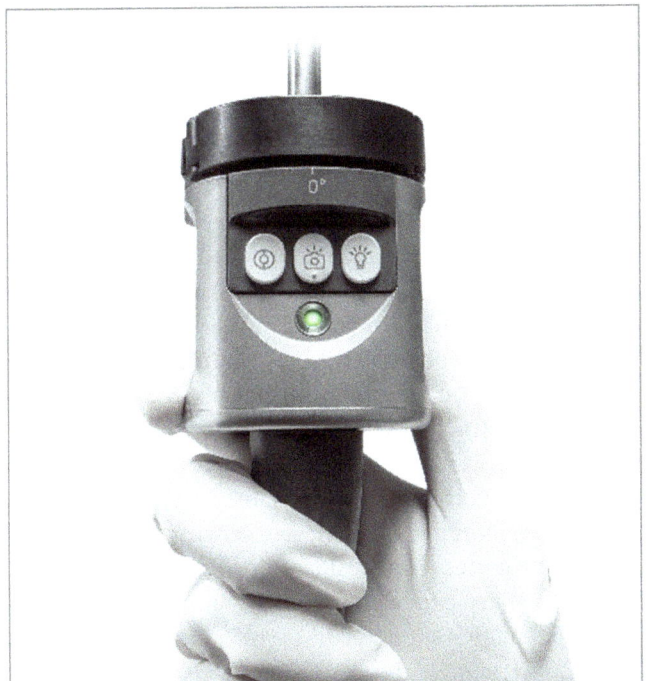

Fig. 5: Firefly fluorescence imaging system integrated in the scope of Da Vinci Xi system by Intuitive Surgical.

Technique

Indocyanine green is administered through intravenous access (a peripheral wide-bore cannula or a central venous catheter) or into the tissue directly based on the desired outcome.

After reconstitution of the drug using distilled water (10 mL sterile distilled water + 25 mg dry lyophilized powder = 2.5 mg of ICG/mL), a test dose of ICG (0.5 mL) is given via the provided filter. The imaging surgical system unit is switched on, and the assembly is prepared. Importantly, it is mandatory to turn off the background white light of the operating room when the drug is about to be injected to prevent white light interference with the fluorescence.

For intravenous use, a prepared weight-scaled dose of ICG solution is injected into the central or peripheral line as a tight bolus followed by a bolus of 10–12 mL of normal saline. The fluorescence imaging and angiography are performed, and the image is visualized on the monitor screen.[8]

SURGICAL APPLICATIONS

Role of Indocyanine Green in Liver Surgery

Dynamic Assessment of Liver Function

According to the clearance principle, hepatic clearance for any individual is calculated as follows:

$Cl = Q \times Ex$

Cl: Hepatic clearance

Ex: Liver extraction capacity

Q: Liver blood flow

Drugs and compounds are classified as high or low extraction substances based on their hepatic extraction capacity. The hepatic extraction rate of high extraction substances is an indirect measure of the liver blood flow. The opposite is true for substances with a low extraction rate. Clearance of these compounds, independent of the hepatic blood flow, is an indirect measure of metabolism or elimination processes. A key aspect of this principle is that the intrinsic hepatic clearance (Cl_{int}) becomes a measure of the capacity of the liver to remove substances when blood flow is not limited. Worldwide, ICG clearance is the most easy, reliable, and popularly used test for the perioperative dynamic assessment of liver function in case of major hepatic surgeries (liver resection or liver transplantation) and in the hepatology intensive care unit (ICU). The absence of metabolism and enterohepatic recirculation supports the correlation between ICG elimination kinetics and liver function.[9]

The conventional standardized technique of determination of ICG clearance (ICG_{Cl}) relies upon a rather complex ex vivo photometric analysis of multiple arterial blood samples obtained in a short time frame (15 minutes) after the intravenous administration. In spite of being the historical gold standard technique, it is used for research purposes only.

The novel noninvasive transcutaneous pulse dye densitometry (PDD) devices that can measure ICG concentrations are more commonly used in clinical practice. Among them are LiMon (Pulsion Medical System, Germany)

TABLE 1: Quantitative indocyanine green (ICG) kinetics variables.[10]

Variable	Denomination	Unit	Normal value
ICG_{PDR}	ICG plasma disappearance rate	%/min	>18–24%/min
ICG_{R15}	ICG retention ratio after 15 minutes	%	<10%
$ICG_{t1/2}$	ICG half-life	Minutes	3–5 minutes
ICG_{Cl}	ICG clearance	mL/min/kg	6–12 mL/min/kg

and DDG 2001 (Nihon Kohden, Japan). The use of these devices is validated in studies, and their interpretation results are comparable to the conventional techniques.[10-12]

Indocyanine green elimination is expressed as ICG plasma disappearance rate (ICG_{PDR}) or retention rate at 15 minutes (ICG_{R15}), assessing relative ICG concentration changes in the plasma.

The most commonly assessed ICG clearance parameters are as follows **(Table 1)**:
- Plasma disappearance rate—ICG_{PDR}
- Retention rate at 15 minutes—ICG_{R15}
- Disappearance rate constant (or elimination rate constant) (K constant)—ICG_K
- ICG clearance—ICG_{Cl}

Out of these, ICG_{PDR} and ICG_{R15} are the two most frequent kinetic parameters in clinical practice for dynamic assessment of liver function.[13-15] Major indications include the following:
- Assessment of the liver functional reserve before hepatic resection, particularly in cirrhotic patients. While computed tomography (CT) volumetry provides an idea of the volume of future liver remnant (FLR), ICG clearance estimates the functional capacity of the FLR, which is important particularly when planning major resections in cirrhotic and chronic liver disease (CLD) patients **(Flowchart 1)**.
- In liver transplantation, ICG is commonly used to assess the function of the graft [especially in case of extended criteria donors or suboptimal (marginal) graft]. Occasionally, it is used intraoperatively for sequential assessments of the graft during various phases of liver transplantation. It is more commonly used in the early postoperative period (post-transplantation) for dynamic assessment of the recovery of the graft.
- Biliary tree anomalies are quite common, and this remains the Achilles' heel of liver transplant. Donor hepatectomy involves visualization of the biliary anatomy and anomalies of the hepatic ducts that are surrounded by dense fibrous Glisson's sheath at the hilum. Magnetic resonance cholangiopancreatography (MRCP) provides a good preoperative road map of the biliary tree and its anomalies; however, it is not suitable for

Flowchart 1: Makuuchi decisional algorithm to select liver resection procedures in cirrhotic patients according to liver functional reserve.[9]

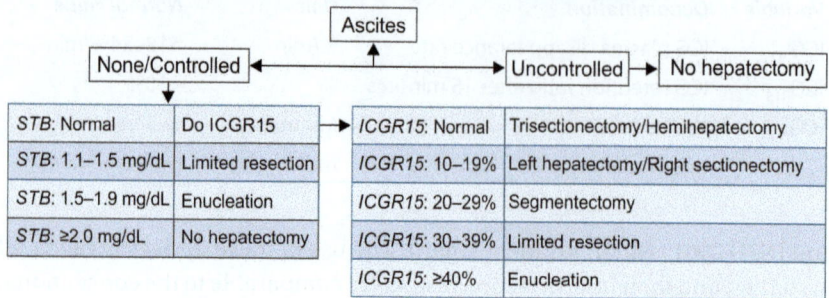

(ICGR: indocyanine green retention rate; STB: serum total bilirubin)

real-time visualization during surgery. Intraoperative cholangiography (IOC) is commonly used for this purpose. However, it is invasive, carries a risk of cholangitis, and requires fluoroscopy leading to radiation exposure. Intrabiliary injection of ICG aids in real-time visualization of the bile ducts around the hilar plate and in determining the optimal site for bile duct division, especially during minimally invasive surgery.[16]

- Post hepatectomy, assessment, and functional evaluation of the remnant liver in both cirrhotic and noncirrhotic patients.

  Note: The interpretation of the test result might be altered in the following situations:
  - The results must be interpreted with caution in the presence of hyperbilirubinemia and biliary obstruction as the ICG excretion process is significantly altered.
  - In case of repeated administrations, if the time interval between sequential doses of ICG is too short (<30 minutes), residual ICG may change the baseline drift and the ICG clearance parameters might be altered.
  - Stable hemodynamic conditions are imperative for a reliable test result. Systemic or local conditions that can affect hepatic blood flow (low cardiac output inducing hepatosplanchnic hypoperfusion or hepatic artery thrombosis and abdominal hypertension, respectively) reduce the ICG extraction and clearance. On the contrary, splanchnic hyperperfusion increases ICG extraction, in turn producing (falsely) high ICG_{PDR} readings.

- Fluorescence imaging for hepatic tumors, multifocal lesions, and hepatic metastatic lesions: Well-differentiated hepatocellular carcinomas take up ICG normally but retain the same for a prolonged time due to an impaired biliary tree excretion mechanism. This helps in visualization of fluorescence in tumor tissue intraoperatively after washout from the normal surrounding hepatic parenchyma. This also enables visualization of tiny multifocal lesions that are difficult to visualize and locate by the naked eye. For this indication, ICG must be given intravenously within 7–14 days before surgery, which ensures complete washout from the normal hepatic parenchyma. Preoperative liver function assessment can be carried out at the same time. On the other hand, poorly differentiated hepatic tumors or metastatic liver lesions do not take up and retain ICG; however, the compressed adjacent nontumorous hepatic parenchyma surrounding these lesions retain ICG due to impaired morphology and physiology. This leads to visualization of a rim of fluorescence around these lesions intraoperatively.[17]

ICG-guided Liver Resection for Anatomical Delineation (Open/Minimally Invasive Surgery)

- The segmental anatomy of liver with their boundaries can be delineated by injecting 0.25–2.5 mg/mL ICG into the portal vein or by injecting 2.5 mg ICG intravenously following closure of the proximal portal pedicle of hepatic regions planned for resection. This technique is useful when an anatomical resection is planned.

  It was later refined by increasing the dilution of ICG solution used for fluorescence and using an imaging system that enables superimposition of fluorescence images on colored images. Injection of indigo carmine solution with ICG concomitantly enhances the success rate of hepatic segment identification, especially in patients with cirrhosis with/without dense perihepatic fibrosis (reoperative surgery).[18,19]

- In addition to the positive staining technique described above, hepatic segments can also be identified by observing the fluorescence of the normal hepatic parenchyma planned to be preserved. Closure/division of the corresponding portal pedicle supplying the segments planned for resection becomes ischemic and appears as dark areas (negative staining technique). This can be achieved by intravenous injection of ICG. The latter technique is especially useful in laparoscopic hepatic segmentectomy, in which injection of ICG solution into the portal vein is technically difficult.[18-20]

- ICG is also useful for estimation of portal uptake function in veno-occlusive regions of the liver during hepatectomy or living-donor liver transplantation, by measuring trends of fluorescence intensity of the hepatic regions following ICG injection.[18-20]

Role of Indocyanine Green in Surgery of the Biliary Tract (Indocyanine Green Fluorescence Cholangiography)

Delineation of Biliary Anatomy

During laparoscopic cholecystectomy: Injury to the biliary tree during laparoscopic cholecystectomy was traditionally attributed to the initial learning curve of a surgeon. Subsequently, misinterpretation of biliary anatomy during dissection was found to be the primary cause. IOC is often used by surgeons in difficult cases. It can detect bile duct injuries on the table. However, IOC is invasive, can cause postoperative cholangitis, and itself requires access to the biliary tree (gallbladder/cystic duct).[21]

Fluorescence cholangiography with ICG, on the other hand, uses intravenous access to visualize the biliary tree, thus eliminating the risk of cholangitis and opening the bile duct. ICG is administered 30 minutes before surgery and is excreted in bile without any metabolism by the liver. The excitation of protein-bound ICG by NIR light leads to emission of fluorescence, thereby delineating the biliary tree intraoperatively. Fluorescence imaging is achieved through a system consisting of a small control unit, a CCD camera, a xenon light source, and a 10-mm laparoscope containing specially coated lenses that transmit NIR light.[4,21]

An alternative method of visualizing the biliary tree is by direct intrabiliary injection of ICG via a preexisting percutaneous transhepatic biliary catheter or direct injection into the extrahepatic biliary tree using a fine needle.[22] Combined fluorescence angiography (FA) and cholangiography can delineate the cystic artery and hepatic artery as well during cholecystectomy. This is especially useful in cases with difficult/frozen Calot's triangle, acute cholecystitis, suspicion of anomalous biliary anatomy, cholecystectomy for obese patients, and completion cholecystectomy for residual gallbladder **(Figs. 6A and B)**. To some extent, fluorescence cholangiography also has the ability to identify biliary stones in the cystic duct and common bile duct (CBD) as well as detect bile leak intraoperatively; however, the data available is limited.[23]

Identification of Hilar biliary anatomy during Benign biliary stricture repair: Benign biliary stricture (BBS) repair following iatrogenic bile duct injuries with or without a biliary fistula is often associated with dense scarring and adhesions present at the hilum. Identification of the bile duct with altered biliary anatomy at the hepatic hilum remains a challenge. Moreover, a higher level of injuries and associated hepatic changes (atrophy-hypertrophy complex) due to prolonged biliary obstruction leads to rotation of the hilar anatomy.

The bile duct at the hilum is conventionally identified by the "Hepp-Couinaud" technique of lowering the hilar plate and aspiration of bile using a syringe and needle. However, this is a blind and crude technique and has an associated risk of bleeding. It becomes even more difficult in type 4/5 strictures. Fluorescence cholangiography by administration of ICG 30–60 minutes prior to surgery or intrabiliary administration via a preexisting percutaneous transhepatic biliary tube clearly delineates the biliary anatomy and the bile duct at the hilum. It is noninvasive and mitigates the chances of

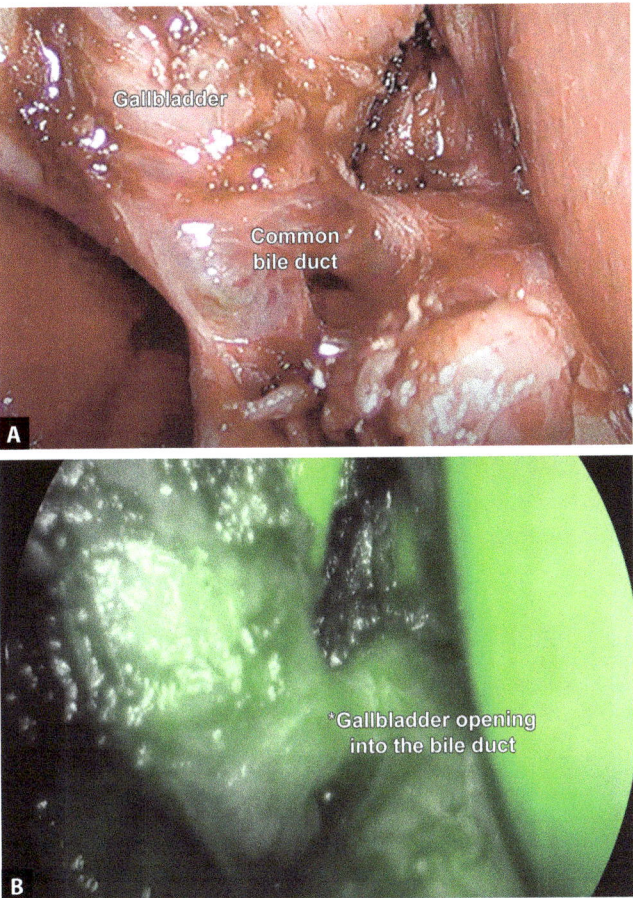

Figs. 6A and B: Indocyanine green (ICG) fluorescence delineating the gallbladder with obscured cystic duct and common bile duct junction during laparoscopy. (A) White light and (B) near-infrared (NIR) mode with ICG fluorescence.

trauma to the surrounding structures and major vessels. Surgeons attempting minimally invasive repair for BBS also find fluorescence cholangiography useful for intraoperative identification of the bile ducts. It also helps to identify aberrant sectoral ducts and/or right and left ducts in case of high complex injuries.[21-25]

Indocyanine Green Fluorescence Angiography for Real-time Assessment of Tissue Perfusion

Assessment of Vascularity of Colorectal Anastomosis

Anastomotic leak is one of the most dreaded complications following colorectal surgery. Tissue perfusion of the bowel ends plays an integral role in anastomotic healing. Traditionally, intraoperative vascularity of the bowel is assessed subjectively by color, peristalsis, and arterial pulsations, which lack predictive accuracy.[26,27]

An array of more objective modalities of assessment of perfusion is available such as Doppler flowmetry, pH measurement, and even an on-table angiography. They all have one or the other limitation: Difficult to use in the operating room, time consuming, inaccurate, and/or costly. Standardization and reproducibility of these techniques are other issues.[8]

Fluorescence angiography utilizing ICG allows for real-time intraoperative evaluation of bowel perfusion. Advantages of this technique include its ease of application, quick results, inexpensive, and excellent visualization and reproducibility.

Intraoperatively, ICG-FA is performed after bowel transection and also after the completion of anastomosis **(Figs. 7 and 8)**. The resection margins are revised in case of reduced fluorescence, and anastomosis is performed on a well-perfused zone. Not only the visualization of fluorescence, but the time to appearance of fluorescence is equally important as a marker

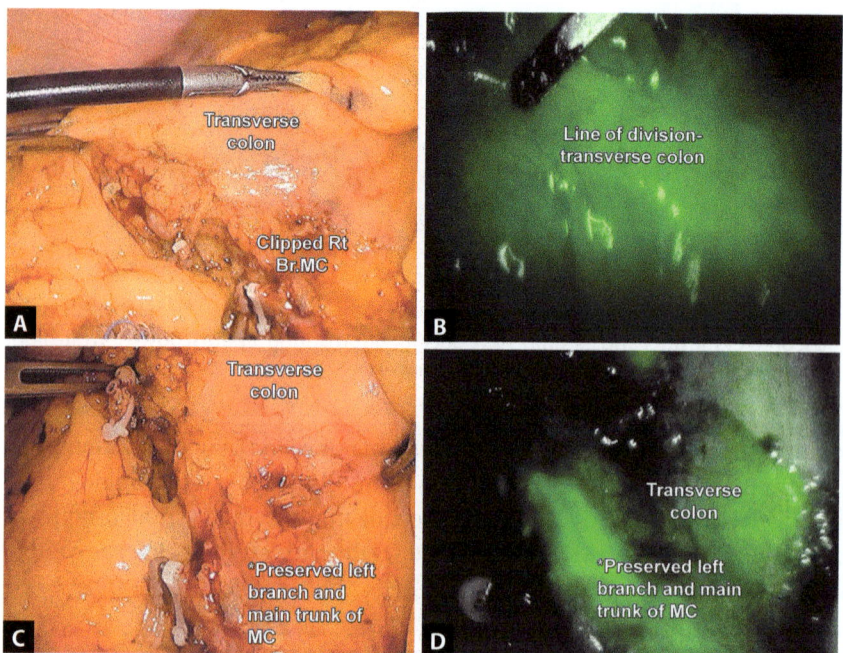

Figs. 7A to D: (A) Transverse colon after clipping and division of right branch of middle colic vessels prior to division during a laparoscopic right hemicolectomy; (B) Near-infrared (NIR) mode with indocyanine green-fluorescein angiography (ICG-FA) showing enhancement of the transverse colon with good vascularity in the planned area for division; (C) Transverse mesocolon with middle colic trunk and its preserved left branch; (D) ICG-FA enhancement of the mesocolon with preserved middle colic pedicle and adjacent transverse colon.

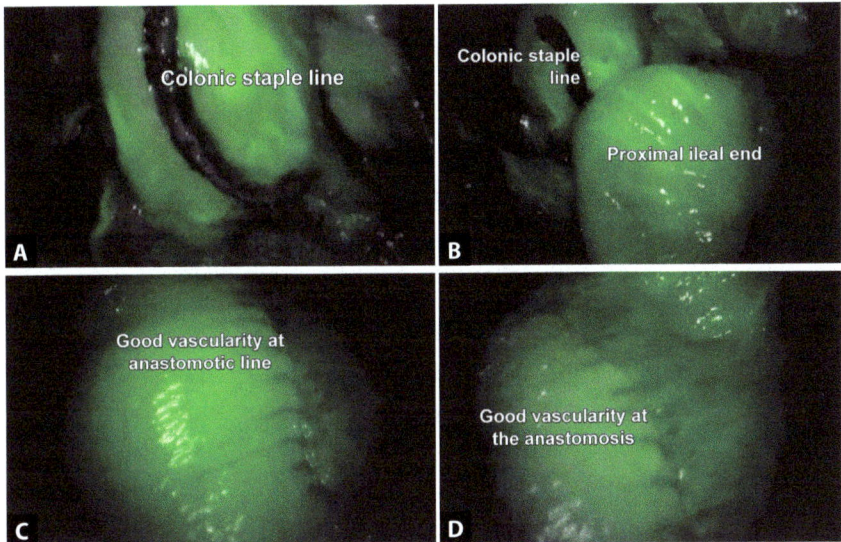

Figs. 8A and B: Good vascularity seen in the large bowel after resection: (A) Before anastomosis—colonic staple line and ileal end; (B) After anastomosis—vascularity along the anastomotic line.

of good vascularity. If the time to fluorescence is within 60–90 seconds of administration of ICG, the bowel segment is considered to have good vascularity and is safe for anastomosis. However, this technique needs further validation through prospective studies and randomized trials.[8,26,27]

Gastric Conduit Formation Following Esophagectomy

Similar to colorectal surgery, anastomotic leak is one of the important causes of death in esophageal surgeries. The anastomotic leak rate varies from 6.2 to 27%. Among several factors responsible for a safe anastomosis, ensuring an adequate blood supply is the most important. Stomach is frequently used for construction of a conduit following esophagectomy. The gastric conduit made is based on the right gastroepiploic vessels with or without preservation of the right gastric artery. The base of the conduit is generally well perfused compared to the tip (the site of anastomosis). Perfusion at the tip of the conduit is generally dependent on the intramural collateral capillary network of the stomach and is the most important factor for a satisfactory, well-perfused anastomosis. Moreover, when the conduit is taken to the neck, kinking, malalignment, or stretch on the supplying pedicle can compromise the vascularity of the conduit tip.[28-32]

Indocyanine green FA intraoperatively can be performed after step 1: construction of the conduit, step 2: after migration of the conduit to the anastomotic site, and step 3: after construction of the anastomosis. The fluorescence can be compared to that of the base of the conduit and the time to fluorescence can be noted (<90 seconds is good vascularity), and the anastomosis is fashioned in the well-perfused zone safely. The final real-time perfusion of the anastomosis can also be assessed intraoperatively.[31,33]

Surgery for Mesenteric Arterial Ischemia

Intestinal ischemia develops as a consequence of severe hypoperfusion of the bowel caused by various reasons. It leads to transmural necrosis of the bowel wall followed by perforation, peritonitis, sepsis, and organ failure if not diagnosed and treated early. Even with the best of management, the mortality exceeds 60%. At operation, determination of adequate bowel perfusion is extremely vital and, in presence of areas of frank ischemia, the judgment of appropriate resection margins is crucial. Extensive resections should be carefully considered as they can result in short bowel syndrome (SBS) with subsequent intestinal failure. This is associated with poor quality of life and significant morbidity. An extremely conservative approach may leave ischemic bowel in situ necessitating reoperation with an increased risk of postoperative mortality. Most appropriate extent of resection may be difficult to predict as a wide range of variables including hemodynamic instability and vasopressor support coexist. Also, a surgeon's experience becomes equally important.[34]

Intraoperative, real-time FA is a promising technique that has shown value for evaluation of adequacy of bowel perfusion. It can act as a guide to intraoperative decisions when there is a doubt regarding bowel viability. It may help reduce extensive resections, reoperations, and prevent SBS; however, more evidence is needed before it can be called a standard technique.[34]

Note: The findings of FA in acute/emergency situations may be altered and may not be reliable due to hemodynamic instability and use of vasopressors. Hence, it cannot be considered as a standard of care in this situation.

Use for Sentinel Lymph Node Mapping

Indocyanine green solution is injected subcutaneously around the tumor at 3, 6, 9, and 12 o'clock in cases of cutaneous melanoma or in the periareolar region in cases of breast cancer. Near about 5 mg of ICG is required for the procedure. It can also be used in surgery for gastric or colorectal malignancies to aid in lymphadenectomy by visualizing the lymphatic drainage basin of the tumor.

Technique Used in Breast Surgery

Sentinel lymph node mapping (SLNM) is done when breast conservation surgery is planned in cases of carcinoma breast. The operating room is darkened during axillary surgery. Repeated switching from "normal" to NIR light allows visualizing anatomy and fluorescence, respectively. Lymphatic vessels containing ICG are visualized transcutaneously, followed to the axillary region through an approximately 4-cm longitudinal incision on the skin along the anterior axillary line. The transcutaneous visibility of the lymphatic vessels is helpful to determine the exact site for skin incision. When lymph vessels are not seen transcutaneously, skin incision is made in the anterior axillary line to locate them. These lymph vessels lead to the ICG-positive nodes (sentinel nodes). In order to avoid leakage of ICG from the lymphatic system, which can discolor the surgical field and interfere with the color in lymph nodes, dissection along lymphatics is preferred over dividing them along the course. All ICG-positive nodes are sampled. Dissection is finished when no fluorescent lymph vessels or nodes are seen.[35,36]

Use of Indocyanine Green in Endocrine Surgery

Thyroid Surgery

During thyroidectomy, especially during minimally invasive approach or redo surgery, ICG is commonly used for the following indications:
- To identify the parathyroid glands (PTGs) before dissection of the thyroid gland with the use of intraoperative fluorescent imaging. It potentially reduces the chances of injury or contamination in the bloodstream as the area of dissection in relation to the thyroid gland can be visualized accurately.
- To objectively evaluate the viability of PTGs following total thyroidectomy. Four varying degrees of ICG fluorescence have been noted in PTGs following thyroidectomy.[37]

Parathyroid Surgery

During parathyroidectomy, ICG is used for the following indications:
- Identification and localization of pathologic PTGs in primary hyperparathyroidism, especially in redo operation.
- Evaluation of perfusion of preserved PTGs and prediction of its function postoperatively with the aim to avoid long-term hypoparathyroidism after subtotal parathyroidectomy.[37-39]

Use for Ureter Identification

When a colonic/colorectal resection is being performed or during a gynecologic procedure requiring extensive pelvic dissection, ICG fluorescence helps in identification and prevention of ureteric injuries **(Fig. 9)**. This can be done using cystoscopy and catheterization of the ureter followed by direct instillation of ICG into the ureter prior to the planned resection. Ureters

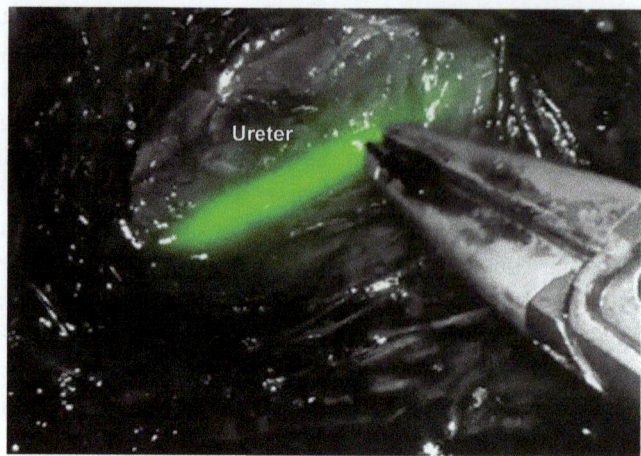

Fig. 9: Fluorescence seen in ureter after instillation of indocyanine green (ICG) via cystoscopy directly into the ureter during anterior resection in a case of carcinoma rectum.

course posteriorly in the retroperitoneum closely to the dissection field down into the pelvis and can easily be injured during mobilization of the colon and rectum or performing pelvic dissection. The placement of ureteral stents to assist in the identification process during surgery is quite common, especially in pelvic reoperative surgery. However, the placement of stents is invasive and is not without associated complications. It is more time consuming, costly, and subsequently requires an additional procedure for removal of the stent. Thus, ICG fluorescence is a convenient intraoperative method to recognize ureters during surgery.[40,41]

Use in Neurosurgery

For Cerebrovascular Surgery

Intraoperative digital subtraction angiography (DSA) is the gold standard technique for vascular interventions; however, it needs a radiology expert, is time consuming, expensive, involves radiation exposure, and requires a hybrid operation room. ICG video angiography (ICG-VA) is replacing it at many neurosurgical centers because it is simple, rapid, affordable, and reliable. It generates real-time images with good quality and high spatial resolution. The main purpose of aneurysm surgery is complete exclusion of the aneurysm from circulation while preserving the parent, perforating, and branching vessels.

In aneurysm surgery, ICG-VA gives adequate information about the clipped neck and parent/branching artery involvement in >90% of cases. Even the perforators of 0.5 mm diameter can be picked up effectively with this technique. But the residuals at the neck located behind the aneurysm cannot be detected by ICG-VA. ICG fluorescence may also be affected by calcifications, thick wall atherosclerotic vessels, and thrombosed aneurysms. Intraoperative DSA still remains the method of choice for such cases as well as for giant, complex aneurysms and aneurysms in deeper locations.[42-44]

In arteriovenous malformations (AVM) surgery, though neuronavigation can identify the nidus, it cannot assess the flow of AVMs. By using ICG-VA, we can identify the blood flow in arterialized veins and the residual nidus as well, especially in diffuse-type AVMs. But in deep-seated AVMs, we cannot rely only on this method and we may require intraoperative DSA to confirm the findings. In extracranial–intracranial (EC-IC) bypass, ICG-VA gives exact information about the anastomotic site so that early bypass graft failure can be avoided.[42-44]

Fluorescence-guided Brain Tumor Surgery

In the early 2000s, ICG was primarily used in neurosurgery as an angiography tool. In 2016, a novel technique named second-window ICG (SWIG) was developed using ICG fluorescence. This technique involves infusion of a high dose of ICG (5.0 mg/kg) in patients 24 hours prior to surgery. The tumor-targeting mechanism behind SWIG is known as the enhanced permeability and retention (EPR) effect, which stipulates that vascular permeability around solid tumors is pathologically enhanced due to structural breakdown, impaired lymphatic drainage, and increased permeability mediators. This leads to prolonged retention of ICG by the tumor mass. The fluorescence is directly related to the gadolinium enhancement of the tumor on T1-weighted magnetic resonance imaging (MRI). Hyperintensity with gadolinium on MRI is the strongest predictor of positive fluorescence, whereas nonenhancing tumors do not fluoresce, providing insight into the mechanism of ICG localization. To date, applications of SWIG have been reported in patients with high-grade gliomas, meningiomas, brain metastases, pituitary adenomas, craniopharyngiomas, chordomas, and pinealomas.[45]

Use in Cardiothoracic Surgery

For Early Graft Patency Assessment Post Coronary Artery Bypass Grafting

Early graft patency is a major determinant of morbidity and mortality following coronary artery bypass surgery. Intimal hyperplasia and atherosclerosis cause long-term graft failure, while early failure is usually attributed in part to technical errors during surgery. The need for intraoperative graft evaluation is paramount to determining the need for revision and ensuring future patency and functioning grafts.

The procedure begins after the distal anastomosis is complete. The NIR light source and camera source are positioned over the heart and activated just prior to the first ICG bolus. ICG is injected into the central venous system either via a central line or injection into the inferior vena cava in cases of off-pump coronary artery bypass grafting (CABG). For on-pump CABG, it is administered through the cardiopulmonary bypass oxygenator or into the ascending aorta. ICG is safe, rapid, and convenient to use intraoperatively.[46]

The limitations of this technique are that it is a qualitative assessment and the fluorescence and transit time of ICG across the graft cannot be measured. Each graft has to be evaluated and requires 3-4 minutes, which prolongs operative time. Pedicled conduits usually have poor visualization when compared to skeletonized conduits, making this technique of limited value in the former case. For adequate imaging, the heart needs to be rotated as the assessment is not possible when the heart is in its native position. There is a possibility of graft crimping when the heart is repositioned, and this can prove to be deleterious.[46] Hence, this technique requires further refinement, and more data is required before it can be considered as a standard technique for evaluation of anastomosis following CABG.

Use in Plastic Surgery

ICG Lymphangiography for Staging and Treatment of Lymphedema

Around 0.5 mL of the ICG solution is injected via the skin or subcutaneous tissue into a webspace or adjacent to a flexural crease. The region of interest is then illuminated with a light source after 60 seconds. Dermal and subdermal lymphatics can be identified to an approximate depth of 15 mm. Both static and dynamic protocols can be used. In the dynamic protocol, the patient receives manual lymphatic massage during imaging to qualitatively evaluate the capacity for drainage in individual lymphatic channels.

Indocyanine green lymphangiography findings are classified into two patterns: The normal "linear" pattern and the abnormal "dermal backflow (DB)" pattern. The DB pattern can be subdivided into "reticular", "splash", "stardust", and "diffuse" patterns. This is especially used in patients with primary and secondary lymphedema for mapping the lymphatic vessels and the regional lymph nodes to plan further surgical management.[47,48]

ICG Microangiography for Preoperative Perforator Mapping in Reconstructive Surgeries and for Intraoperative/Postoperative Assessment of Perfusion of Free Flaps, Pedicle Flaps, and Large Skin Paddle Flaps

Similar to ICG angiography, fluorescence microangiography is used to assess the microcirculation network of the skin and the soft tissue. In reconstructive surgery, successful outcomes are mainly dependent on the perfusion of the flap through the pedicle or feeding perforator vessels after isolation and transfer to the target site. It not only provides information about the flow through pedicle vessels, the enhancement also denotes the well-perfused and poorly perfused areas of the flap guiding early intraoperative corrective measures.[49]

To Assess the Vascularity of Skin Flaps Raised during Anterior Component Separation (Abdominal Wall Reconstruction for Ventral Hernia Repair) or During Modified Radical Mastectomy for Breast Cancer

While raising skin flaps for reconstruction surgery, excessive undermining of the flaps can compromise the vascularity of the skin and subcutaneous tissue and, in turn, lead to flap necrosis. Hence, ICG fluorescence is used to assess the perfusion of the skin flaps intraoperatively using the normal skin fluorescence as control and can guide the surgeon to take early corrective measures if required during the procedure itself.[49]

Estimation of the Depth and Grading of Burn Wounds

In burn wounds, the depth of involvement varies with the degree of damage to the microcirculation, and impaired microcirculation is directly associated with the degree of tissue necrosis. Hence, using the fluorescence seen in the normal unburned skin as control, ICG-FA is used to assess the depth of the burn wounds and, in turn, predict the possible viability of the skin and soft tissue.[49]

■ ADVANTAGES AND DISADVANTAGES

Since its inception, ICG has found an array of applications in various medical and surgical procedures. The advantages of ICG fluorescence imaging are as follows:
- *Patient safety:* Nontoxic and nonionizing
- *Ideal for angiography:* Binds efficiently to blood lipoproteins, i.e., it does not leak from circulation.
- Short life span in blood circulation allowing repeated applications
- *Good contrast:* There is not much NIR autofluorescence in tissue, giving a low noise background.
- *Deep imaging:* Operates in tissue optical window (NIR)
- Simple and cheap imaging method

However, like any other imaging modality, ICG carries a few drawbacks too:
- ICG is very recent in many applications such as cancer surgery, CABG, and reconstructive surgery, and further refinement in techniques and devices is required.

- ICG needs special equipment and camera for real-time fluorescence imaging.
- ICG has nonlinear fluorescence quantum yield versus the concentration used; hence, it is a qualitative rather than a quantitative assessment.
- ICG injection solution contains some sodium iodide; thus, an allergic reaction is possible and has been reported as well.
- ICG is unstable in solutions (beyond 10 hours) and when exposed to light. Hence, it needs to be freshly prepared for use.

■ FUTURE PROSPECTS

Having numerous applications, ICG fluorescence imaging and angiography are still in their nascent stages. ICG-mediated fluorescence in combination with technical advances in image-guided surgery and interventional procedures has the potential to create new functional imaging procedures which can expand or even replace the existing established surgical techniques. Though it is not considered as a standard of care in current surgical practice, with further refinement in the technique and imaging acquisition equipment, it can overcome its shortcomings. The development of quantitative methods to estimate the fluorescence and other new refinements in the technique may further widen the horizon for the application of ICG in clinical practice. Integration of ICG fluorescence with artificial intelligence in the future may also assist in standardized interpretation of the results of fluorescence imaging and may help in decision-making during the procedure. Artificial intelligence may also enable superimposition of fluorescence imaging on the normal anatomical image of the organ of interest to better interpret the results during a procedure. Many areas are yet to be explored, and further ongoing improvisation in the technique of ICG-FGS may increase its application in various fields and also make it a standard of care and modality of choice for real-time FGS in near future.

■ CONCLUSION

ICG-fluorescence imaging is relatively safe, sensitive, and nonspecific fluorophore-based navigation tool widely used in monitoring real-time organ perfusion and function. Developments in existing systems are continually being made to define standards, quantify fluorescent signals, and discover new prospective tracers. Additionally, a successful program for the development and application of FGS would require solid collaboration with optical engineers (for the development of hardware), computer scientists (for the development of the software), chemists (for the engineering of fluorophores), and medical professionals to enable clinical translation. Further research, including prospective trials and randomized controlled trials will provide robust evidence for both surgeons and patients in expanding the clinical utility of ICG.

REFERENCES

1. Stewart HL, Birch DJS. Fluorescence guided surgery. Methods Appl Fluoresc. 2021;9(4).
2. Alander JT, Kaartinen I, Laakso A, Pätilä T, Spillmann T, Tuchin VV, et al. A review of indocyanine green fluorescent imaging in surgery. Int J Biomed Imaging. 2012;2012:940585.
3. Bertani C, Cassinotti E, Della Porta M, Pagani M, Boni L, Baldari L. Indocyanine green: a potential to explore: narrative review. Ann Laparosc Endosc Surg. 2022;7:9.
4. Boni L, David G, Mangano A, Dionigi G, Rausei S, Spampatti S, et al. Clinical applications of indocyanine green (ICG) enhanced fluorescence in laparoscopic surgery. Surg Endosc. 2015;29(7):2046-55.
5. Cherrick GR, Stein SW, Leevy CM, Davidson CS. Indocyanine green: observations on its physical properties, plasma decay, and hepatic extraction. J Clin Invest. 1960;39(4):592-600.
6. Topaloglu N, Gulsoy M, Yuksel S. Antimicrobial photodynamic therapy of resistant bacterial strains by indocyanine green and 809-nm diode laser. Photomed Laser Surg. 2013;31(4):155-62.
7. Hope-Ross M, Yannuzzi LA, Gragoudas ES, Guyer DR, Slakter JS, Sorenson JA, et al. Adverse reactions due to indocyanine green. Ophthalmology. 1994;101(3):529-33.
8. Gilshtein H, Yellinek S, Wexner SD. The evolving role of indocyanine green fluorescence in the treatment of low rectal cancer. Ann Laparosc Endosc Surg. 2018;3:85-5.
9. Imamura H, Sano K, Sugawara Y, Kokudo N, Makuuchi M. Assessment of hepatic reserve for indication of hepatic resection: decision tree incorporating indocyanine green test. J Hepatobiliary Pancreat Surg. 2005;12(1):16-22.
10. Vos JJ, Wietasch JKG, Absalom AR, Hendriks HGD, Scheeren TWL. Green light for liver function monitoring using indocyanine green? An overview of current clinical applications. Anaesthesia. 2014;69(12):1364-76.
11. Wagener G. Assessment of hepatic function, operative candidacy, and medical management after liver resection in the patient with underlying liver disease. Semin Liver Dis. 2013;33(3):204-12.
12. Halle BM, Poulsen TD, Pedersen HP. Indocyanine green plasma disappearance rate as dynamic liver function test in critically ill patients. Acta Anaesthesiol Scand. 2014;58(10):1214-9.
13. Seyama Y, Kokudo N. Assessment of liver function for safe hepatic resection. Hepatol Res. 2009;39(2):107-16.
14. Mazza E, Prosperi M, DeGasperi A, Reggiori G, Corti A, Grugni C, et al. Plasma disappearance rate of indocyanine green after liver transplantation: always a reliable tool to predict graft function and outcome? Liver Transpl. 2008;14:S201:LB476.
15. Mizuguchi T, Kawamoto M, Meguro M, Hui TT, Hirata K. Preoperative liver function assessments to estimate the prognosis and safety of liver resections. Surg Today. 2014;44:1-10.

16. Mizuno S, Isaji S. Indocyanine green (ICG) fluorescence imaging-guided cholangiography for donor hepatectomy in living donor liver transplantation. Am J Transplant. 2010;10(12):2725-6.
17. Kokudo N, Ishizawa T. Clinical application of fluorescence imaging of liver cancer using indocyanine green. Liver Cancer. 2012;1(1):15-21.
18. Nomi T, Hokuto D, Yoshikawa T, Matsuo Y, Sho M. A novel navigation for laparoscopic anatomic liver resection using indocyanine green fluorescence. Ann Surg Oncol. 2018;25(13):3982.
19. Urade T, Sawa H, Iwatani Y, Abe T, Fujinaka R, Murata K, et al. Laparoscopic anatomical liver resection using indocyanine green fluorescence imaging. Asian J Surg. 2020;43(1):362-8.
20. Ishizawa T, Saiura A, Kokudo N. Clinical application of indocyanine green-fluorescence imaging during hepatectomy. Hepatobiliary Surg Nutr. 2016;5(4):322-8.
21. Pesce A, Piccolo G, La Greca G, Puleo S. Utility of fluorescent cholangiography during laparoscopic cholecystectomy: a systematic review. World J Gastroenterol. 2015;21(25):7877-83.
22. Husarova T, MacCuaig WM, Dennahy IS, Sanderson EJ, Edil BH, Jain A, et al. Intraoperative imaging in hepatopancreatobiliary surgery. Cancers (Basel). 2023;15(14):3694.
23. de'Angelis N, Catena F, Memeo R, Coccolini F, Martínez-Pérez A, Romeo OM, et al. 2020 WSES guidelines for the detection and management of bile duct injury during cholecystectomy. World J Emerg Surg. 2021;16:30.
24. Gao Y, Li M, Song ZF, Cui L, Wang BR, Lou XD, et al. Mechanism of dynamic near-infrared fluorescence cholangiography of extrahepatic bile ducts and applications in detecting bile duct injuries using indocyanine green in animal models. J Huazhong Univ Sci Technol Med Sci. 2017;37(1):44-50.
25. Figueiredo JL, Siegel C, Nahrendorf M, Weissleder R. Intraoperative near-infrared fluorescent cholangiography (NIRFC) in mouse models of bile duct injury. World J Surg. 2010;34(2):336-43.
26. Shen Y, Yang T, Yang J, Meng W, Wang Z. Intraoperative indocyanine green fluorescence angiography to prevent anastomotic leak after low anterior resection for rectal cancer: a meta-analysis. ANZ J Surg. 2020;90(11):2193-200.
27. Su H, Wu H, Bao M, Luo S, Wang X, Zhao C, et al. Indocyanine green fluorescence imaging to assess bowel perfusion during totally laparoscopic surgery for colon cancer. BMC Surg. 2020;102.
28. Shimada Y, Okumura T, Nagata T, Sawada S, Matsui K, Hori R, et al. Usefulness of blood supply visualization by indocyanine green fluorescence for reconstruction during esophagectomy. Esophagus. 2011;8(4):259-66.
29. Koyanagi K, Ozawa S, Oguma J, Kazuno A, Yamazaki Y, Ninomiya Y, et al. Blood flow speed of the gastric conduit assessed by indocyanine green fluorescence: new predictive evaluation of anastomotic leakage after esophagectomy. Medicine (United States). 2016;95(30):e4386.
30. Slooter MD, de Bruin DM, Eshuis WJ, Veelo DP, van Dieren S, Gisbertz SS, et al. Quantitative fluorescence-guided perfusion assessment of the gastric conduit to predict anastomotic complications after esophagectomy. Dis Esophagus. 2021;34(5):1-8.

31. Luo RJ, Zhu ZY, He ZF, Xu Y, Wang YZ, Chen P. Efficacy of indocyanine green fluorescence angiography in preventing anastomotic leakage after McKeown minimally invasive esophagectomy. Front Oncol. 2021;10:619822.
32. Karampinis I, Ronellenfitsch U, Mertens C, Gerken A, Hetjens S, Post S, et al. Indocyanine green tissue angiography affects anastomotic leakage after esophagectomy. A retrospective, case-control study. Int J Surg. 2017;48:210-4.
33. Kumagai Y, Hatano S, Sobajima J, Ishiguro T, Fukuchi M, Ishibashi KI, et al. Indocyanine green fluorescence angiography of the reconstructed gastric tube during esophagectomy: efficacy of the 90-second rule. Dis Esophagus. 2018;31(12).
34. Joosten JJ, Longchamp G, Khan MF, Lameris W, van Berge Henegouwen MI, Bemelman WA, et al. The use of fluorescence angiography to assess bowel viability in the acute setting: an international, multi-centre case series. Surg Endosc. 2022;36(10):7369-75.
35. Ballardini B, Santoro L, Sangalli C, Gentilini O, Renne G, Lissidini G, et al. The indocyanine green method is equivalent to the 99mTc-labeled radiotracer method for identifying the sentinel node in breast cancer: a concordance and validation study. Eur J Surg Oncol. 2013;39(12):1332-6.
36. Grischke EM, Röhm C, Hahn M, Helms G, Brucker S, Wallwiener D. ICG fluorescence technique for the detection of sentinel lymph nodes in breast cancer: results of a prospective open-label clinical trial. Geburtshilfe Frauenheilkd. 2015;75(9):935-40.
37. Zaidi N, Bucak E, Yazici P, Soundararajan S, Okoh A, Yigitbas H et al. The feasibility of indocyanine green fluorescence imaging for identifying and assessing the perfusion of parathyroid glands during total thyroidectomy. J Surg Oncol. 2016;113:775-8.
38. Spartalis E, Ntokos G, Georgiou K, Zografos G, Tsourouflis G, Dimitroulis D, et al. Intraoperative indocyanine green (ICG) angiography for the identification of the parathyroid glands: current evidence and future perspectives. In Vivo. 2020;34(1):23-32.
39. Jitpratoom P, Anuwong A. The use of ICG enhanced fluorescence for the evaluation of parathyroid gland preservation. Gland Surg. 2017;6(5):579-86.
40. Yeung TM, Volpi D, Tullis ID, Nicholson GA, Buchs N, Cunningham C, et al. Identifying ureters in situ under fluorescence during laparoscopic and open colorectal surgery. Ann Surg. 2016;263(1):e1-2.
41. Siddighi S, Yune JJ, Hardesty J. Indocyanine green for intraoperative localization of ureter. Am J Obstet Gynecol. 2014;211:436.e1-2.
42. Balamurugan S, Agrawal A, Kato Y, Sano H. Intraoperative indocyanine green video-angiography in cerebrovascular surgery: an overview with review of literature. Asian J Neurosurg. 2011;6(2):88-93.
43. Norat P, Soldozy S, Elsarrag M, Sokolowski J, Yağmurlu K, Park MS, et al. Application of indocyanine green videoangiography in aneurysm surgery: evidence, techniques, practical tips. Front Surg. 2019;6:34.
44. Della Puppa A, Rossetto M, Volpin F, Rustemi O, Grego A, Gerardi A, et al. Microsurgical clipping of intracranial aneurysms assisted by neurophysiological monitoring, microvascular flow probe, and ICG-VA: outcomes and intraoperative data on a multimodal strategy. World Neurosurg. 2018;113:e336-44.

45. Teng CW, Huang V, Arguelles GR, Zhou C, Cho SS, Harmsen S, et al. Applications of indocyanine green in brain tumor surgery: review of clinical evidence and emerging technologies. Neurosurg Focus. 2021;50(1):1-10.
46. Ohmes LB, Di Franco A, Di Giammarco G, Rosati CM, Lau C, Girardi LN, et al. Techniques for intraoperative graft assessment in coronary artery bypass surgery. J Thorac Dis. 2017;9(Suppl. 4):S327-32.
47. Liu M, Liu S, Zhao Q, Cui Y, Chen J, Wang S. Using the indocyanine green (ICG) lymphography to screen breast cancer patients at high risk for lymphedema. Diagnostics (Basel). 2022;12(4):983.
48. Burrows PE, Gonzalez-Garay ML, Rasmussen JC, Aldrich MB, Guilliod R, Maus EA, et al. Lymphatic abnormalities are associated with *RASA1* gene mutations in mouse and man. Proc Natl Acad Sci U S A. 2013;110(21):8621-6.
49. Holm C. Clinical applications of ICG fluorescence imaging in plastic and reconstructive surgery. Open Surg Oncol J. 2010;2:37-47.

CHAPTER 3

Third-space Endoscopy

Arunima Verma, Rahul, Saurabh Bokade, Sunil Kumar

■ INTRODUCTION

Conventional endoscopic interventions are carried out within the lumen of the gastrointestinal tract (GIT). This is termed first-space endoscopy and includes diagnostic endoscopy, polypectomy, biopsy, variceal ligation, dilatation, and so on. The gastroenterologists with experience and expertise ventured the peritoneal cavity through natural orifice transluminal endoscopic surgery (NOTES). It was first described in an animal model by Anthony Kalloo at Johns Hopkins in the year 2000. He demonstrated successful transgastric liver biopsy in a porcine model. This was followed by few reports on transgastric appendicectomy, cholecystectomy, peritoneal biopsy, and tubal ligation in humans using flexible scopes. The biggest advantage is a scarless surgery, a perfect procedure from cosmetic standpoint.[1,2] However, it has remained an experimental procedure till date and is still not a curriculum in clinical practice. The risk of nonhealing of iatrogenic perforation created during the procedure, followed by sepsis, remains high, apart from the difficulty in dissection.

In the last decade, a new concept of submucosal endoscopy has evolved. It involves raising a mucosal flap, creating a tunnel in the submucosal plane, and addressing the pathologies in deeper layers of GIT. It was introduced by Sumiyama et al. in 2007 when they used this route to enter the peritoneal cavity. The name "third-space endoscopy (TSE)" was christened by Khashab and Pasricha in 2013. Pasricha et al. described the first transmucosal myotomy in a porcine model. However, Inoue et al. documented the first peroral endoscopic myotomy (POEM) in humans in 2010.[2-4] The success of POEM paved the path for multiple TSE procedures. In this chapter, the authors will critically discuss the various TSE procedures, their feasibility, and applicability.

In nutshell, the gastrointestinal lumen is the first space where conventional endoscopies are performed. The second space is the peritoneal cavity, which has been surgeon's forte, and the third space is the intramural space or the submucosal space.

TECHNIQUE AND INSTRUMENTS FOR THIRD-SPACE ENDOSCOPY

The basic steps of all TSE procedures include **(Figs. 1A to C)**:
- A submucosal cushion is raised 4–5 cm proximal to the area of interest.
- Mucosal incision is placed on the raised cushion to raise a flap and fashion a linear submucosal tunnel beyond the pathology to secure enough working place. This is done by carbon dioxide insufflation.
- Desired procedure (myotomy, tumor excision) is performed away from the mucosal entry site.
- The mucosal defect is closed with endoclips, sutures, or endoloops.

Instruments required for TSE include high-definition endoscopes, carbon dioxide insufflator, electrosurgical unit, and endoscopic devices (electrosurgical knives with water jet, hemostatic forceps, and clips and endoloops).[5]

Procedures described under TSE are performed under general anesthesia. They are enlisted in **Table 1**.

PERORAL ENDOSCOPIC MYOTOMY

Peroral endoscopic myotomy is a minimally invasive endoscopic procedure that involves creating a myotomy across the inner circular muscle layer of the esophagus. POEM has gained popularity as an effective and safe treatment for achalasia cardia, offering shorter hospital stays, faster recovery, and lower complication rates compared to traditional surgical approaches. Long-term studies have shown excellent symptomatic relief and esophageal emptying.[5]

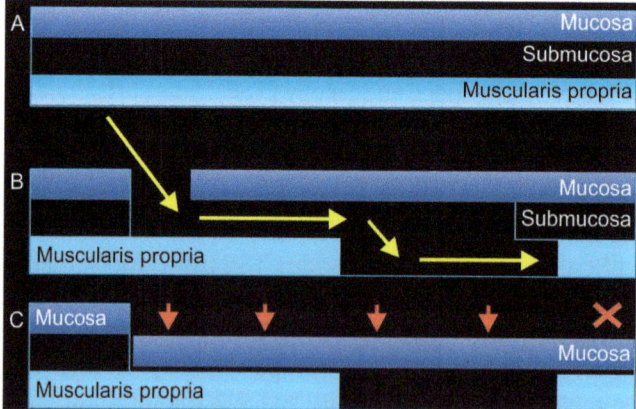

Figs. 1A to C: Principle of third-space endoscopy: (A) Gastrointestinal tract has three layers; (B) Mucosal is breached 5–10 cm proximal to the area of interest and then approached through a submucosal tunnel. Procedure is completed; (C) Mucosal defect is closed and remains away from the intervention site.[6]

TABLE 1: Third-space endoscopy procedures.

Name of the procedure	Indications
Peroral endoscopic myotomy (POEM)	• Achalasia • Diffuse esophageal spasm • Jackhammer esophagus • Gastroesophageal junction outflow obstruction
Gastric-POEM or peroral pyloromyotomy (G-POEM or POP)	Gastroparesis
Zenker-POEM or submucosal tunneling endoscopic septum division (Z-POEM/STESD)	Zenker's diverticulum
Peroral endoscopic tunneling for restoration of the esophagus (POETRE)	Complete esophageal obstruction/stricture
Per-rectal endoscopic myotomy (PREM)	Hirschsprung's disease
Submucosal tunneling endoscopic dissection (STER)	Submucosal tumors [leiomyoma, gastrointestinal stromal tumor (GIST)]

Peroral endoscopic myotomy was first introduced as treatment for achalasia in humans by Inoue et al. in 2010. This approach aimed to club the advantages of a minimally invasive endoscopic approach and the long-term efficacy of surgical myotomy. POEM is generally performed as a five-step procedure **(Box 1)**.

The Japan Esophageal Society has provided descriptive rules for diagnosing achalasia cardia on endoscopy. They are as follows:
- Dilatation of the esophageal lumen
- Abnormal retention of food and/or liquid remnants in the esophagus
- Whitish change and thickening of the esophageal mucosal surface
- Functional stenosis of the esophagogastric junction (EGJ), in which the endoscope passes through the stenotic segment and the EGJ fails to dilate by insufflation
- Abnormal contraction waves of the esophagus.

Only about half of the patients show characteristic endoscopic features; therefore, caution should be taken not to exclude the diagnosis of achalasia in patients with normal findings on endoscopy. Several endoscopic features have been described as highly suggestive of achalasia cardia, including pinstripe pattern, rosette-like folds, and Champagne glass appearance **(Figs. 2 and 3)**.[7]

The patient shows improvement in a pinstripe pattern after POEM but has developed post-treatment gastroesophageal reflux (GERD) disease.

Peroral endoscopic myotomy is a promising therapeutic modality for achalasia patients who have failed to respond to pneumatic dilation (PD) therapy.

BOX 1: Steps of peroral endoscopic myotomy.
1. Entry into the submucosal space at 14–15 cm proximal to esophagogastric junction (EGJ) either at 2 o'clock or at 5–6 o'clock position
2. Submucosal tunneling is done by combination of electrocautery dissection, injection of saline with dye, and carbon dioxide insufflation. The dissection is carried out till 2–3 cm beyond EGJ. Use of an ultraslim endoscope makes the procedure less invasive. The EGJ is identified by submucosal space widening in the cardia or by distance from the incisors. Other methods include fluoroscopy (distance between the tip of endoscope in submucosal plane and a radiopaque marker at EGJ placed at the start is estimated) and second endoscope (retroflex view by a second endoscope allows real-time assessment of cardia)
3. Endoscopic myotomy—anterior or posterior. The anterior myotomy is preferred at 2 o'clock position as it is in line with the anterior aspect of lesser curvature. The posterior myotomy is performed at 5–6 o'clock position, especially in patients with failed laparoscopic Heller's myotomy (HM) in order to avoid scarred tissue anteriorly. Selective division of circular muscle fibers in the esophagus is the key. Longitudinal layer is divided only at EGJ and the cardia. Selective division of circular muscles in esophagus prevents leakage of carbon dioxide into the mediastinum
4. Adequacy of the myotomy is assessed at the end of the procedure—subjective relaxation of EGJ
5. Closure of the mucosal entry by endoclip or sutures

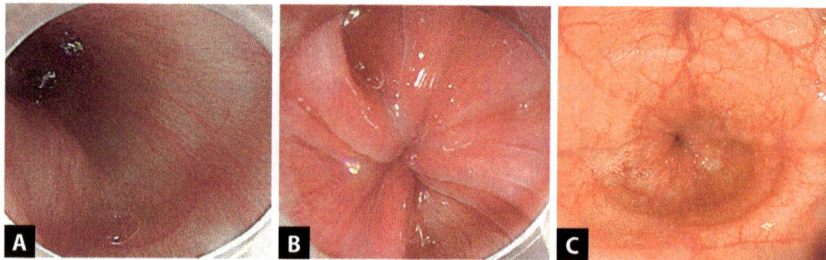

Figs. 2A to C: Endoscopic features in achalasia cardia: (A) Pinstripe pattern; (B) Rosette-like esophageal folds; (C) Champagne glass sign.

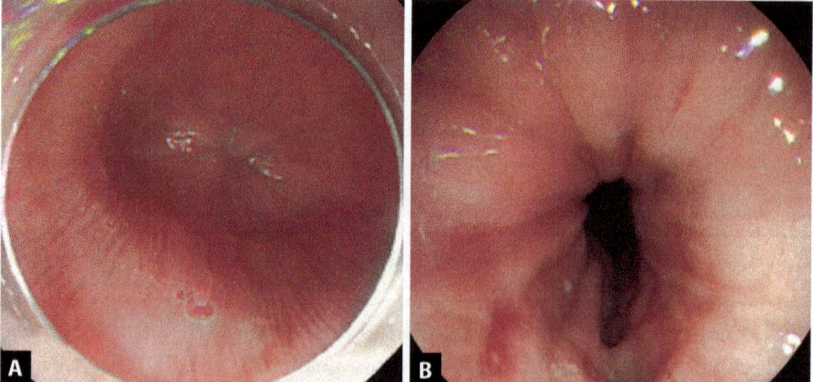

Figs. 3A and B: Endoscopic images of a patient with achalasia (A) before POEM and (B) after POEM. (POEM: peroral endoscopic myotomy)

Previous dilation procedures have no obvious influence on the efficacy of POEM surgery.[8] Werner et al. published a multicenter, open-label, prospective, randomized controlled noninferiority trial comparing POEM and laparoscopic Heller myotomy (HM) with Dor's fundoplication. The primary outcome was post-treatment clinical efficacy at 24 months. Out of 211 patients, 108 underwent POEM and the rest ($n = 103$) underwent HM. The clinical efficacy (symptom relief) was comparable in the two groups at 24 months follow-up (82.4 vs. 80.6%); however, the GERD was significantly higher in patients who underwent POEM.[9]

A recent meta-analysis by Schlottmann et al. analyzed the response rates of 7,782 patients in 24 studies who underwent either laparoscopic HM, the present gold standard for achalasia ($n = 5,834$), or POEM ($n = 1,958$). Symptom improvement in dysphagia was observed in 93.5% of the patients who underwent POEM and 91.0% of those who underwent HM at 12-month follow-up and in 92.7 and 90.0% at 24-month follow-up, respectively. However, POEM was associated with a significantly higher incidence of pathological reflux as evidenced by pH monitoring.[10]

A multicenter comparative study by Kumbhari et al. compared the treatment outcomes of POEM with those of HM in patients with type III achalasia. POEM showed better clinical outcomes, with a response rate of 98.0% in comparison to 80.8% with HM.[11] POEM and HM had similar long-term (4-year) efficacy with similar adverse event and reflux rates, but POEM was associated with greater efficacy in type III achalasia.[12]

A total of 564 patients were included in a study conducted by Quan-Lin Li. After a median follow-up of 49 months (range, 3–68 months), the Eckardt score and lower esophageal sphincter (LES) pressure were significantly decreased [median Eckardt score, 8–2 ($p < 0.05$); median LES pressure, 29.7–11.9 mm Hg ($p < 0.05$)]. Fifteen failures occurred within 3 months, 23 between 3 months and 3 years, and 10 after 3 years. The estimated clinical success rates at 1, 2, 3, 4, and 5 years were 94.2%, 92.2%, 91.1%, 88.6%, and 87.1%, respectively. Multivariate Cox regression revealed long disease duration (≥10 years) and history of prior interventions to be risk factors for recurrence. Clinical reflux occurred in 37.3% of patients (155/416). POEM is a highly safe and effective treatment for achalasia cardia with favorable long-term outcomes.[13]

Peroral endoscopic myotomy is associated with a short-term clinical response of 82–100% in treatment of patients with achalasia. The patients had a minimum of 4 years of follow-up. Clinical response was defined by an Eckardt score ≤3. A total of 146 patients were included from 11 academic medical centers in this study conducted by Brewer Gutierrez et al., which showed POEM as a durable and safe procedure with an acceptably low adverse event rate and an excellent long-term clinical response.[14]

Peroral endoscopic myotomy is a safe, effective, and durable treatment for achalasia in children. Prior treatment does not affect the outcomes of

POEM in children.[15] POEM allows for a longer myotomy than laparoscopic HM, which may result in improved clinical outcomes. Hence, POEM appears to be an effective and safe alternative in patients with type III achalasia.[11]

A total of 2,342 patients {age 48.1 [standard deviation (SD) 6.8] years; 50.1% males} with a median follow-up of 48 months (interquartile range 45–60) were analyzed by Vespa et al. This study consolidated long-term clinical efficacy of POEM with achalasia. Post-POEM symptomatic reflux remained stable over time. The risk for Barrett's esophagus and peptic strictures appeared minimal.[16]

Although acid reflux increases after POEM, majority are mild and respond to medications (proton-pump inhibitors). The incidence of reflux (12–21%) does not differ with the site of myotomy (anterior or posterior).[17] Two mechanisms have been proposed to decrease the chances of reflux: Limiting the myotomy on stomach to <2 cm, and at the EGJ, perforator vessels should be identified, and the plane of myotomy is kept to the right of it in order to avoid injury to the sling fibers. Recently, POEM with fundoplication has been advocated by few, where fundoplication is added to anterior myotomy. This significantly decreases the rate of reflux, according to few short-term studies.[18] Further prospective studies with large cohorts are required to establish the role of endoscopic fundoplication in patients undergoing POEM.

Incidence of major adverse events after POEM is relatively uncommon (<1%). Capnoperitoneum and capnothorax can occur, but in majority, they resolve spontaneously. Technical failure is reported to be <1%, with the most common causes being submucosal fibrosis, multiple interventions, and long-standing disease with sigmoid esophagus. Bleeding complication in one large study was reported to be 0.9% and mucosal perforation was 2.8%.[19] Overall, POEM is a safe procedure.

GASTRIC PERORAL ENDOSCOPIC MYOTOMY OR PERORAL PYLOROMYOTOMY

Delayed gastric emptying in the absence of mechanical obstruction is termed gastroparesis. It is a complex disorder usually seen in patients with prolonged diabetes (autonomic neuropathy causes gastric dysmotility) and following upper gastrointestinal surgery (vagotomy causes pylorospasm). Medical treatment includes dietary modifications and use of prokinetics. Metoclopramide [approved by the Food and Drug Administration (FDA)] is effective in certain patients but may cause extrapyramidal side effects with prolonged use.[20,21] Endoscopic dilatation for pylorospasm and botulinum injection have been tried but have failed to show improvement in symptoms.[22] Laparoscopic pyloromyotomy, although effective, is an invasive method. Endoscopic stenting can be used for symptom relief but cannot be used as a permanent solution. Stent migration is a common problem.[23]

A novel technique in the form of gastric peroral endoscopic myotomy (G-POEM) or peroral pyloromyotomy (POP) was first described by Khasab et al. in 2013.[24] It works on the principles of POEM, wherein mucosal entry is fashioned 5 cm proximal to the pyloric channel, submucosal tunnel is created, and pyloric muscle ring is identified and divided to a length of 2–3 cm (distal to proximal direction), avoiding injury to the duodenal mucosa. In cases of difficulty in identification of pyloric ring, authors have used fluoroscopy as a guide to improve accuracy. Lesser curvature approach is superior to greater curvature approach in terms of technical success and ease of procedure. Most common complications include capnoperitoneum, bleeding, and ulceration, majority of which can be managed conservatively.[25] Several studies have shown satisfactory technical success (95–100%) of G-POEM; however, they do not match the clinical results of POEM done for achalasia cardia. One of the important explanations is the complex nature of the disease (gastroparesis). The results are better in patients with gastroparesis following surgery (pylorospasm) and short duration of symptoms. Outcomes are variable in patients with delayed gastric emptying due to poor motility (diabetic autonomic neuropathy) or long-standing disease leading to gastric dilatation.[26,27]

In a study by Gonzalez et al., diabetes and female gender were associated with inferior outcomes. The benefit in terms of relief of symptoms and gastric emptying was highest when the etiology was not known (idiopathic) and worst for gastroparesis due to diabetes (92 vs. 43% at 6 months following G-POEM in favor of idiopathic gastroparesis).[28] Hence, patients should be selected wisely for optimum results.

■ ZENKER'S PERORAL ENDOSCOPIC MYOTOMY

Zenker diverticulum (ZD), also called pharyngeal pouch, occurs due to mucosal herniation through cricopharyngeus muscle. It is an uncommon clinical condition caused by impaired relaxation or paradoxical spasm of cricopharyngeus muscle during the act of swallowing. Treatment options are endoscopic division of septum using stapler or diverticulectomy/diverticulopexy with cricopharyngeal myotomy. Endoscopic treatment is preferred; however, it is associated with high recurrence rates to the tune of 10–12%.[29] Surgery provides complete myotomy, thus decreasing the recurrence, but carries its own set of complications. With the advent of TSE, a minimally invasive endoscopic technique with high clinical success rate can be performed. This is termed submucosal tunneling endoscopic septum division (STESD) or Zenker's peroral endoscopic myotomy (Z-POEM).

The procedure is done under general anesthesia using a therapeutic endoscope. Mucosa is incised proximal to the septum, and a tunnel is fashioned on both sides of the septum (diverticular side and esophageal side) till the base. The septum is divided completely. Esophageal myotomy is done to a length of around 2 cm. The mucosal opening is finally clipped.

Being a rare disease, the literature on Z-POEM is limited to case reports and few case series. In a series by Juliana et al., the success rate of Z-POEM was >95%. However, long-term follow-ups and comparative studies are needed to establish the efficacy. Being more invasive than endoscopic stapling, the procedure should be cautiously used in elderly patients with multiple comorbidities.[30]

PERORAL ENDOSCOPIC TUNNELING FOR RESTORATION OF ESOPHAGUS

Chemoradiotherapy and/or surgery in advanced esophageal malignancy may result in tight stricture(s) causing complete esophageal obstruction. Strictures spanning >3 cm are not amenable for endoscopic dilatation, even by a transillumination-guided rendezvous technique (combined approach—antegrade with retrograde endoscopy through the gastrostomy). As a replacement for morbid surgical procedures in such situations, peroral endoscopic tunneling for restoration of esophagus (POETRE) has shown promise in salvaging these patients.[31,32] The procedure is again based on the principles of TSE. Mucosal is incised 5 cm from the stricture in a prograde or retrograde fashion based on the position of the stricture. A submucosal tunnel is dissected across the stricture. The length of the tunnel is guided by illumination or fluoroscopy from the opposite end (through gastrostomy). Once the endoscopes from the two sides meet, a guidewire is negotiated across the submucosal tunnel into the lumen on the opposite side. Over the guidewire, dilatation is done and a covered metallic stent is placed across the stricture.[33] The technical success rate, as described by different authors, is high. The patients required regular dilatation of the neo-esophagus after stent removal. However, due to the rarity of this disease, literature search on POETRE is limited to case reports and small case series.[34] Multicenter studies are required to bring forth the nuances of the procedure.

PER-RECTAL ENDOSCOPIC MYOTOMY

Per-rectal endoscopic myotomy (PREM) was first described by Bapaye et al. for Hirschsprung's disease (HD) in 2016.[35] HD is a rare congenital disorder, wherein the submucosal and myenteric ganglion cells are absent in the rectosigmoid region for a variable length. The diseased segment remains spastic, while proximal normal colon becomes distended. Patients present with functional large bowel obstruction in infancy. Few with short segment involvement manifest late in adulthood with constipation.

Conventional treatment of HD is pull-through of the normal colon to fashion a colon anal anastomosis, bypassing the spastic segment, but it is associated with high morbidity. PREM is a novel technique and is based on the concepts of POEM. Submucosal tunnel is fashioned beyond the spastic segment through an incision just above the dentate line. Posterior complete myotomy is done in a cranial to caudad direction. Near the anorectal junction, internal sphincter fibers are selectively divided, and external sphincter fibers are preserved. The length of myotomy is predetermined by endoscopy, manometry, and fluoroscopy, usually ranging from 5 to 8 cm. The maximum length of myotomy in a case series was up to 20 cm for an aganglionic segment of 15 cm.[36] Technical success rates are high, with few complications. Clinical efficacy (improvement in manometry and decrease in requirement of laxatives) on short-term and mid-term follow-up is encouraging. Further validation is required to establish PREM as a standard procedure for HD.

■ SUBMUCOSAL TUNNELING ENDOSCOPIC RESECTION

Submucosal tunneling endoscopic resection (STER) is a technique that allows resection of submucosal tumors or subepithelial tumors (SETs) following the principles of TSE. Mucosa is incised 5 cm proximal to the lesion, and a submucosal tunnel is created as described earlier. The site of incision is determined based on the endoscopic finding of a submucosal bulge or, in small lesions, with the help of an endoscopic ultrasound. Once a space is created by insufflation, the lesion is carefully dissected off the surrounding tissue (mucosa, deeper muscle layers) with the use of electrosurgical knives or snare. The lesion is removed in a net and sent for histopathology. The mucosal defect is closed after ensuring hemostasis using techniques (endoclips or sutures) as described earlier before removal of the scope. The procedure duration is variable (15–360 minutes) and depends on the size and location of the tumor. The average postprocedure hospital stay is 4 days.[37]

The first successful STER procedure was described by Inoue et al. in 2012. A meta-analysis of 16 studies was published in 2016. This included 703 patients with 736 subepithelial lesions, the most common being leiomyoma, followed by gastrointestinal stromal tumor, schwannoma, and fibrous tumor. En bloc resection was possible in approximately 95%, and complete resection was reported in around 100%.[38] Chances of failure of STER or prolonged procedure duration was more in tumors with irregular margin, size >3.5 cm, and those located along lesser curvature or in fundus of the stomach. For small esophageal tumors, STER has been shown to be better than thoracoscopic enucleations. In a study by Li et al., where the mean size of the lesion was ~2 cm, STER was associated with shorter operative time, shorter hospital stays, and slightly better complete enucleation rate. STER may replace thoracoscopy in future, especially for small lesions (<30 mm).[39]

■ TRAINING IN THIRD-SPACE ENDOSCOPY

Technical success in TSE procedures depends on the availability of specialized instruments and expertise. The learning curve is usually long

(25–100 cases). POEM being the most common procedure, majority of data is based on this procedure. In a large study on >1,000 procedures, the learning curve to achieve competency was described as 100 cases, and the threshold to decrease the procedure time was 70 cases.[40] Currently, few centers and clinicians around the world have managed to cross this threshold. Rarity of the diseases addressed by TSE and the long learning curves are major roadblocks to training aspiring endoscopists. Authors have suggested training sessions on cadavers and animals to help improve skills and attain proficiency in TSE.

■ CONCLUSION

Third-space endoscopy continues to evolve in the field of gastrointestinal endoscopy. In the last decade, it has emerged as a promising technique with high safety profile for multiple upper gastrointestinal disorders (achalasia cardia, Zenker's diverticulum, gastroparesis, submucosal tumors) and few rectal pathologies. Large studies with long-term results in comparison to established standard procedures are needed to better describe the efficacy of TSE. Presently, these procedures are limited to few specialized centers. Structured training programs can be helpful to overcome the steep learning curve and help this technique to evolve further.

■ REFERENCES

1. Kalloo AN. Natural orifice transluminal endoscopic surgery (NOTES). Gastroenterol Hepatol (NY). 2007;3(3):183-4.
2. Inoue H, Minami H, Kobayashi Y, Sato Y, Kaga M, Suzuki M, et al. Peroral endoscopic myotomy (POEM) for esophageal achalasia. Endoscopy. 2010; 42(4):265-71.
3. Sumiyama K, Gostout CJ, Rajan E, Bakken TA, Knipschield MA, Marler RJ. Submucosal endoscopy with mucosal flap safety valve. Gastrointest Endosc. 2007;65:688-94.
4. Pasricha PJ, Hawari R, Ahmed I, Chen J, Cotton PB, Hawes RH, et al. Submucosal endoscopic esophageal myotomy: a novel experimental approach for the treatment of achalasia. Endoscopy. 2007;39:761-4.
5. Tang X, Gong W, Deng Z, Zhou J, Ren Y, Zhang Q, et al. Comparison of conventional versus Hybrid knife peroral endoscopic myotomy methods for esophageal achalasia: a case-control study. Scand J Gastroenterol. 2016;51:494-500.
6. Bapaye A, Korrapati SK, Dharamsi S, Dubale N. Third space endoscopy: lessons learnt from a decade of submucosal endoscopy. J Clin Gastroenterol. 2020;54(2):114-29.
7. Han SY, Youn YH. Role of endoscopy in patients with achalasia. Clin Endosc. 2023; 56:537-45.
8. Ling T, Guo H, Zou X. Effect of peroral endoscopic myotomy in achalasia patients with failure of prior pneumatic dilation: a prospective case-control study. J Gastroenterol Hepatol. 2014;29(8):1609-13.

9. Werner YB, Hakanson B, Martinek J, Repici A, von Rahden BHA, Bredenoord AJ, et al. Endoscopic or surgical myotomy in patients with idiopathic achalasia. N Engl J Med. 2019;381:2219-29.
10. Schlottmann F, Luckett DJ, Fine J, Shaheen NJ, Patti MG. Laparoscopic heller myotomy versus peroral endoscopic myotomy (POEM) for achalasia: a systematic review and meta-analysis. Ann Surg. 2018;267(3):451-60.
11. Kumbhari V, Tieu AH, Onimaru M, El Zein MH, Teitelbaum EN, Ujiki MB, et al. Peroral endoscopic myotomy (POEM) vs. laparoscopic Heller myotomy (LHM) for the treatment of type III achalasia in 75 patients: a multicenter comparative study. Endosc Int Open. 2015;3(3):195-201.
12. Podboy AJ, Hwang JH, Rivas H, Azagury D, Hawn M, Lau J, et al. Long-term outcomes of per-oral endoscopic myotomy compared to laparoscopic Heller myotomy for achalasia: a single-center experience. Surg Endosc. 2021;35(2):792-801.
13. Li QL, Wu QN, Zhang XC, Xu MD, Zhang W, Chen SY, et al. Outcomes of per-oral endoscopic myotomy for treatment of esophageal achalasia with a median follow-up of 49 months. Gastrointest Endosc. 2018;87(6):1405-12.e3.
14. Brewer Gutierrez OI, Moran RA, Familiari P, Dbouk MH, Costamagna G, Ichkhanian Y, et al. Long-term outcomes of per-oral endoscopic myotomy in achalasia patients with a minimum follow-up of 4 years: a multicenter study. Endosc Int Open. 2020;8(5):E650-5.
15. Rolland S, Paterson W, Bechara R. Achalasia: current therapeutic options. Neurogastroenterol Motil. 2023;35(1):e14459.
16. Vespa E, Pellegatta G, Chandrasekar VT, Spadaccini M, Patel H, Maselli R, et al. Long-term outcomes of peroral endoscopic myotomy for achalasia: a systematic review and meta-analysis. Endoscopy. 2023;55(2):167-75.
17. Khashab MA, Sanaei O, Rivory J, Eleftheriadis N, Chiu PWY, Shiwaku H, et al. Peroral endoscopic myotomy: anterior versus posterior approach. A randomized single-blinded clinical trial. Gastrointest Endosc. 2020;91(2):288-97.e7.
18. Isomoto H, Ikebuchi Y. Japanese guidelines for peroral endoscopic myotomy: 1st edition. Dig Endosc. 2019;31:27-9.
19. Haito-Chavez Y, Inoue H, Beard KW, Draganov PV, Ujiki M, Rahden BHA, et al. Comprehensive analysis of adverse events associated with per oral endoscopic myotomy in 1826 patients: an international multicenter study. Am J Gastroenterol. 2017;112:1267-76.
20. Camilleri M, Parkman HP, Shafi MA, Abell TL, Gerson L, American College of Gastroenterology. Clinical guideline: management of gastroparesis. Am J Gastroenterol. 2013;108:18-37; quiz 38.
21. Camilleri M, Bharucha AE, Farrugia G. Epidemiology, mechanisms, and management of diabetic gastroparesis. Clin Gastroenterol Hepatol. 2011;9:5-12; quiz e7.
22. Friedenberg FK, Palit A, Parkman HP, Hanlon A, Nelson DB. Botulinum toxin A for the treatment of delayed gastric emptying. Am J Gastroenterol. 2008;103:416-23.
23. Clarke JO, Sharaiha RZ, Kord Valeshabad A, Lee LA, Kalloo AN, Khashab MA. Through-the-scope transpyloric stent placement improves symptoms and gastric emptying in patients with gastroparesis. Endoscopy. 2013;45(Suppl. 2): E189-90.
24. Khashab MA, Stein E, Clarke JO, Saxena P, Kumbhari V, Chander Roland B, et al. Gastric peroral endoscopic myotomy for refractory gastroparesis: first human endoscopic pyloromyotomy (with video). Gastrointest Endosc. 2013;78:764-8.

25. Allemang MT, Strong AT, Haskins IN, Rodriguez J, Ponsky JL, Kroh M. How I do it: per-oral pyloromyotomy (POP). J Gastrointest Surg. 2017;21:1963-8.
26. Bapaye A. Third-space endoscopy—can we see light at the end of the tunnel? Endoscopy. 2018;50:1047-8.
27. Mekaroonkamol P, Patel V, Shah R, Li T, Li B, Tao J, et al. 838 duration of the disease, rather than the etiology of gastroparesis, is the key predictive factor for clinical response after gastric per oral endoscopic pyloromyotomy (GPOEM). Gastrointest Endosc. 2018;87:119-20.
28. Gonzalez JM, Benezech A, Vitton V, Barthet M. G-POEM with antro-pyloromyotomy for the treatment of refractory gastroparesis: mid-term follow-up and factors predicting outcome. Aliment Pharmacol Ther. 2017;46:364-70.
29. Albers DV, Kondo A, Bernardo WM, Sakai P, Moura RN, Silva GL, et al. Endoscopic versus surgical approach in the treatment of Zenker's diverticulum: systematic review and meta-analysis. Endosc Int Open. 2016;4:E678-86.
30. Yang J, Novak S, Ujiki M, Hernández Ó, Desai P, Benias P, et al. An international study on the use of peroral endoscopic myotomy in the management of Zenker's diverticulum. Gastrointest Endosc. 2020;91(1):163-8.
31. Goguen LA, Norris CM, Jaklitsch MT, Sullivan CA, Posner MR, Haddad RI, et al. Combined antegrade and retrograde esophageal dilation for head and neck cancer-related complete esophageal stenosis. Laryngoscope. 2010;120:261-6.
32. Babich JP, Diehl DL, Entrup MH. Retrograde submucosal tunneling technique for management of complete esophageal obstruction. Surg Laparosc Endosc Percutan Tech. 2012;22:e232-5.
33. Perbtani Y, Suarez AL, Wagh MS. Emerging techniques and efficacy of endoscopic esophageal reconstruction and lumen restoration for complete esophageal obstruction. Endosc Int Open. 2016;4:E136-42.
34. Wagh MS, Draganov PV. Per-oral endoscopic tunneling for restoration of the esophagus: a novel endoscopic submucosal dissection technique for therapy of complete esophageal obstruction. Gastrointest Endosc. 2017;85:722-7.
35. Bapaye A, Wagholikar G, Jog S, Kothurkar A, Purandare S, Dubale N, et al. Per rectal endoscopic myotomy for the treatment of adult Hirschsprung's disease: first human case (with video). Dig Endosc. 2016;28:680-4.
36. Bapaye A, Dashatwar P, Biradar V, Biradar S, Pujari R. Initial experience with per-rectal endoscopic myotomy for Hirschsprung's disease: medium- and long-term outcomes of the first case series of a novel third-space endoscopy procedure. Endoscopy. 2021;53(12):1256-60.
37. Inoue H, Ikeda H, Hosoya T, Onimaru M, Yoshida A, Eleftheriadis N, et al. Submucosal endoscopic tumor resection for subepithelial tumors in the esophagus and cardia. Endoscopy. 2012;44:225-30.
38. Jain D, Desai A, Mahmood E, Singhal S. Submucosal tunneling endoscopic resection of upper gastrointestinal tract tumors arising from muscularis propria. Ann Gastroenterol. 2017;30:262-72.
39. Li QY, Meng Y, Xu YY, Zhang Q, Cai JQ, Zheng HX, et al. Comparison of endoscopic submucosal tunneling dissection and thoracoscopic enucleation for the treatment of esophageal submucosal tumors. Gastrointest Endosc. 2017;86:485-91.
40. Liu Z, Zhang X, Zhang W, Zhang Y, Chen W, Qin W, et al. Comprehensive evaluation of the learning curve for peroral endoscopic myotomy. Clin Gastroenterol Hepatol. 2018;16:1420-6.e2.

CHAPTER 4

Acute Appendicitis: Recent Concepts

R Kalayarasan, S Suresh Kumar, Vikram Kate, N Ananthakrishnan

■ INTRODUCTION

Acute appendicitis (AA) is the most common cause of an acute surgical abdomen, with a lifetime risk of 7–8%, particularly common between 10 and 30 years of age. The incidence decreases with age, with only 15% occurring above 50 years of age, compared to 30% in younger patients. The lifetime risk of developing AA is higher in males compared to females (8.6 vs. 6.7%, ratio 1.4:1). Nevertheless, the risk of undergoing appendectomy is higher among females (23%) compared to male patients (12%), perhaps due to a mistaken diagnosis in the presence of pelvic inflammatory disease or incidental appendicectomy during pelvic procedures, leading to a 26% negative appendectomy rate in females of the reproductive age group.[1]

The diagnosis of AA is made difficult because of other conditions in the abdomen that mimic the clinical features, particularly in pregnancy and the elderly, wherein an atypical clinical history and clinical findings lead to a delay in diagnosis with higher morbidity. Even with current diagnostic and therapeutic modalities, AA is associated with 10% morbidity and a mortality rate of 1–5%, which is increased in the elderly due to a higher frequency of complicated appendicitis (18–70%) compared to younger patients (3–29%). There are geographical variations in presentation, severity, and diagnostic workup modalities in different countries, which makes generalization of guidelines for the diagnosis and management of AA problematic.[2]

■ DIAGNOSIS OF ACUTE APPENDICITIS: LIMITATIONS IN CLINICAL EXAMINATION

The diagnosis of AA is usually based on a careful clinical history correlated with physical examination findings, supported by laboratory investigations, without the need for sophisticated imaging. The accuracy of clinical diagnosis is largely dependent on the seniority of the surgeon and tends to fall in inexperienced hands. The accuracy of diagnosis is up to 90% in typical presentation, with significant false negatives in women of childbearing age, elderly, and preschool children due to atypical symptoms and signs. Several methods have been studied to increase the accuracy of clinical diagnosis, including assessment by senior surgeons, combining laboratory investigations, and several scoring systems. Clinical prediction rules (CPR), also known as clinical scoring systems (CSS), are used to increase diagnostic accuracy.[3]

Clinical Scoring for Diagnosing Acute Appendicitis

The term CSS is a misnomer since it often combines investigations with clinical findings. CSS help in establishing the diagnosis of AA with sufficient certainty for decision-making. These scoring systems are derived from a large clinical database from patients with suspected and later confirmed diagnosis of AA by analyzing multiple variables that were either individually or collectively associated with the diagnosis or exclusion of AA with predictable certainty. Many scoring methods have been described and validated in the last four decades, starting from the Alvarado scoring to the recent adult appendicitis score (AAS) by Sammalkorpi et al.[4] However, the best CSS for clinical use is yet to be clearly established. More often, the higher cut-off scores in most of the CSS increase specificity and positive predictive value, with a significant fall in the sensitivity. Hence, often these CSS are used to rule out rather than to confirm the diagnosis. Among the many validated CPRs, Alvarado scoring method, appendicitis inflammatory response (AIR) score, AAS, and Raja Isteri Pengiran Anak Saleha Appendicitis (RIPASA) are the most validated in adult patients.[3-6] The pediatric appendicitis score (PAS) was developed for the pediatric population as the application of other scoring methods is often difficult due to inadequate history and limited examination findings in children. The commonly used CSS comprises similar clinical and laboratory variables **(Table 1)**[4-8] with varying weightage on the individual parameters **(Table 2)**.

Alvarado Score

Alvarado score, first proposed by Alvarado in 1986 after retrospectively analyzing 305 patients admitted with abdominal pain suggestive of AA, also known as MANTRELS score, is the most commonly used and the most validated scoring system for AA.[5] Based on univariate analysis, Alvarado proposed six clinical parameters, including migratory pain, anorexia, nausea or vomiting, tenderness in the right iliac fossa, rebound tenderness, and elevated temperature >37.5°C, and two laboratory parameters, including leukocytosis and a shift to the left. All variables are given a score of 1 except right lower quadrant tenderness and leukocytosis, which are given 2 each. A score of 7 or more was considered to suggest AA. With the originally recommended cut-off score of 7, further studies showed a sensitivity and specificity ranging from 67.65 to 96.3% and 58.18 to 89.39%, respectively. The area under the curve (AUC) ranged from 0.74 to 0.88 with a cut-off of 7. A higher cut-off score (≥8) improved the specificity up to 97% with an AUC

TABLE 1: Parameters included in the most commonly used clinical prediction rules (CPRs).

		Alvarado score[5]	AIR score[6]	AAS score[4]	RIPASA score[7]	PAS score[8]
Clinical history	Anorexia	1			1	1
	Nausea or vomiting	1			1	
	Vomiting		1			1
	Migration of pain to the right iliac fossa	1		2	0.5	1
	Pain in right iliac fossa	2	1	2	0.5	
Clinical signs	RIF tenderness			3: Women >50 years or men (any age) 1: Women <50 years	1	2
	Rebound tenderness or muscular guarding	1	1: Light 2: Medium 3: Strong	2: Mild 4: Moderate to severe	1: Rebound tenderness 2: Muscular guarding	
	Cough/percussion/hopping tenderness in right lower quadrant					2
	Rovsing's sign				2	
Body temperature		1: >37.5°C	1: ≥38.5°C		1: >37 and ≤39°C	1: ≥38°C
Laboratory investigations	WBC count: ×10⁹/L	2: >10	1: 10–14.9 2: ≥15	1: ≥7.2 and <10.9 2: ≥10.9 and <14 3: ≤14	1	

Contd...

Contd...

	Alvarado score[5]	AIR score[6]	AAS score[4]	RIPASA score[7]	PAS score[8]
Leukocytosis shift (shift to left)	1				
Polymorphonuclear leukocytes %		1: 70–84 2: >85	2: ≥62 and <75 3: ≥75 and <83 4: ≥83		1: >75%
Negative urine analysis				1	
Inflammatory marker					
CRP		1: 10–49 mg/L 1: ≥50 mg/L	Symptoms <24 hours + 1: CRP: 4–10 2: CRP: 11–24 3: CRP: 25–82 1: CRP: >83 Symptoms >24 hours + 2: CRP: 12–52 2: CRP: 53–151 1: CRP: >152		
Gender				0.5: Female 1: Male	
Age				1: <40 2: >40	
Duration of symptoms				1: <48 hours 2: >48 hours	

(AAS: adult appendicitis score; AIR: appendicitis inflammatory response; PAS: pediatric appendicitis score; RIF: right iliac fossa; RIPASA: Raja Isteri Pengiran Anak Saleha Appendicitis; WBC: white blood cell)

	Alvarado score[5]	AIR score[6]	AAS score[4]	RIPASA score[7]	PAS score[8]
Total parameters	8	7	7	15	
Total score	10	12	23		
Not likely appendicitis	0–4	0–4	0–10	<5	≤5
Equivocal	5–6	5–8	11–15	5–7.5	
Probably appendicitis	7–8			7.5–12	
Highly likely appendicitis	9–10	9–12	≥16	>12	≥6

TABLE 2: Score cut-off for various commonly used clinical prediction rules (CPRs).

(AAS: adult appendicitis score; AIR: appendicitis inflammatory response; PAS: pediatric appendicitis score; RIPASA: Raja Isteri Pengiran Anak Saleha Appendicitis)

of 8.4 with a simultaneous drop in sensitivity to 37–44%. The advantage of Alvarado scoring includes a limited number of variables with a score of 1 or 2 per variable, which is easier to calculate compared to multiple parameters and decimal scoring points of other methods.[7,8] However, some authors have expressed difficulty in including a shift to left of neutrophils due to variations in the interpretation of the same. To overcome this shortfall, Kalan et al. proposed a modified Alvarado scoring method with seven parameters after removing the left shift.[9] This modified Alvarado scoring reached lesser sensitivity (53.8–97.6%), specificity (28.57–80%), and an AUC (0.69) for the same cut-off value and hence is not commonly used.[10]

Appendicitis Inflammatory Response Score

This is more user-friendly and has better sensitivity, specificity, and AUC compared to the Alvarado score. It was proposed by Andersson et al. in 1997 after studying data of 316 patients admitted with suspected AA using multivariate logistic regression analysis of the variables rather than the univariate analysis of Alvarado.[6]

The AIR consists of seven variables, including four clinical parameters, namely vomiting, pain in the right iliac fossa, rebound tenderness in the right iliac fossa, and temperature >38.5°C, and three laboratory parameters, including white blood cell (WBC) count, proportion of polymorphonuclear leukocytes, and C-reactive protein (CRP) levels. The individual score for each parameter ranges from 1 to 3, with a total possible score of 12. A score of >8 indicates a high probability, 5–8 indicates an intermediate probability, and <5 indicates a low probability of AA. With the original cut-off of >8, the AIR score showed low sensitivity (11–30%) and high specificity (84–99%). When the cut-off was lowered to >5, the sensitivity increased (84–97%) with an acceptable specificity (56–69%). The score has shown good performance with an AUC of 0.8–0.97.[8] However, some authors have expressed concern regarding the grading of rebound tenderness to light, medium, and strong as this may be subjective. Nonetheless, the AIR has been shown to perform best in terms of sensitivity, specificity, and AUC in a recent systematic analysis that included 12 derivation studies and 22 validation studies.

Adult Appendicitis Score

The inherent fallacy of the Alvarado score and the AIR lies in including only patients with a histologically confirmed AA and excluding those with a clinical diagnosis of AA but managed conservatively, thus raising the possibility of bias. To address this issue, Sammalkorpi et al. in 2014 proposed a scoring system by prospectively analyzing 829 patients attending emergency medical services (EMS) with pain in the right iliac fossa.[4] After multivariate logistic regression, seven variables with four clinical parameters, including pain in right iliac fossa, relocation of pain, right lower quadrant guarding, and three laboratory parameters, including leukocyte count, proportion of neutrophils, and CRP, were included. The score for each parameter ranged from 1 to 3, with a total score of 23. Sammalkorpi et al. proposed a cut-off of ≥16 to predict a high probability, ≤10 to predict low probability, and 11–15 for an intermediate probability for diagnosis of AA.[4] With the proposed cut-off, the AAS showed 58% sensitivity, 92% specificity, and an AUC of 0.88. Subsequent studies showed better sensitivity (90–96%) and AUC (0.83) with a cut-off score of 8, however, with a fall in specificity (61–64%). Subdivisions based on the grading of clinical signs, differential score based on gender, and level of laboratory parameters with the duration of symptoms make the scoring method difficult and more time consuming.[9]

RIPASA Score

After analyzing preoperative and operative data of 400 patients who underwent appendectomy, Chong et al. derived a CSS with 15 variables, including various demographic parameters such as age, gender, duration of symptoms, and clinical signs and laboratory parameters.[7] A meta-analysis of 12 studies comparing RIPASA with Alvarado score has shown excellent sensitivity (94%) at a cut-off of 7.5 with an AUC of 0.94, with a low specificity (55%) compared to the Alvarado score. The high number of parameters with decimal point scores for many parameters, the RIPASA scoring is very difficult and time consuming and hence has not been validated by many studies.[3,9,10]

Scoring Methods for Pediatric Patients

Acute appendicitis remains the most common surgical emergency in the pediatric population. Difficulty in getting a reliable clinical history and clinical examination makes it challenging to use available CSS in the pediatric population. Samuel's PAS and Alvarado score are the most commonly used.[5,8-11] In addition to all parameters of Alvarado, the PAS score also includes right lower quadrant pain on coughing, hopping, and percussion. In a systematic review by Kulik et al., the sensitivity of PAS was shown to be 80-100% with a likelihood ratio of 0-0.27, compared to 72-93% and 0.09-0.3, respectively, for Alvarado.[11] The review also showed that PAS and Alvarado scoring methods overdiagnose AA by 35% and 32%, respectively. The application of PAS and Alvarado scoring in preschool children is even more difficult due to atypical presentation and a higher rate of complications developing within a short interval after the onset of symptoms. A retrospective analysis by Mecco et al. of 747 children showed AIR to be better for predicting AA in children compared to Alvarado and PAS.[12] This study showed that the AIR scores had better AUC (0.9) compared to PAS (0.82) and Alvarado (0.87) scores. With a false-negative rate of 14% compared to 7% for Alvarado and 18% for PAS, the AIR outperformed the two scores in terms of specificity and positive predictive value, possibly due to inclusion of CRP and grading for laboratory parameters such as CRP, WBC count, and proportion of neutrophils. Chung et al. studied the Alvarado score in predicting complicated appendicitis in children and showed that rebound tenderness has the highest positive predictive value in diagnosing complicated AA in children.[13] Though CSS are useful tools in diagnosing pediatric AA, considering the unreliable clinical history, atypical clinical signs, and rapid progression to complications, it is not recommended to make a diagnosis of AA in children solely based on the CPR.

Scoring Methods for Females in the Reproductive Age Group or with Pregnancy

Pelvic inflammatory disease, ovarian cyst with or without torsion, and genitourinary infections are the frequently encountered conditions that, at times, are mistaken for AA in women. Pregnant patients present with atypical symptoms and restricted physical examination due to the gravid uterus. Nausea, vomiting, tachycardia, and elevated WBC, which occur due to the physiological changes in pregnancy, make these parameters unreliable for diagnosis of AA. Limitations on use of imaging studies due to risk of radiation add to diagnostic difficulty. Higher rate of preterm labor and abortion is reported in pregnant patients diagnosed with AA. Also, complicated appendicitis significantly increases fetal and maternal mortality. Hence, there is a need for a suitable CSS that addresses variations in physiology during pregnancy. Tatli et al., in a retrospective analysis of pregnant patients with AA, showed that the Alvarado score at a cut-off of ≥7 has a sensitivity and specificity of 78.9 and 80%, respectively.[14] Montoglu et al. validated nine CSS in 79 pregnant patients admitted with suspected AA. The study included 79 nonpregnant females of the reproductive age group (20-45 years) who underwent appendectomy as controls and showed that with a sensitivity of 78.46%, specificity of 78.57%, positive predictive value of 94.4, and AUC of 0.8, the RIPASA scoring performed best in the pregnant patients for a cut-off score of 8.5.[15] In a nonpregnant patient, Tzanakis et al. scoring performed best with a sensitivity and specificity of 87.8 and 53.8%, respectively, and a PPV of 90.6 and an AUC of 0.79. In the absence of further studies, one may require laboratory parameters, inflammatory markers, and nonradiation imaging modalities in addition to CSS.[16]

ROLE OF LABORATORY INVESTIGATIONS AND INFLAMMATORY MARKERS AS INDEPENDENT PREDICTORS

White blood cell count, proportion of neutrophils, and CRP are among the most commonly used laboratory parameters in the diagnosis of AA. While these laboratory parameters, in combination, significantly reduced the need for imaging and helped stratify patients, they have failed to attain sufficient sensitivity and specificity to be used as independent risk predictors for AA. Zouari et al. have shown that a CRP >10 mg/L and WBC >16,000/mL strongly predict AA in children with acute abdominal pain.[17] Higher WBC and CRP levels correlated with the diagnosis of complicated AA.[17] Zani et al. showed that 58% of patients with complicated AA had a CRP >40 mg/L compared to only 37% of patients with uncomplicated AA.[18] Huckins et al. prospectively evaluated a panel including WBC, CRP, and calprotectin in 422 patients with suspected AA and showed a sensitivity of 97.5% and a negative predictive value of 98.4%. With exclusion of calprotectin, the other achieved the same sensitivity and negative predictive value.[19] Though procalcitonin has been shown to have less diagnostic accuracy than CRP and WBC, it has been shown to be significantly associated with complicated appendicitis in a recent meta-analysis. Various inflammatory biomarkers such as CRP, WBC, calprotectin, *APPY1* panel of biomarkers, absolute neutrophil count (ANC), and procalcitonin were evaluated in a prospective study by Benito et al.[20] In the multivariate regression analysis, only the *APPY1* panel of biomarkers and ANC were found to be significantly associated. Kiliç et al. have shown a significant association between ischemia-modified albumin (IMA) and computed tomography (CT) findings in differentiating complicated AA with uncomplicated AA.[21] Other biomarkers, including leucine-rich alpha-2-glycoprotein (Appendicitis Urinary Biomarker), were also shown to be sensitive in the diagnosis of AA in a few studies. To summarize, laboratory parameters and serum biomarkers have been shown to be useful tools in the diagnosis of AA and help in reducing the need for CT. Current guidelines recommend using biomarkers in the diagnosis of AA in both adults and children. Total WBC count, proportion of neutrophils, and CRP are recommended in all the patients, and in addition, ANC and urine analysis are to be added for pediatric patients.

SUMMARY OF GUIDELINES FOR USING CLINICAL SCORING AND LABORATORY INVESTIGATIONS IN THE DIAGNOSIS OF ACUTE APPENDICITIS

In a recent systematic analysis, Kularatna et al. mentioned the difficulty in meta-analysis due to lack of homogeneity in 12 published and 22 validation studies of CSS.[22] As these scoring methods are only to aid stratifications of risk groups, an individualized approach considering age, comorbidity, risk of anesthesia, risk of radiation exposure, etc., is more important before making a clinical judgment. The Alvarado score, AIR, and AAS are shown to be sufficiently sensitive to rule out AA and to identify patients who do not require hospital admission. They also stratify patients who require imaging and further observation or reevaluation but not for confirming the diagnosis, as per the recent Jerusalem guidelines. The Jerusalem guidelines of 2020 recommend only AIR and AAS to confirm the diagnosis of AA. CSS is not recommended in pregnant patients and pediatric populations by the recent guidelines due to atypical presentation and high risk of complications.[23] The CSS-based diagnostic algorithm is shown in **Flowchart 1**.

RADIOLOGICAL INVESTIGATIONS

Imaging is mainly useful in intermediate-risk patients as low-risk patients may not require further evaluation and high-risk patients will be planned for therapeutic intervention. Ultrasonography (USG) abdomen is the initial investigation of choice. Features suggestive of AA are presence of a dilated appendix >6 mm, noncompressible lumen, wall thickness >2 mm, and increased vascularity. As USG is operator and patient-variability dependent, the reported sensitivity and specificity in various series range from 44 to 100% and 56 to 100%, respectively **(Table 3)**.[24-31] The accuracy to diagnose AA can be increased by using a standardized USG reporting template.

Computed tomography abdomen is indicated in patients with a negative USG finding. CT findings typical of AA are a dilated appendix >6 mm, periappendiceal fat stranding, and presence of phlegmon or abscess in the region of appendix. The accuracy of CT to diagnose appendicitis exceeds 94% and is often used to differentiate complicated from uncomplicated appendicitis. Uncomplicated appendicitis on CT is defined as dilated appendix (>6 mm) with wall thickening or enhancement. Presence of periappendiceal edema with or without minimal periappendiceal fluid does not increase the severity of grading on imaging. However, appendicolith, periappendiceal abscess, enhancement defect in the wall of appendix with phlegmon, and/or extraluminal air on CT are classified

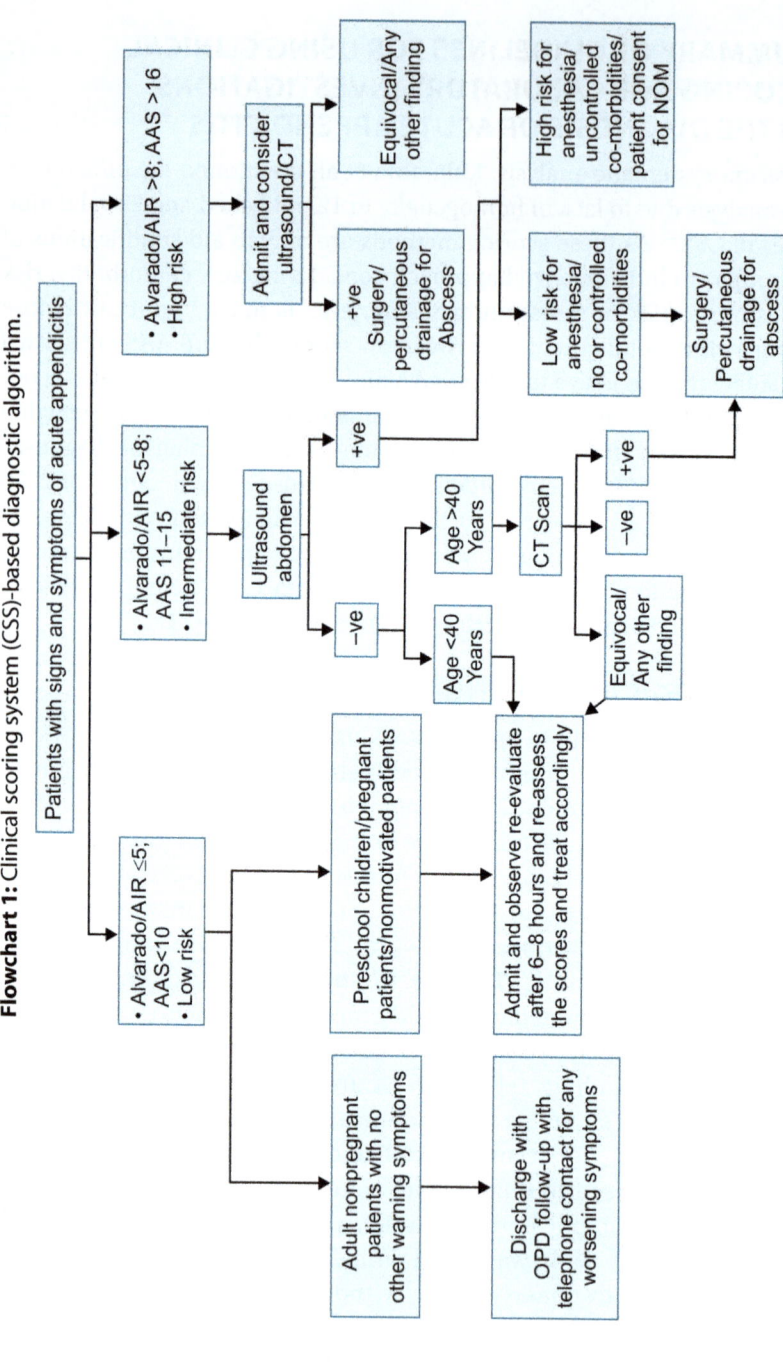

Flowchart 1: Clinical scoring system (CSS)-based diagnostic algorithm.

(AAS: adult appendicitis score; AIR: appendicitis inflammatory response; CT: computed tomography; NOM: nonoperative management; OPD: outpatient department)

TABLE 3: Variable sensitivity and specificity of ultrasound abdomen to diagnose acute appendicitis.

Authors	Year	Number of patients	Study population	Sensitivity (%)	Specificity (%)
Mittal et al.[24]	2013	2,625	Children	72.5	97
Sivit et al.[25]	2000	386	Children	75	89
Garcia et al.[26]	1999	108	Children	44	93
Lowe et al.[27]	2001	67	Children	100	88
Poortman et al.[28]	2003	199	Adults	79	78
Horton et al.[29]	2000	106	Adults	76	90
Bendeck et al.[30]	2002	105	Adults	86	56
Khanzada et al.[31]	2009	238	Adults	98	100

as complicated appendicitis. The OPTICAP (OPTImization of Computed tomography for acute appendicitis) randomized trial reported that use of a low-dose radiation protocol (3.33 vs. 4.44 mSv) contrast-enhanced CT has comparable diagnostic accuracy with less radiation exposure. In adolescents and young adults, the radiation dose could be further reduced to 2 mSv without affecting diagnostic accuracy.[30] Sensitivity is comparable between intravenous (96%), rectal contrast (97%), and intravenous and oral contrast (96%) and is superior to noncontrast CT (91%) to diagnose AA. The sensitivity and specificity of MRI to diagnose appendicitis are comparable to CT and are the preferred first-line imaging in pregnant patients despite higher costs and availability issues. The size criteria for diagnosis are similar to CT, and T2-weighted images show high signal intensity fluid in the appendiceal lumen. In pregnant patients, the main drawback of USG is nonvisualization of appendix, ranging from 34.1 to 71%. The nonvisualization rate is higher during the third trimester, and MRI is the gold standard investigation in this group of patients.

To summarize, USG abdomen is the recommended first-line investigation for patients in whom imaging is indicated based on clinical assessment. Cross-sectional imaging is recommended in patients with persistent right iliac fossa pain and indeterminate USG findings. CT is the commonly used cross-sectional imaging, except in pediatric and pregnant patients. Also, with emerging evidence for nonoperative treatment, the role of CT is increasing to differentiate uncomplicated from complicated appendicitis. In patients with a negative cross-sectional imaging finding, nonoperative treatment is appropriate. However, if the abdominal pain persists or increases in severity, diagnostic laparoscopy is recommended to establish the correct diagnosis.

MANAGEMENT

Treatment of Uncomplicated Appendicitis: Surgery Versus Conservative Treatment

Appendectomy has been the first-line treatment of AA since its first description in 1735 by Claudius Amyand. Reginald Fitz, the originator of the term appendicitis, hypothesized that untreated appendicitis progressed from acute disease to perforation based on longer duration of symptoms in patients with appendicular perforation compared to those without perforation. However, Fitz's other observation, that pathological evidence of spontaneously resolved appendicitis was noted in one-third of the population undergoing autopsy in the preappendectomy era, suggests that surgery may not be required in all patients. Also, the evidence from submarine crew who developed appendicitis while at sea and treated successfully with antibiotics without an increased risk of perforation supported the role of conservative treatment.[32]

Eriksson and Granstrom published the first randomized controlled trial (RCT) comparing surgery with conservative treatment in 40 patients and reported that antibiotic treatment was as effective as surgery.[33] While subsequent RCTs supported the safety of antibiotic treatment, they were limited by small sample size, reliance on clinical parameters for diagnosis of AA, and unclear determination of the primary endpoint. The landmark Appendicitis Acuta (APPAC) multicenter, noninferiority trial from Finland randomized 530 adult patients with CT-confirmed uncomplicated AA to surgical treatment ($n = 273$) or medical therapy with antibiotics ($n = 257$). Successful completion of an appendectomy was the primary endpoint in the surgery group, whereas hospital discharge without the need for appendectomy and no recurrent appendicitis till 1 year after the initial episode was taken as the primary endpoint in the hospital group. While the 27.3% failure rate in the antibiotic-treated group exceeded the prespecified 24% noninferiority margin, a success rate of 72.7% in patients in the conservative arm underscores the role of nonoperative treatment in AA. Also, none of the patients who required delayed appendectomy in the antibiotic arm developed any major complications.

In the APPAC 5-year follow-up study, an additional 30 patients in the antibiotics group required surgery between 1 and 5 years.[34] The authors concluded that the 39.1% recurrence rate within 5 years supports the use of medical treatment as an alternative to surgical therapy for uncomplicated AA. A meta-analysis of 20 studies comparing antibiotic and surgical treatment for image-proven uncomplicated AA concluded that antibiotic therapy is a feasible treatment option with 8.5% index admission antibiotic treatment failure rate and 19.2% recurrence at 1-year follow-up in antibiotic-treated patients.

Despite high-level evidence supporting the role of antibiotic therapy, it is still not widely accepted as the first-line therapy by patients and surgeons. Of the 1,738 respondents who participated in an anonymous Internet-based survey, the majority (90.7%) chose laparoscopic (85.8%) or open (4.9%) appendectomy, and <10% preferred antibiotics alone. Prompt treatment, avoidance of recurrence, and related complications were the reasons proposed by the respondents to prefer surgical treatment. Also, most surgeons who participated in the survey chose appendectomy over antibiotic treatment for uncomplicated AA. In the APPAC trial, at 7 years follow-up, long-term quality of life of patients included in the appendectomy and antibiotic group were comparable. However, patients who underwent appendectomy after failed antibiotic treatment were less satisfied than patients who had successful medical or surgical therapy. While uncomplicated appendicitis and diverticulitis share similar epidemiological trends, the role of primarily antibiotic therapy has been widely accepted in diverticulitis compared to appendicitis. The differing treatment approaches have more to do with the morbidity of colonic resection compared to appendectomy than differences in the pathological process. The most recent of these trials, published in the NEJM, is a nonblinded, noninferiority, RCT comparing a 10-day course of antibiotics with appendectomy in 1,552 patients. The trial concluded that antibiotics were not inferior to appendectomy. Participants with an appendicolith had a higher probability of appendectomy within 90 days in the antibiotic group.

To enable proper decision-making, patients should be provided with unbiased recent clinical evidence on the management of appendicitis. While RCTs represent a high level of evidence, they have limitations such as use of an open rather than minimally invasive approach in most studies and use of long-course antibiotic therapy. With available evidence, nonoperative management should be offered to children and young adults (<40 years) with uncomplicated AA without appendicolith on imaging. Appendicolith on preoperative imaging is associated with a higher failure rate with antibiotics therapy and appendicular perforation. Similarly, incidental detection of appendicular tumors is more common in older patients presenting with appendicitis. In patients eligible for antibiotic therapy to aid decision-making, it is reasonable to suggest that they have 70% chance of resolution with nonoperative treatment. Patients who wish to avoid surgery and are willing to accept the 30% chance of recurrence will select nonoperative therapy. In all other patient groups, appendectomy is preferred.

Nonoperative Therapy of Uncomplicated Appendicitis: Parenteral or Oral or No Antibiotics?

In most RCTs, in hospital intravenous antibiotics were given for 2–3 days followed by 7–10 days of oral antibiotics in patients randomized to antibiotic therapy. In the APPAC trial, intravenous ertapenem was given for 3 days followed by oral levofloxacin and metronidazole for 1 week. As parenteral antibiotics require hospital admission, Talan et al. assessed the feasibility of outpatient management in patients randomized to antibiotics therapy.[35] Based on the results of the pilot study, APPAC II trial was initiated to assess whether oral antibiotics are as effective as combined intravenous and oral antibiotic therapy. In the oral antibiotics group, moxifloxacin 400 mg once daily would be given for 7 days, and in the combined group, the antibiotic regimen used in the APPAC trial would be given. If the noninferiority of oral antibiotics is proven, utilization of hospital resources would substantially decrease. The results are awaited.

Another limitation of antibiotic therapy in RCTs is the use of broad-spectrum antibiotics to ensure patient safety. However, this increases the possibility of emergence of antimicrobial resistance. Park et al. randomized patients with CT-confirmed appendicitis to no-antibiotic regimen with supportive care (intravenous fluids, analgesics, and antipyretics in the event of fever) or a 4-day course of antibiotics with supportive care.[35] Comparable treatment failure rates among patients receiving supportive care and antibiotics suggest the possibility of spontaneous clinical remission in uncomplicated appendicitis. As this study was a single-blinded RCT, the Finnish group initiated APPAC III multicenter, double-blind, placebo-controlled, superiority RCT to compare antibiotic therapy with placebo. If the results of this trial document the safety of supportive treatment, the strategy of appendectomy for all patients with uncomplicated AA will be difficult to justify. Future evidence can potentially save a significant proportion of patients from unnecessary surgical intervention.

Uncomplicated Appendicitis: Timing of Appendectomy After Admission

As mentioned earlier, perforated appendicitis is pathophysiologically different from uncomplicated appendicitis and untreated appendicitis does not invariably progress to complicated appendicitis. Analysis of the American College of Surgeons National Surgical Quality Improvement Program (NSQIP) database and meta-analysis by van Dijk et al. reported that delaying appendectomy for up to 24 hours after hospital admission does not increase the risk of complicated appendicitis or postoperative morbidity, including surgical site infection.[36] However, it is important to understand that the available evidence does not support delaying surgery in patients in whom surgery is indicated, but rather that a short delay of up to 24 hours due to logistical constraints does not adversely affect postoperative outcomes.[37] Similarly, in pregnant patients with equivocal findings of appendicitis on USG, observation for up to 24 hours, followed by repeat USG and appendectomy, does not adversely affect the maternal and fetal outcomes.

Laparoscopic versus Open Appendectomy

Since its first description in 1983 by Kurt Semm, laparoscopic appendectomy has gained wide acceptance and become one of the commonly performed minimally invasive surgical procedures. However, initial RCTs comparing open and laparoscopic appendectomy reported a high incidence of intra-abdominal abscess in patients undergoing laparoscopic appendectomy. Ukai et al. conducted a meta-analysis of 64 RCTs comparing laparoscopic and open appendectomy published between 1991 and 2014.[38] Cumulative analysis of RCTs published before 2001 reported that laparoscopic appendectomy was associated with an increased risk of intra-abdominal abscess (cumulative odds ratio 2.35). However, this difference became insignificant when the trials published after 2001 were included in the analysis (cumulative odds ratio 1.32). Improvement in surgical skills, laparoscopic instrumentation, and more complete aspiration of periappendiceal fluid contributed to decreased intra-abdominal abscess after laparoscopic appendectomy. Recent meta-analysis reported that postoperative pain, wound infection, and hospital stay were less in adult patients undergoing laparoscopic appendectomy, with a more rapid return to normal activities. Outpatient laparoscopic appendectomy can be safely performed in selected uncomplicated AA patients with reduction in overall cost. Also, RCTs have documented the safety and superiority of laparoscopic appendectomy in patients with complicated appendicitis and patients with high-risk features such as obesity, advanced age, and pregnancy. In patients undergoing laparoscopic appendectomy for complicated appendicitis, irrigation of peritoneal cavity with saline does not reduce the incidence of intra-abdominal abscess compared to suction alone. However, the irrigant fluid should be completely aspirated to minimize postoperative intra-abdominal abscess. While single-incision laparoscopic appendectomy is safe and feasible, it is associated with longer operative time, higher analgesic requirement, and wound infection rate compared to conventional three-port technique. There is no significant difference in the postoperative outcomes between different techniques described for mesoappendix dissection. While monopolar and bipolar energy devices are commonly used and cost-effective, other devices such as ultrasonic shears and advanced vessel sealing devices can be used depending on the intraoperative findings, surgeon's judgment, and availability of resources.[38] To summarize, laparoscopic appendectomy using a conventional three-port technique is preferred over open appendectomy in patients with uncomplicated and complicated appendicitis, including high-risk groups, provided laparoscopic equipment and expertise are available.

Intraoperative Grading of Acute Appendicitis

As intraoperative findings dictate postoperative management with antibiotics and outcomes such as complications, grading systems for AA have been

TABLE 4: Various systems for intraoperative grading of acute appendicitis.

Grade	AAST grading[39]	Golmes et al.[40]	WSES[41]
0	–	Normal-looking appendix	Normal-looking appendix (endoappendicitis/periappendicitis)
1	Acutely inflamed appendix, intact	Hyperemia and edema	Inflamed appendix (hyperemia, edema ± fibrin without or little pericolic fluid)
2	Gangrenous appendix, intact	Fibrinous exudate	• *2A:* Segmental necrosis (without or little pericolic fluid) • *2B:* Base necrosis (without or little pericolic fluid) • Inflammatory tumor
3	Perforated appendix with local contamination	• *3A:* Segmental necrosis • *3B:* Base necrosis	• *3A:* Phlegmon • *3B:* Abscess <5 cm without peritoneal free air • *3C:* Abscess >5 cm without peritoneal free air
4	Perforated appendix with periappendiceal phlegmon or abscess	• *4A:* Abscess • *4B:* Regional peritonitis	*Perforated:* Diffuse peritonitis with or without peritoneal free air
5	Perforated appendix with generalized peritonitis	Diffuse peritonitis	–

(AAST: American Association for the Surgery of Trauma; WSES: World Society of Emergency Surgery)

proposed for standardization **(Table 4)**.[39-41] Also, grading facilitates uniform patient stratification for research in appendicitis. American Association for the Surgery of Trauma (AAST) and Gome's grading are based on intraoperative findings, whereas the World Society of Emergency Surgery (WSES) grading incorporates clinical, imaging, and intraoperative findings. These grading systems have been prospectively validated, and, in general, postoperative antibiotics are required in patients with grade 3 and above appendicitis. Also, postoperative complications are more common in patients with grade 3 or more appendicitis. Sartelli et al. reported that WSES grade 3c–4 appendicitis is an independent risk factor for postoperative mortality.[41]

Whether macroscopically normal appendix should be removed during laparoscopy performed for a patient with suspected appendicitis is a controversial topic. When other pathologies such as Meckel's diverticulitis is identified as a cause for the abdominal pain, then normal-appearing appendix need not be removed. However, when alternate pathology is not identified, there are no uniform guidelines on whether appendectomy should be performed. Strong et al. performed a multicenter audit of 3,138 patients who underwent appendicectomy with a documented pathological specimen.[42] Of the 496 patients in whom appendix was assessed as normal by the surgeon, pathological evidence of appendicitis was observed in 138 (27.8%) patients. Of the 2,642 patients documented to have an inflamed appendix by the surgeon, a normal appendix on pathological assessment was observed in 254 (9.6%) patients. As overall disagreement was observed in 392 (12.5%) patients, authors recommended appendectomy in patients with a macroscopically normal-looking appendix. On the other hand, Sørensen et al., in a retrospective study of 271 patients who underwent laparoscopy for suspected appendicitis but did not undergo appendectomy since it appeared grossly normal, reported that 56 (20.7%) patients were readmitted with similar complaints after a median duration of 10 months. Eighteen patients underwent a laparoscopic appendectomy after radiological evaluation, of which pathological evidence of appendicitis was observed in only one patient. Hence, the authors concluded that it is not necessary to remove a macroscopically normal appendix during laparoscopy for clinically suspected AA. While the European Association of Endoscopic Surgery 2016 guidelines recommend appendectomy, Dutch guidelines recommend against removal of a normal-appearing appendix.[43] The Society of American Gastrointestinal and Endoscopic Surgeons guidelines recommend individualized decision-making. All the guidelines are based on low-quality evidence and the strength of recommendation is categorized as weak. In the current scenario, with improvement in clinical scores and imaging technology, the possibility of detecting an intraoperative normal appendix has reduced to about 5%. In the absence of high-level evidence, the surgeon has to decide on the removal of a normal-looking appendix based on the perceived risk–benefit ratio for an individual patient.

MANAGEMENT OF PERFORATED APPENDICITIS WITH ABSCESS

The optimal management of complicated AA with abscess or phlegmon is a matter of debate. Both nonoperative treatment (percutaneous drainage + antibiotics) and surgical treatment with appendectomy have merits and pitfalls. While surgery offers one-time treatment with the potential for quick recovery and short postoperative stay, periappendiceal adhesions increase the technical difficulty and complications. For percutaneous drainage of abscess, although less invasive, an optimum window may not be available in a significant proportion of patients. Andersson and Petzold, in a meta-analysis of 61 studies published between January 1964 and December 2005 comparing nonoperative and surgical treatment of appendiceal abscess, reported that immediate surgery is associated with a higher morbidity compared with nonsurgical treatment (odds ratio 3.3).[44] With the widespread use of the laparoscopic approach, early appendectomy has been evaluated in multiple comparative studies and RCTs. In a recent RCT, Mentula et al. reported that patients who underwent early laparoscopic appendectomy had fewer readmissions (3 vs. 27%) and additional interventions (7 vs. 30%) compared to nonoperative treatment.[45] However, the need for bowel resection in 10% of patients and a 13% risk of incomplete appendectomy underscores the need for experienced laparoscopic surgeons to perform these procedures. Based on the available data, it is reasonable to conclude that nonoperative management with percutaneous drainage and abscess can be considered as first line of treatment, especially in patients with a high surgical risk.[43] In centers with experienced laparoscopic surgeons, laparoscopic appendectomy is a safe alternative and is associated with less readmissions and additional interventions compared to conservative treatment, with a comparable hospital stay.

During appendectomy for complicated appendicitis, if the base of the appendix is healthy, endoloops/suture ligation or polymeric clips are commonly used for stump closure. In patients with unhealthy base, use of endostaplers is preferred. Inversion of appendiceal stump is no longer recommended. Routine use of drains is not recommended as it does not reduce the incidence of intra-abdominal abscess and prolongs hospital stay.

ROLE OF INTERVAL APPENDECTOMY AFTER INITIAL SUCCESSFUL NONOPERATIVE TREATMENT

The 12–24% recurrence rate after initial nonoperative treatment of complicated appendicitis has led to advocacy for routine interval appendectomy. While interval appendectomy is a safe procedure, it can be associated with nonnegligible morbidity of approximately 10% and increased readmission and hospital costs. Hall et al. randomized 106 patients to interval appendectomy and active observation.[46] The authors reported that 12% of patients under the active observation arm developed histologically proven recurrent AA and 6% of patients who underwent interval appendicectomy developed severe complications related to surgery. Hence, the authors recommended against routine interval appendectomy and reserved it only for patients who develop recurrent symptoms. Recently, Peri-Appendicitis Acuta RCT from the Finnish group, comparing interval appendectomy and follow-up with MRI after initial successful nonoperative treatment of complicated appendicitis, was prematurely terminated as the interim analysis revealed evidence of appendiceal neoplasm in 12 of the 60 patients included in the trial. Further, all patients who developed neoplasms were older than 40 years. Hence, based on the current evidence, it is reasonable to conclude that in patients younger than 40 years, interval appendectomy should be performed only in those with recurrent symptoms. In patients older than 40 years, colonoscopy and contrast-enhanced CT abdomen should be performed for evaluation of colon cancer followed by routine interval appendectomy.[44]

■ CONCLUSION

Acute appendicitis is the most common surgical emergency. Hence, a standard approach to diagnosis and management is essential. A clinical scoring system based diagnostic algorithm provided in this chapter will help in choosing appropriate line of management. While appendectomy remains first-line therapy for acute appendicitis, non-operative treatment with antibiotics is a viable treatment option in selected patients with uncomplicated appendicitis.

■ REFERENCES

1. Cervellin G, Mora R, Ticinesi A, Meschi T, Comelli I, Catena F, et al. Epidemiology and outcomes of acute abdominal pain in a large urban emergency department: retrospective analysis of 5,340 cases. Ann Transl Med. 2016;4:362.
2. Viniol A, Keunecke C, Biroga T, Stadje R, Dornieden K, Bösner S, et al. Studies of the symptom abdominal pain—a systematic review and meta-analysis. Fam Pract. 2014;31:517-29.
3. Frountzas M, Stergios K, Kopsini D, Schizas D, Kontzoglou K, Toutouzas K. Alvarado or RIPASA score for diagnosis of acute appendicitis? A meta-analysis of randomized trials. Int J Surg. 2018;56:307-14.
4. Sammalkorpi HE, Mentula P, Leppäniemi A. A new adult appendicitis score improves diagnostic accuracy of acute appendicitis—a prospective study. BMC Gastroenterol. 20141;14:11.
5. Alvarado A. A practical score for the early diagnosis of acute appendicitis. Ann Emerg Med. 1986;15:557-64.
6. Andersson M, Andersson RE. The appendicitis inflammatory response score: a tool for the diagnosis of acute appendicitis that outperforms the Alvarado score. World J Surg. 2008;32:1843-9.
7. Chong CF, Adi MI, Thien A, Suyoi A, Mackie AJ, Tin AS, et al. Development of the RIPASA score: a new appendicitis scoring system for the diagnosis of acute appendicitis. Singapore Med J. 2010;51:220.
8. Samuel M. Pediatric appendicitis score. J Pediatr Surg. 2002;37:877-81.
9. Kalan M, Talbot D, Cunliffe WJ, Rich AJ. Evaluation of the modified Alvarado score in the diagnosis of acute appendicitis: a prospective study. Ann R Coll Surg Engl. 1994;76:418-9.
10. Meltzer AC, Baumann BM, Chen EH, Shofer FS, Mills AM. Poor sensitivity of a modified Alvarado score in adults with suspected appendicitis. Ann Emerg Med. 2013;62:126-31.
11. Kulik DM, Uleryk EM, Maguire JL. Does this child have appendicitis? A systematic review of clinical prediction rules for children with acute abdominal pain. J Clin Epidemiol. 2013;66:95-104.
12. Macco S, Vrouenraets BC, de Castro SM. Evaluation of scoring systems in predicting acute appendicitis in children. Surgery. 2016;160:1599-604.
13. Chung PHY, Dai K, Yang Z, Wong KKY. Validity of Alvarado score in predicting disease severity and postoperative complication in pediatric acute appendicitis. World J Pediatr Surg. 2019;2:e000003.
14. Tatli F, Yucel Y, Gozeneli O, Dirican A, Uzunkoy A, Yalçın HC, et al. The Alvarado score is accurate in pregnancy: a retrospective case-control study. Eur J Trauma Emerg Surg. 2019;45:411-6.

15. Mantoglu B, Gonullu E, Akdeniz Y, Yigit M, Firat N, Akin E, et al. Which appendicitis scoring system is most suitable for pregnant patients? A comparison of nine different systems. World J Emerg Surg. 2020;15:1-8.
16. Tzanakis NE, Efstathiou SP, Danulidis K, Rallis GE, Tsioulos DI, Chatzivasiliou A, et al. A new approach to accurate diagnosis of acute appendicitis. World J Surg. 2005;29:1151-6.
17. Zouari M, Louati H, Abid I, Ben Abdallah AK, Ben Dhaou M, Jallouli M, et al. C-reactive protein value is a strong predictor of acute appendicitis in young children. Am J Emerg Med. 2018;36:1319-20.
18. Zani A, Teague WJ, Clarke SA, Haddad MJ, Khurana S, Tsang T, et al. Can common serum biomarkers predict complicated appendicitis in children? Pediatr Surg Int. 2017;33:799-805.
19. Huckins DS, Copeland K, Self W, Vance C, Hendry P, Borg K, et al. Diagnostic performance of a biomarker panel as a negative predictor for acute appendicitis in adult ED patients with abdominal pain. Am J Emerg Med. 2017;35:418-24.
20. Benito J, Acedo Y, Medrano L, Barcena E, Garay RP, Arri EA. Usefulness of new and traditional serum biomarkers in children with suspected appendicitis. Am J Emerg Med. 2016;34:871-6.
21. Kiliç MÖ, Güldoğan CE, Balamir İ, Tez M. Ischemia-modified albumin as a predictor of the severity of acute appendicitis. Am J Emerg Med. 2017;35:92-5.
22. Kularatna M, Lauti M, Haran C, MacFater W, Sheikh L, Huang Y, et al. Clinical prediction rules for appendicitis in adults: which is best? World J Surg. 2017;41:1769-81.
23. Di Saverio S, Podda M, De Simone B, Ceresoli M, Augustin G, Gori A, et al. Diagnosis and treatment of acute appendicitis: 2020 update of the WSES Jerusalem guidelines. World J Emerg Surg. 2020;15:1-42.
24. Mittal MK, Dayan PS, Macias CG, Bachur RG, Bennett J, Dudley NC, et al. Performance of ultrasound in the diagnosis of appendicitis in children in a multicenter cohort. Acad Emerg Med. 2013;20:697-702.
25. Sivit CJ, Applegate KE, Stallion A, Dudgeon DL, Salvator A, Schluchter M, et al. Imaging evaluation of suspected appendicitis in a pediatric population: effectiveness of sonography versus CT. AJR Am J Roentgenol. 2000;175:977-80.
26. Garcia Peña BM, Mandl KD, Kraus SJ, Fischer AC, Fleisher GR, Lund DP, et al. Ultrasonography and limited computed tomography in the diagnosis and management of appendicitis in children. JAMA. 1999;282:1041-6.
27. Lowe LH, Penney MW, Stein SM, Heller RM, Neblett WW, Shyr Y, et al. Unenhanced limited CT of the abdomen in the diagnosis of appendicitis in children: comparison with sonography. AJR Am J Roentgenol. 2001;176:31-5.
28. Poortman P, Lohle PN, Schoemaker CM, Oostvogel HJ, Teepen HJ, Zwinderman KA, et al. Comparison of CT and sonography in the diagnosis of acute appendicitis: a blinded prospective study. AJR Am J Roentgenol. 2003;181:1355-9.
29. Horton MD, Counter SF, Florence MG, Hart MJ. A prospective trial of computed tomography and ultrasonography for diagnosing appendicitis in the atypical patient. Am J Surg. 2000;179:379-81.
30. Bendeck SE, Nino-Murcia M, Berry GJ, Jeffrey Jr RB. Imaging for suspected appendicitis: negative appendectomy and perforation rates. Radiology. 2002;225:131-6.

31. Khanzada TW, Samad A, Sushel C. Negative appendectomy rate: can it be reduced? J Liaquat Univ Med Health Sci. 2009;8:19-22.
32. Fitz R. Perforating inflammation of the vermiform appendix. Am J Med Sci. 1886;92:321-46.
33. Eriksson S, Granstrom L. Randomized controlled trial of appendicectomy versus antibiotic therapy for acute appendicitis. Br J Surg. 1995;82:166-9.
34. Salminen P, Tuominen R, Paajanen H, Rautio T, Nordström P, Aarnio M, et al. Five-year follow-up of antibiotic therapy for uncomplicated acute appendicitis in the APPAC randomized clinical trial. JAMA. 2018;320:1259-65.
35. Talan DA, Saltzman DJ, Mower WR, Krishnadasan A, Jude CM, Amii R, et al. Antibiotics-first versus surgery for appendicitis: a US pilot randomized controlled trial allowing outpatient antibiotic management. Ann Emerg Med. 2017;70:1-11.e9.
36. Park HC, Kim MJ, Lee BH. Randomized clinical trial of antibiotic therapy for uncomplicated appendicitis. Br J Surg. 2017;104:1785-90.
37. van Dijk ST, van Dijk AH, Dijkgraaf MG, Boermeester MA. Meta-analysis of in-hospital delay before surgery as a risk factor for complications in patients with acute appendicitis: In-hospital delay before surgery and complications after appendicectomy. Br J Surg. 2018;105:933-45.
38. Ukai T, Shikata S, Takeda H, Dawes L, Noguchi Y, Nakayama T, et al. Evidence of surgical outcomes fluctuates over time: results from a cumulative meta-analysis of laparoscopic versus open appendectomy for acute appendicitis. BMC Gastroenterol. 2016;16:37.
39. Shafi S, Aboutanos M, Brown CVR, Ciesla D, Cohen MJ, Crandall ML, et al. Measuring anatomic severity of disease in emergency general surgery. J Trauma Acute Care Surg. 2014;76:884-7.
40. Gomes CA, Sartelli M, Di Saverio S, Ansaloni L, Catena F, Coccolini F, et al. Acute appendicitis: proposal of a new comprehensive grading system based on clinical, imaging and laparoscopic findings. World J Emerg Surg. 2015;10:60.
41. Sartelli M, Baiocchi GL, Di Saverio S, Ferrara F, Labricciosa FM, Ansaloni L, et al. Prospective observational study on acute appendicitis worldwide (POSAW). World J Emerg Surg. 2018;13:19.
42. Strong S, Blencowe N, Bhangu A, National Surgical Research Collaborative. How good are surgeons at identifying appendicitis? Results from a multi-centre cohort study. Int J Surg. 2015;15:107-12.
43. Gorter RR, Eker HH, Gorter-Stam MAW, Abis GS, Acharya A, Ankersmit M, et al. Diagnosis and management of acute appendicitis. EAES consensus development conference 2015. Surg Endosc. 2016;30:4668-90.
44. Andersson RE, Petzold MG. Nonsurgical treatment of appendiceal abscess or phlegmon: a systematic review and meta-analysis. Ann Surg. 2007;246:741-8.
45. Mentula P, Sammalkorpi H, Leppäniemi A. Laparoscopic surgery or conservative treatment for appendiceal abscess in adults? A randomized controlled trial. Ann Surg. 2015;262:237-42.
46. Hall NJ, Eaton S, Stanton MP, Pierro A, Burge DM, CHINA study collaborators and the Paediatric Surgery Trainees Research Network. Active observation versus interval appendicectomy after successful non-operative treatment of an appendix mass in children (CHINA study): an open-label, randomised controlled trial. Lancet Gastroenterol Hepatol. 2017;2:253-60.

CHAPTER 5

Neuroendocrine Tumors of the Gastroenteropancreatic System

Gurudutt P Varty, Vikram A Chaudhari, Manish S Bhandare, Shailesh V Shrikhande

■ INTRODUCTION

Neuroendocrine tumors (NETs) arise from the diffuse neuroendocrine cell system. Most frequently, these neoplasms occur in the gastrointestinal system followed by the lung.[1] Historically, these tumors were described by various terms such as APUDomas, Kulchitsky cell tumors, argentaffinomas, carcinoid tumors, and pancreatic islet tumors. In the year 2000, the World Health Organization (WHO) developed a universal nomenclature and classification system labeling them as neuroendocrine tumors. Currently, the 2019 WHO classification is widely accepted for classifying NETs and guiding management. Gastroenteropancreatic neuroendocrine tumors (GEP-NETs) are a group of tumors originating from enterochromaffin (neuroendocrine) cells of the gut.[2]

■ EPIDEMIOLOGY

Annual incidence and prevalence of GEP-NETs are rising steadily around the world in recent years. According to the Surveillance, Epidemiology, and End Results (SEER) data, the age-adjusted incidence of GEP-NETs has increased from 1.05 to 5.45 cases/100,000 population in the USA between 1975 and 2015 with an annual percentage change of 4.98%.[3] In Europe, the incidence of GEP-NETs currently ranges between 1.33 and 2.33/100,000 population; however, this data is heterogeneous and retrospective.[1] Multicenter longitudinal NET registry from India reported 407 GEP-NET patients in 2017 wherein data was collected from 2001 to 2016 from six tertiary care centers. Even though the exact incidence was not reported, the rising incidence of GEP-NETs was noted since the initiation of the registry.[4] Widespread use of cross-sectional imaging, availability of sensitive diagnostic tools, and higher awareness among clinicians seem to contribute to the rise in GEP-NETs incidence.

Men are affected marginally more frequently than women.[1] GEP-NETs usually occur sporadically. Around 5–25% of the cases are associated with some familial or genetic predisposition. Familial syndromes associated with GEP-NETs [particularly pancreatic neuroendocrine tumors (Pan-NETs)] are described in **Table 1**.

TABLE 1: Hereditary syndromes associated with NETs.

Syndrome	Gene associated	NET manifestation
MEN1 (Werner syndrome)	MENIN	Parathyroid hyperplasia, pituitary adenoma, and gastroenteropancreatic NETs [Zollinger–Ellison syndrome, insulinoma, VIPoma, thymic, and/or bronchial tube endocrine tumors (foregut carcinoid tumors)]
MEN2 (2A, 2B)	RET	Medullary thyroid carcinoma (MEN2A and 2B), pheochromocytoma (MEN2A and 2B), primary hyperparathyroidism (MEN2A), neuromas of the tongue, ganglioneuromas of the intestine, and a marfanoid habitus (MEN2B)
MEN4	CDKN1B	Parathyroid adenoma/hyperplasia, pituitary adenoma, gastroenteropancreatic NETs
von Hippel–Lindau (VHL)	VHL	Pheochromocytoma/paraganglioma, pancreatic NETs
Neurofibromatosis type I (Recklinghausen disease)	NF1	Pheochromocytoma, duodenal NETs
Tuberous sclerosis	TSC1, TSC2	Pancreatic NETs

(MEN1: multiple endocrine neoplasia type 1; MEN2A: multiple endocrine neoplasia type 2A; MEN2B: multiple endocrine neoplasia type 2B; MEN4: multiple endocrine neoplasia type 4; NET: neuroendocrine tumor)

■ PATHOLOGY AND CLASSIFICATION

Histological diagnosis can be obtained from either the resected specimen or core biopsies. Fine-needle aspiration may not provide sufficient tissue for accurate diagnosis and calculation of the proliferation index. The neuroendocrine nature of the tumor is confirmed by the immunohistochemical detection of neuroendocrine markers such as synaptophysin and chromogranin A (CgA). Tumor grade and differentiation are the key factors to determine the clinical behavior of GEP-NETs. The grade refers to the proliferative activity of neoplastic cells, which is measured by the Ki-67 (MIB1) index and the mitotic rate, whereas the differentiation refers to the extent to which tumor cells resemble their normal counterparts. Neuron-specific enolase (NSE) and CD56 are other nonspecific markers that are often positive in GEP-NETs.

Gastroenteropancreatic neuroendocrine tumors are currently classified according to the WHO Classification of Digestive System Tumors, 2019, and staged according to the Union for International Cancer Control/American Joint Committee on Cancer (UICC/AJCC) tumor, node, and metastasis (TNM) staging system or the European Neuroendocrine Tumor Society (ENETS) TNM classification. As per the 2019 WHO classification, GEP-NETs are divided into well-differentiated (WD) NETs grades 1, 2, and 3 and poorly differentiated neuroendocrine carcinomas (NECs) **(Table 2 and Figs. 1A to D)**.

TABLE 2: The WHO 2019 classification for gastroenteropancreatic NETs.

Morphology	Grade	Mitotic count/2 mm²	Ki-67 index (%)
Well-differentiated NET	G1	<2	<3
Well-differentiated NET	G2	2–20	3–20
Well-differentiated NET	G3	>20	>20
Poorly-differentiated NET • Small cell • Large cell	G3	>20	>20
MiNEN			
Tumor-like lesions			

(MiNEN: mixed neuroendocrine non-neuroendocrine neoplasm; NET: neuroendocrine tumor; WHO: World Health Organization)

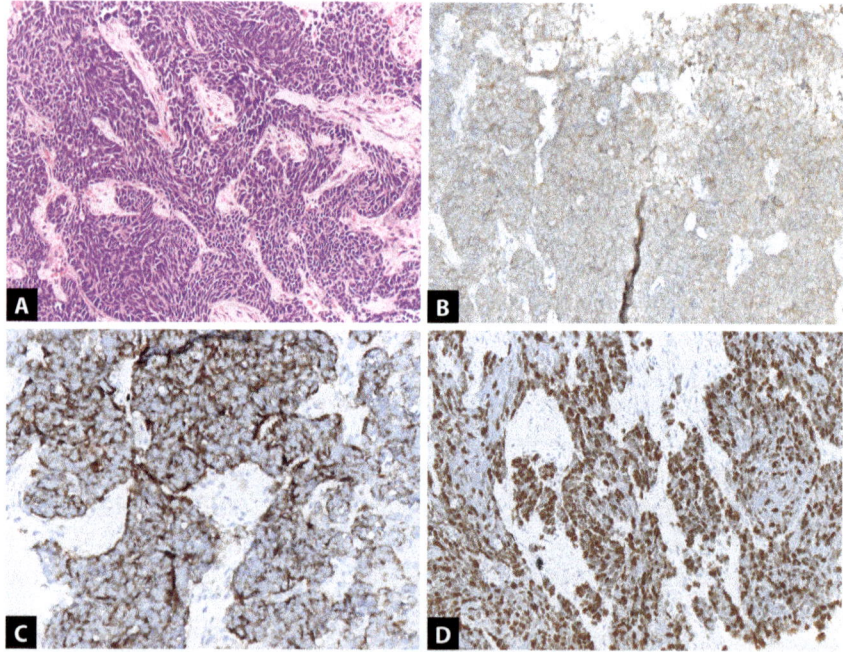

Figs. 1A to D: *Neuroendocrine carcinoma.* Histology shows a tumor arranged in the interconnected thick fascicles with intervening fibrous stroma. The tumor cells are spindle to epithelioid with hyperchromatic nuclei and scant cytoplasm. Tumor molding is seen (A). By immunohistochemistry, the tumor cells are diffusely and strongly positive for synaptophysin (B) and chromogranin (C). The MIB1 labeling index is 85–90% in the highest proliferating areas (D).

Poorly differentiated NECs are further classified into small-cell and large-cell NECs. Another notable change was the introduction of the term mixed neuroendocrine non-neuroendocrine neoplasms (MiNENs) to include other non-neuroendocrine histological variants apart from adenocarcinoma. MiNENs comprise both neuroendocrine and non-neuroendocrine components (>30% of either one). These were earlier classified as mixed adenoneuroendocrine carcinoma (MANEC). For staging, the TNM staging system proposed by ENETS was recently widely adopted by the eighth edition of the UICC/AJCC staging system for various types of GEP-NETs.[5] For all NECs, the staging system of adenocarcinomas is applicable.[5]

■ CLINICAL EVALUATION, DIAGNOSIS, AND WORKUP

Evaluation for GEP-NETs can be broadly divided into:
- History and physical examination
- Biochemical testing
- Imaging
- Biopsy

History and Physical Examination

The incidence of carcinoid syndrome is around 19% in patients with NETs.[6] Intestinal NETs with carcinoid syndrome present with flushing, diarrhea, wheezing or fatigue, and shortness of breath secondary to heart failure, whereas those without carcinoid syndrome present with nonspecific vague abdominal pain. Similarly, functioning Pan-NETs usually have symptoms that fit into one of the syndromes such as Zollinger–Ellison syndrome (ZES), WDHA (watery diarrhea, hypokalemia, and achlorhydria), and Cushing's syndrome, whereas nonfunctional (NF) Pan-NETs present with nonspecific abdominal pain or, rarely, jaundice and weight loss. NETs of the gastroduodenal region can present with gastric outlet obstruction or bleeding (hematemesis, melena). Thus, the symptoms related to GEP-NETs mainly depend on the size and location of the tumor apart from its functional status. A detailed family history needs to be elucidated, especially in <40-year-old patients, to rule out familial syndromes such as multiple endocrine neoplasia type 1 (MEN1), multiple endocrine neoplasia type 2 (MEN2), neurofibromatosis type 1 (NF1), von Hippel–Lindau (VHL), and tuberous sclerosis.

Biochemical Testing

Twenty-four-hour urinary 5-hydroxy indoleacetic acid (5-HIAA) is the gold standard biochemical test for small intestinal neuroendocrine tumors (SI-NETs) (sensitivity—73%, specificity—100%).[7] An acceptable alternative is plasma 5-HIAA levels (sensitivity—89%, specificity—97%). Serum CgA is commonly found to be elevated in the majority of patients of GEP-NETs.

However, it is not an ideal biomarker for screening as its specificity is affected by various other factors such as the use of proton-pump inhibitors (PPIs), chronic atrophic gastritis, kidney, liver, and heart failure, and several other non-neuroendocrine malignancies. Furthermore, normal serum CgA levels can also be found in GEP-NETs. However, serum CgA is specific and sensitive for tumor progression, and basal levels of serum CgA can predict overall survival (OS). It is important to note that serum CgA alone is inadequate to predict tumor progression and on follow-up, it must always be used in conjunction with imaging. Serum measurements of insulin, gastrin, glucagon, cholecystokinin, cortisol, vasoactive intestinal peptide (VIP), and insulin-like growth factor-1 (IGF-1) need to be done in the appropriate clinical setting. N-terminal pro-brain natriuretic peptide (NT-proBNP) is a useful biomarker in the diagnosis of carcinoid heart disease secondary to carcinoid syndrome. Another tumor marker elevated in 30–50% of GEP-NETs is NSE (sensitivity—38%, specificity—73%).[8] Elevated preoperative NSE does have prognostic implications but is currently not widely favored because of low sensitivity.

Imaging

Indications of radiological imaging in GEP-NETs are:
- Localization and characterization of primary tumor
- Assessment of locoregional spread of primary tumor
- Staging and evaluation of metastatic disease
- Treatment planning
- Follow-up

Contrast-enhanced Computed Tomography

Contrast-enhanced computed tomography (CECT) is the first investigation of choice for the assessment, staging, and surgical planning of GEP-NETs. GEP-NETs intensely enhance in the arterial phase on CECT scan as they are hypervascular tumors **(Figs. 2A and B)**.[9] The tumor size, presence of calcification and necrosis along with the pattern of enhancement are important radiological features that differentiate malignant from benign tumors. CECT scan has a sensitivity of 70–80% in the detection of a primary tumor.[9] Poor soft-tissue resolution making it difficult to differentiate between reactive and metastatic nodal tissue and exposure to ionizing radiation are the main disadvantages of CT scan.

Magnetic Resonance Imaging

Gastroenteropancreatic neuroendocrine tumors are T1 hypointense, T2 hyperintense, and brightly enhancing on postcontrast sequences **(Figs. 3A and B)**. Diffusion-weighted imaging assigns an apparent diffusion

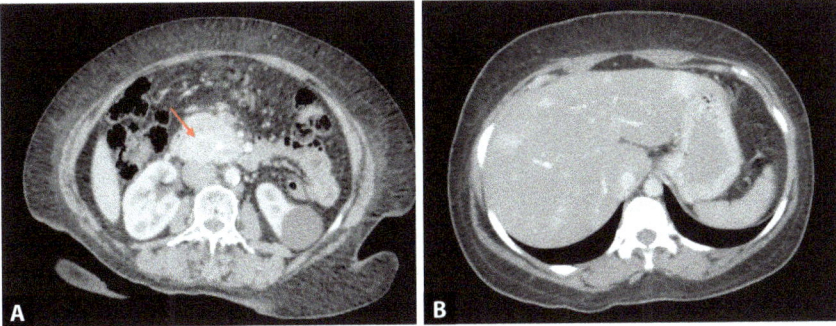

Figs. 2A and B: *Pancreatic neuroendocrine tumor (NET) with liver metastasis.* (A) Contrast-enhanced computed tomography (CECT) axial image showing a hyperenhancing mass (red arrow) arising from the pancreatic head and uncinate process with internal calcification; (B) CECT axial image showing hyperenhancing multiple bilobar liver metastasis.

coefficient (ADC), which helps to differentiate between well- and poorly-differentiated lesions.[10] Magnetic resonance imaging (MRI) is generally used when other imaging findings are equivocal. It is somewhat superior when compared to CECT in the evaluation of neuroendocrine liver metastasis (NELM) and subcentimetric liver lesions and also plays an important role in differentiating liver metastasis from other benign hepatic lesions.[9]

Endoscopic Ultrasound

A high-frequency ultrasound (US) probe (7.5–10 mHz) can be used taking advantage of the close proximity of the transducer to the pancreas. This results in improved image resolution and increased sensitivity (79–100%) for the detection of small and multiple Pan-NETs.[11] A major advantage of endoscopic ultrasound (EUS) is obtaining tissue biopsy during the same setting. EUS is an operator-dependent test. It is technically challenging and it requires specialized training. It may increase the cost of evaluation and may not be widely available.

Nuclear Medicine-based Functional Imaging

Somatostatin-based nuclear imaging has a very important role in the primary diagnosis as well as staging of GEP-NETs. They are equally important in the post-treatment follow-up and response evaluation after therapy.[12] One of the main characteristics inherent to the NETs is the overexpression of somatostatin receptors (SSTRs) on its cell surface, which enables imaging with somatostatin analogs labeled with different radionuclides. Functional imaging utilizes various compounds tagged with another radioactive substance that emits radiation, which, in turn, is captured by either a gamma camera or a positron emission tomography (PET) machine.

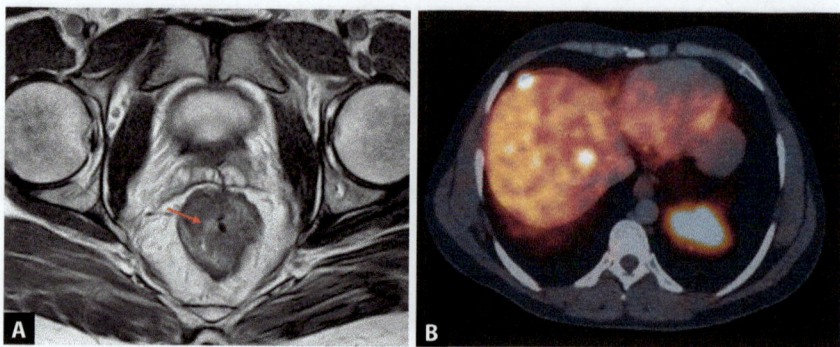

Figs. 3A and B: *Rectal neuroendocrine tumor (NET) with liver metastasis.* (A) Magnetic resonance imaging (MRI) T2-weighted (T2W) axial image showing circumferential growth (red arrow) in the lower rectum; (B) DOTA computed tomography (CT) showing two metastatic lesions in segments VIII and IVA of the liver.

Somatostatin Receptor—Single Photon Emission Computed Tomography

^{111}Indium (^{111}In)-labeled or ^{99m}technetium (^{99m}Tc)-labeled somatostatin analogs (SSAs) are commonly used radiotracer agents. ^{111}In-pentetreotide is the most commonly used radiotracer agent. ^{99m}Tc-depreotide and ^{99m}Tc-EDDA/HYNIC-Tyr3-octreotide (^{99m}Tc-EDDA/HYNIC-TOC) are the most commonly used ^{99m}Tc-labeled SSAs.[12] ^{111}In- and ^{99m}Tc-labeled SSTR analogs have similar sensitivity in the detection of GEP-NETs due to the nonspecific abdominal tracer accumulation.[13] Their usage has decreased after the widespread availability of gallium-68 (^{68}Ga) DOTA-PET scan.

Somatostatin Receptor—Positron Emission Tomography-computed Tomography (SSTR PET-CT)

Image quality with a positron-emitting radionuclide labeled compound is superior as compared to the image quality with a gamma camera including single photon emission computed tomography (SPECT) in the diagnosis and staging of the primary lesion, as well as nodal, bone, and liver metastasis. Furthermore, PET has the capability to quantify the tracer uptake, which is expressed as the standardized uptake value (SUV). This plays an important role in the planning of peptide receptor radionuclide therapy (PRRT). SSAs are labeled with the positron emitter ^{68}Ga for PET imaging.[12] ^{68}Ga-DOTATOC, ^{68}Ga-DOTANOC, and ^{68}Ga-DOTATATE are the most commonly used SSAs labeled with ^{68}Ga.[12] Geijer and Breimer reported a sensitivity of 93% and a specificity of 95% of SSTR-PET in their meta-analysis.[14] SSTR PET-CT imaging is the current "gold standard" for the diagnosis and staging of WD grade 1 and grade 2 GEP-NETs. It also plays a key role in directing the choice of systemic therapy (e.g., appropriate patient selection for PRRT) in grade 3 NETs **(Fig. 4)**.

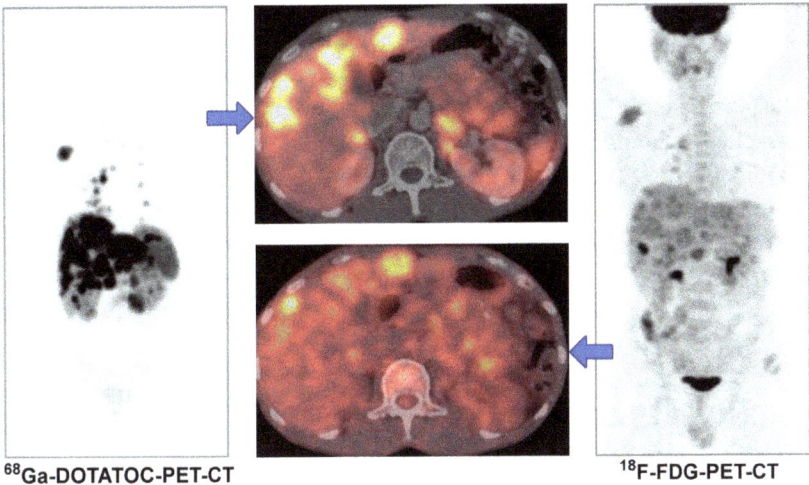

⁶⁸Ga-DOTATOC-PET-CT   ¹⁸F-FDG-PET-CT

Fig. 4: *Dual-tracer imaging (⁶⁸Ga-DOTANOC and ¹⁸FDG).* A 47-year-old gentleman presented with pain in the abdomen associated with generalized weakness and weight loss. Biopsy—WHO well-differentiated grade 2 NET, MIB1 index—8–10%. DOTA PET—MIP image shows multiple foci of tracer uptake in the region of liver, lungs, and right axillary nodes, which on fused PET/CT image corresponds to multiple DOTANOC avid liver metastases. MIP image of FDG-PET shows multiple foci of tracer uptake in liver, lungs, and right axillary nodes. Axial fused PET/CT image shows FDG avid liver metastatic lesions. *Thus, there is dual-tracer uptake on ⁶⁸Ga-DOTANOC PET/CT and FDG-PET/CT images.* This patient was managed by PRRT along with chemotherapy (capecitabine + temozolomide). (CT: computed tomography; FDG: fluorodeoxyglucose; ⁶⁸Ga: gallium-68; MIP: maximum intensity projection; NET: neuroendocrine tumor; PET: positron emission tomography; PRRT: peptide receptor radionuclide therapy; WHO: World Health Organization)

There is a direct correlation between the degree of SSTR expression and the SUV on DOTA-PET imaging. As a result, this can be used as an accurate imaging marker for measuring the treatment response following chemotherapy or PRRT. A modified Krenning scale scoring system is used for uptake interpretation, which compares SSTR expression at the disease site with physiological tracer uptake in the liver and spleen as follows:
- *Grade 1*: Uptake less than normal liver uptake
- *Grade 2*: Uptake equal to normal liver uptake
- *Grade 3*: Uptake greater than normal liver uptake
- *Grade 4*: Uptake more than spleen

As we progress through the spectrum of the grade of GEP-NETs (well differentiated to poorly differentiated), tumors lose their differentiation, which leads to a substantially increased expression of glucose transporter (GLUT). Thus, combined dual imaging with SSTR-PET and fluorodeoxyglucose (FDG)-PET is beneficial for metastatic WD NETs, especially in patients with Ki-67 index between 5 and 20% or those with Ki-67 <5% and have progressed in a short span of <6 months. Also, in cases of metastatic GEP-NETs, dual imaging is important to understand the tumor heterogeneity and characterization of metastatic disease, which has important treatment implications. The utility of dual PET imaging as a baseline imaging modality in metastatic GEP-NETs provides exciting prospect as a prognostic marker as well as establishing treatment protocols. The "NETPET" score combines the complexity of dual PET imaging and combines it into a single parameter.[15] PET using other radiotracers such as ^{18}F-DOPA has a role in high serotonin production and SSTR-negative lesions, whereas ^{68}Ga-Exendin-4 PET has shown superiority in the detection of insulinomas.

PRINCIPLES OF MANAGEMENT OF GASTROENTEROPANCREATIC NEUROENDOCRINE TUMORS

It is recommended that GEP-NET cases be managed in a high-volume center with adequate experience in dealing with GEP-NETs. Management options available range from observation to liver transplantation and should be discussed and agreed upon in a multidisciplinary team comprising specialties regularly dealing with the management of GEP-NETs. Various modalities available for NETs in the armamentarium are surgery, SSAs, cytotoxic chemotherapy, molecular targeted therapy, and PRRT.

Surgery

Surgery remains the mainstay of the treatment for localized or locoregional GEP-NETs. The type and extent of surgery depend on the organ involved and the disease burden. In general, oncological resection with regional lymphadenectomy is recommended. Resection of the primary tumor and/or debulking surgery is beneficial for the local control as well as for mitigating the endocrine symptoms even when R0 resection cannot be achieved. Chemotherapy or PRRT can also be used as a neoadjuvant strategy in a few cases for downstaging the tumor to attain resectability.[16] Surgical management of site-specific GEP-NETs will be considered in the respective sections.

Somatostatin Analogs

Majority of GEP-NETs (>90%) express SSTRs. SSAs—octreotide and lanreotide—are used for symptomatic as well as in the antiproliferative treatment of GEP-NETs. Although SSAs were developed primarily for symptomatic control of NETs because of their antisecretory effect, the results of the PROMID, CLARINET, and CLARINET OLE studies confirm that SSAs do have a positive impact on the progression-free survival (PFS) as well as with their antiproliferative effects.[17-19] In the PROMID study, median PFS was significantly longer in the octreotide long-acting repeatable (LAR) arm as compared to the placebo (14.3 months vs. 6 months). Similarly, in the CLARINET study, which included nonfunctioning NETs, median PFS was found to be significantly longer with the lanreotide as compared to placebo (38.5 months vs. 18 months). Thus, SSA treatment is recommended in metastatic GEP-NETs with a low Ki-67 index (<10%). In the NETTER-1 study, patients with SI-NET who progressed on standard SSA dose were randomized to either PRRT or SSA dose escalation. Although PRRT was found to be superior, the higher dose of SSA did result in an additional 9 months of stabilization of the disease.[20] Abdominal pain, flatulence, diarrhea, injection site subcutaneous nodules, nausea, and development of cholelithiasis are the common side effects of SSAs. Short-acting formulations are especially useful in preventing and treating perioperative carcinoid crisis and in the management of carcinoid syndrome, and may also have a role as rescue medication in refractory carcinoid syndrome.

Peptide Receptor Radionuclide Therapy

Peptide receptor radionuclide therapy is a targeted radionuclide therapy that involves systemic administration of therapeutic peptides labeled with radionuclides that selectively target cancer cells. The preferred choice for PRRT is radiolabeled SSAs. The primary indication for PRRT is locally advanced or metastatic GEP-NETs that demonstrate a high tumor uptake on somatostatin receptor imaging (SSI) **(Fig. 5)**. Yttrium-90 (^{90}Y) and lutetium-177 (^{177}Lu) are the most commonly used radioisotopes with ^{177}Lu preferred over ^{90}Y due to a better toxicity profile. The NETTER-1 study compared PRRT versus high dose of SSA therapy in SI-NETs. At the end of 20 months, 65% of patients in the PRRT arm were without progression compared to 11% in the SSA arm.[20] Currently, PRRT is mainly used for advanced SSTR positive, WD GEP-NETs. PRRT is indicated not only in grades 1 and 2 NETs but also in grade 3 tumors having high SSTR uptake. However, careful patient selection and prospective trials are needed to further elucidate the role of PRRT in grade 3 GEP-NETs. The NETTER-2 trial is currently underway to address this issue. PRRT is administered as three to four cycles of ^{177}Lu-DOTATATE/DOTATOC with an 8-week interval between two cycles. In order to keep the SSTRs unblocked, long-acting SSAs are stopped 4–6 weeks prior to the initiation of PRRT. Side effects of PRRT include nausea, vomiting, pain, marrow depression, and renal impairment, which is usually reversible. Some of the future perspectives in PRRT are as follows:
- Role of PRRT as first-line therapy as explored by NETTER-2 trial. The NETTER-2 trial, which is currently underway, compares PRRT with SSAs versus high-dose SSAs in metastatic or locally advanced inoperable G2

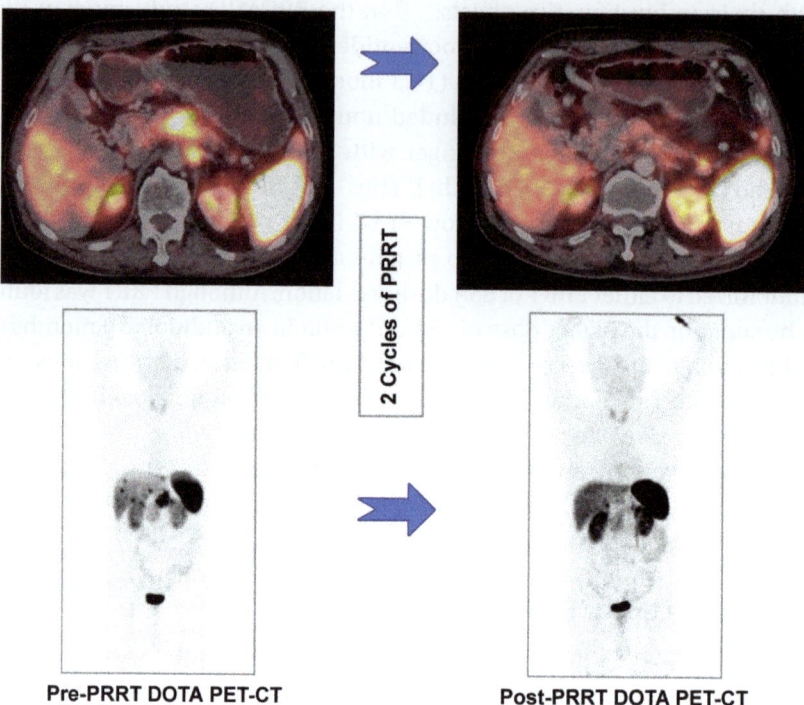

Fig. 5: *Response to PRRT.* A 63-year-old gentleman presented with decreased appetite and weight loss. Pretreatment DOTA PET-CT (MIP and axial fused) showing DOTA avid pancreatic body lesion with multiple liver metastasis. Biopsy from liver lesions was a well-differentiated grade 2 NET with MIB1 of 10%. After two sessions of PRRT, the liver lesions as well as the primary tumor have responded with no DOTA uptake seen on MIP or axial fused PET/CT images. (CT: computed tomography; MIP: maximum intensity projection; NET: neuroendocrine tumor; PET: positron emission tomography; PRRT: peptide receptor radionuclide therapy)

and G3 GEP-NETs with Ki-67 index between 10 and 55% as a first-line therapy.
- Role of PRRT in the neoadjuvant setting in Pan-NETs
- Role of retreatment with PRRT as a salvage therapy
- Role of "Tandem PRRT," which is the combination of ^{90}Y and ^{177}Lu PRRT
- Role of ^{225}actinium/^{213}bismuth/^{211}astatine-based alpha PRRT. Targeted α-particle therapy offers a therapeutic option for patients resistant to the conventional β-irradiation treatments (^{90}Y and ^{177}Lu based).
- Role of intra-arterial PRRT for NET liver metastasis. Intra-arterial PRRT involves the direct administration of radiopharmaceutical agents into the common hepatic artery to increase the site-specific concentration of the drug and avoid the first-pass metabolism due to intravenous administration in standard PRRT.

Chemotherapy

The primary role of systemic chemotherapy is in the management of advanced Pan-NETs and grade 3 GEP-NETs or NECs of any site. Commonly used first-line chemotherapeutic drugs for advanced Pan-NETs are streptozocin/5-fluorouracil (5-FU) or capecitabine (CAP)/temozolomide (TEM). PFS and OS of 23 and 52 months, respectively, have been reported in the treatment of Pan-NETs with streptozocin/5-FU.[21] Similarly, a PFS of 11-20 months but with a slightly higher tumor size response rate is shown by treatment with CAP/TEM.[22] Thus, the combination of capecitabine and temozolomide (CAPTEM) is indicated in progressive WD GEP-NETs, primarily Pan-NETs. The toxicity profile includes nausea and hematological toxicity. Platinum-based chemotherapy with cisplatin/carboplatin plus etoposide is used in the treatment of metastases from high-grade small- or large-cell NEC G3 regardless of the primary tumor origin.

Molecular Targeted Therapy

Everolimus, a mammalian target of rapamycin (mTOR) pathway inhibitor, is approved for advanced, progressive, WD, and nonfunctioning GEP-NETs. In the RADIANT 3 trial, 410 patients with low-intermediate-grade Pan-NETs were randomized to 10 mg everolimus versus placebo. A significant improvement in PFS with everolimus (11 months vs. 4.6 months; $p < 0.001$) was noted.[23] Similar results in other studies (RADIANT 2, RADIANT 4) were also observed with everolimus.[24,25] In the RADIANT 4 study, which included lung and GEP-NET patients, the median PFS was significantly longer in the everolimus arm as compared to the placebo arm (11.0 months vs. 3.9 months).[25]

Because of the significant adverse effects (neutropenia, infections, rash, diarrhea, and hyperglycemia), everolimus is currently reserved for patients who have significant progression of disease on other modalities. Sunitinib, a tyrosine kinase inhibitor, is also approved for use in advanced Pan-NETs. Usually, both everolimus and sunitinib are used after the progression on SSA and chemotherapy.

SITE-SPECIFIC GASTROENTEROPANCREATIC NEUROENDOCRINE TUMORS

Gastroduodenal Neuroendocrine Tumors

Gastric NETs

The origin of gastric NETs is from the enterochromaffin-like cells present in the gastric mucosa. Most gastric NETs are indolent slow-growing tumors; however, some of them can be aggressive resulting in early metastasis. They are classified as types I, II, and III **(Table 3)**. Types I and II gastric

TABLE 3: Classification of gastric NETs.

	Type I	Type II	Type III
Proportion among NETs	70–80	5–6	14–25
Tumor characteristics	Often small (<1–2 cm), multiple in 65% of cases, and polypoid in 78% of cases	Often small (<1–2 cm), multiple, and polypoid	Unique, often large (>2 cm), polypoid, and ulcerated
Associated conditions	Atrophic body gastritis	Gastrinoma/MEN1	None
Pathology	G1–G2 NET	G1–G2 NET	G3 NEC
Serum gastrin levels	↑	↑	Normal
Gastric pH	↑↑	↓↓	Normal
Metastases, %	2–5	10–30	50–100
Tumor-related deaths, %	0	<10	25–30

(MEN1: multiple endocrine neoplasia type 1; NEC: neuroendocrine carcinoma; NET: neuroendocrine tumor)

NETs are usually incidentally found on upper gastrointestinal endoscopy. Type I gastric NETs arise secondary to chronic atrophic gastritis, whereas type II gastric NETs develop in patients with gastrinomas. Gastric NETs are usually <2 cm in size, multiple, and have a Ki-67 index <5%. Tissue diagnosis is achieved by endoscopic biopsy **(Figs. 6A to D)**. Serum CgA and serum gastrin are usually elevated. Gastric acid secretion is low (high pH) in type I tumors, while in type II tumors, acid secretion is high (low pH). For treatment planning, EUS evaluation of the depth of tumor invasion and regional lymph node status is recommended. Single or multiple tumors that are <1 cm can undergo close surveillance as such lesions do not exhibit malignant behavior. A large proportion of these can be kept on surveillance for a prolonged period spanning years owing to their indolent nature. For lesions >1 cm, local excision by endoscopic resection techniques can be performed. However, surgical management is indicated for those with multiple tumors, large lesions, or those invading into and beyond the muscularis propria. Type III gastric NET patients have a propensity for metastasis, usually at the time of diagnosis, and thus warrant systemic therapy. However, type III gastric NET patients with localized disease warrant surgical management, which proceeds in the same manner as for gastric adenocarcinoma (subtotal/total gastrectomy with D2 lymphadenectomy)[26] **(Flowchart 1)**. The 5-year OS in type I and type II gastric NETs is 100 and 95%, respectively, which suggests a favorable overall prognosis, whereas 5-year OS is 50% in type III NETs.

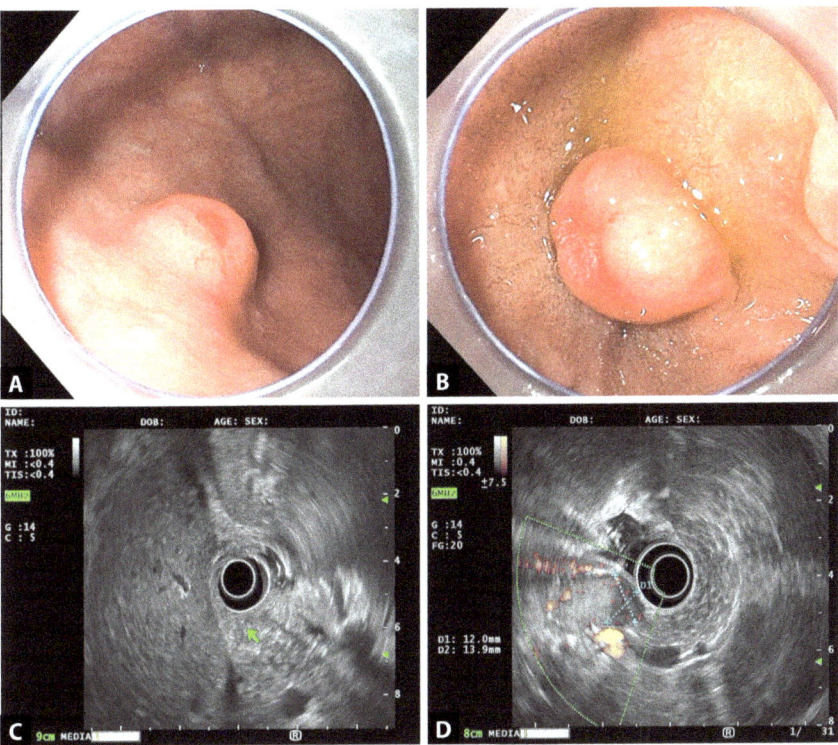

Figs. 6A to D: A 49-year-old lady presented with dyspepsia and diarrhea (six to eight times/day) with serum gastrin levels of 1,200 pg/mL. (A) Endoscopic image of a 1.1 × 1.4 cm nodule along the greater curvature of the stomach in the region of the distal body; (B) Endoscopic image of a 1.2 × 1.2 cm nodule at the D1–D2 junction with central umbilication; (C and D) EUS images of the gastric and duodenal lesion, respectively. The lesion was not found to be invading the submucosa. Biopsy of both the lesions was a well-differentiated grade 1 NET. DOTA CECT scan shows no evidence of metastasis. Patient was managed by endoscopic resection in view of persistent symptoms. (CECT: contrast-enhanced computed tomography; EUS: endoscopic ultrasound; NET: neuroendocrine tumor)

Duodenal NETs

Duodenal NETs are generally diagnosed as an incidental finding during endoscopy, and considerable heterogeneity exists in the presentation, treatment, and outcomes[27] **(Flowchart 2)**. Duodenal NETs can be divided into functioning and nonfunctioning. Nonfunctioning tumors are more common. More than 50% of the patients may have metastatic disease at the time of presentation. Histological diagnosis is achieved by endoscopic biopsy and serum gastrin and CgA may be elevated. Measurement of urinary and serum 5-HIAA levels and serum calcitonin is needed as indicated by the symptoms. CECT/MRI, EUS, and SSI are recommended for staging. As per the ENETS guidelines,[26] endoscopic resection is recommended for duodenal NETs

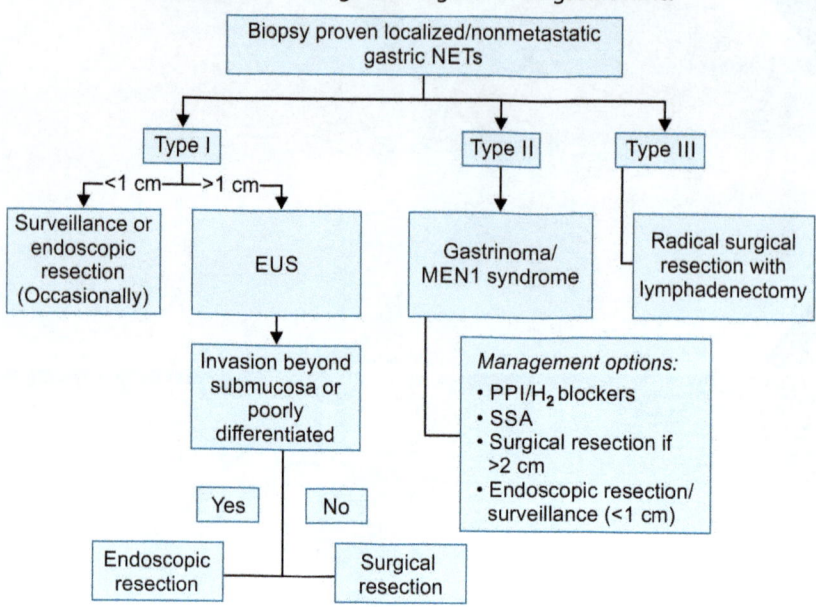

Flowchart 1: Management algorithm for gastric NETs.

(EUS: endoscopic ultrasound; MEN: multiple endocrine neoplasia; NET: neuroendocrine tumor; PPI: proton-pump inhibitor; SSA: somatostatin analog)

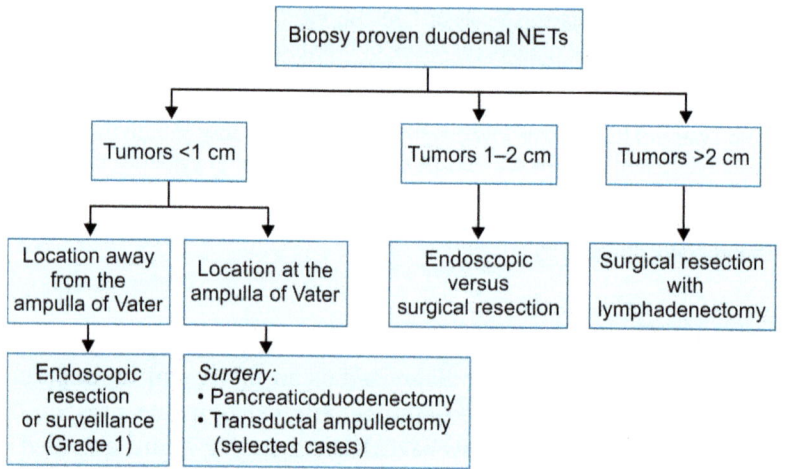

Flowchart 2: Management algorithm for duodenal neuroendocrine tumors (NETs).

≤1 cm in size, confined to the submucosa (T1), and without the evidence of spread to the adjacent lymph nodes or organs. There is no consensus regarding treatment for tumors between 1 and 2 cm without worrisome features, and either surgical or endoscopic approach is justified. Formal staging workup is recommended followed by surgical resection with standard regional lymphadenectomy for tumors >2 cm in size. Another important factor in deciding the treatment for duodenal NETs is its location with relation to the ampulla of Vater. Surveillance is preferred for a grade 1, localized, ≤10 mm, nonfunctioning tumor located away from the ampulla. Larger tumors, which are located away from the ampulla, can be treated with local excision or a pancreas-preserving duodenal resection. Duodenal NETs located at or close to the ampulla of Vater should be resected. Pancreaticoduodenectomy is required for tumors located at or near the ampulla and not amenable to endoscopic resection. A transduodenal ampullectomy can be considered in selected patients.

Pancreatic Neuroendocrine Tumors

The incidence of Pan-NETs is increasing with a reported unfavorable prognosis as compared to other GEP-NETs. The majority of Pan-NETs (80%) are nonfunctional.

Nonfunctional Pancreatic Neuroendocrine Tumors

The majority of patients with NF Pan-NETs are asymptomatic. Nonspecific symptoms such as anorexia, pain, weight loss, nausea, and jaundice may be present in patients with advanced disease at presentation. Serum CgA is the most commonly elevated biomarker utilized in the diagnosis and follow-up of NF Pan-NETs. Triple-phase CECT or contrast-enhanced MRI is essential in accurate diagnosis and disease staging. Tumors are usually small, well delineated, and highly vascularized during the arterial inflow phase of a CECT scan. A CT is also useful in determining the relationship between the tumor and the adjacent organs and a possible vascular infiltration with high accuracy. ^{68}Ga DOTA-PET scan is considered as the gold standard for WD NF Pan-NETs. It is highly accurate in detecting the primary lesion and also the presence of distant metastases. On the other hand, high-grade or poorly differentiated NF Pan-NETs tend to exhibit ^{18}F-FDG-PET avidity than SSTR-PET avidity. Relationship between the tumor and the main pancreatic duct, presence of multifocal disease, possible vascular infiltration, and nodal involvement can be evaluated well with an EUS. Smaller NF Pan-NETs are generally indolent and tend to remain stable during active surveillance, and, therefore, based on this assumption, both the ENETS and the North American Neuroendocrine Tumor Society (NANETs) guidelines advocate conservative management for selected NF Pan-NETs <2 cm in size. The ideal follow-up scheme is still debated; however, a 6-monthly CECT or MRI for the first 2 years and then yearly if the tumor remains stable is recommended. Surgical resection remains the only curative treatment of localized NF Pan-NETs and also has an important role in the management of metastatic disease. Given the risk of nodal involvement, for NF Pan-NETs >2 cm, standard pancreatic resections (pancreaticoduodenectomy/distal pancreatectomy) with lymphadenectomy are preferred to parenchyma-sparing procedures such as enucleation or central/median pancreatectomy.[28] Parenchyma-sparing surgery can be attempted for NF Pan-NET <2 cm. The risk of pancreatic fistula remains high with parenchyma-sparing resections; however, they potentially lower the risk of endocrine and exocrine insufficiency. Minimally invasive approach (laparoscopic or robotic) is feasible for lesions located in the body or tail of pancreas, as well as for those lesions that are amenable to enucleation or central/median pancreatectomy. The long-term benefit of surgery in poorly differentiated grade 3 NF Pan-NETs (or Pan-NECs) is controversial as these patients have a high risk of recurrence after upfront surgery. Such patients may likely benefit from platinum-based perioperative chemotherapy. Radical resections for locally advanced WD grade 1 and grade 2 NF Pan-NETs should be attempted whenever feasible, and these include multivisceral and vascular resections. Preoperative treatment with PRRT may have a role in downsizing the tumor and improving the outcomes after surgery.

Functional Pancreatic Neuroendocrine Tumors (Table 4)

Pancreatic neuroendocrine tumors are classified as functional if they result in symptoms which can be attributed to hormone secretion by the tumor and are generally associated with a more favorable prognosis.

Insulinoma

Patients with insulinoma present with symptoms primarily due to neuroglycopenia (blurred vision, fatigue, confusion, and seizures) and from the excessive catecholamine release secondary to the hypoglycemia (anxiousness, tremor, sweating, palpitation, and weakness). Patients typically describe a history of weight gain, which occurs secondary to increased food intake in order to maintain a normoglycemic state. The classic Whipple's triad consists of symptoms of hypoglycemia, with documented low plasma glucose levels, and the resolution of symptoms after administration of glucose. Evaluation of hypoglycemia should be pursued further only in those patients where a Whipple's triad is documented. Thus, hypoglycemia (blood glucose <55 mg/dL), while the patient is experiencing symptoms and relief after administration of glucose, should be documented first. Inappropriately elevated levels of insulin and C-peptide, while the patient is hypoglycemic, confirms endogenous hyperinsulinemia. If such an episode of hypoglycemia cannot easily be observed, 48–72 hours of supervised fasting is necessary as a confirmatory test. SSTR-PET imaging is limited for insulinomas, with a low specificity, sensitivity, and accuracy of around 25%.[29] However, ^{68}Ga-Exendin PET-CT scans are superior in detecting and staging insulinomas **(Figs. 7A and B)**. Rarely, in situations where the insulinoma remains unlocalized

TABLE 4: Functional pancreatic NETs.

Cell type	Functional Pan-NET	Location	Malignant potential	Decade at diagnosis	M:F	Endocrine medical management for symptom control	Surgery for loco-regional tumor	Perioperative monitoring	5-year survival
Beta	Insulinoma	99% pancreas (equal throughout)	10%	5th	0.7:1	Small frequent meals Diazoxide SSAs	Parenchymal sparing if possible (e.g., enucleation and central pancreatectomy)	Glucose monitoring	80–90%
G	Gastrinoma	90% within "gastrinoma triangle"	60–90%	6th	1.5–2:1	Control acid secretion with PPI SSAs Manage potential anemia from PUD Monitor B_{12} levels	Formal pancreatectomy with lymph node dissection	Continue PPI therapy	50–70% 50–60%
A	Glucagonoma	100% pancreas (equal throughout)	50–80%	5th	1:1	SSAs Manage catabolic state, such as weight loss, malnutrition, electrolyte disturbances, cutaneous breakdown Screen for deep vein thrombosis	Formal pancreatectomy with lymph node dissection	SSAs Nutritional support	40–50%
D1	VIPoma	90% pancreas (75% tail)	40–70%	4th–5th	0.3:1	SSAs Manage consequences of high-volume watery diarrhea, such as hypovolemia, acute kidney injury, and electrolyte disturbance	Formal pancreatectomy with lymph node dissection	SSAs Monitoring of electrolytes	20–40%
D	Somatostatinoma	2/3 pancreas (2/3 head)	60–70%	5th	1:1	SSAs	Formal pancreatectomy with lymph node dissection	SSAs	30–50%

(NET: neuroendocrine tumor; PPI: proton-pump inhibitor; PUD: peptic ulcer disease; SSA: somatostatin analog; VIP: vasoactive intestinal polypeptide)

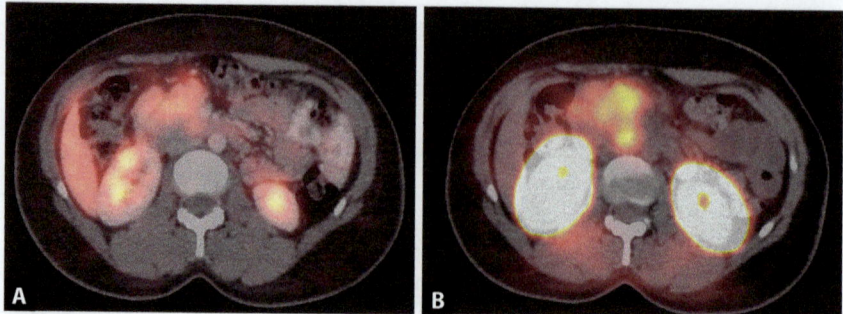

Figs. 7A and B: *Insulinoma*. A 29-year-old female presented with classical "Whipple's triad." (A) *DOTA PET-CT scan*: Axial fused PET/CT image shows DOTANOC uptake in the large pancreatic head lesion (uptake equal to adjacent liver uptake); (B) *Ga-Exendin PET-CT scan*: Axial fused PET/CT shows intense tracer uptake (more than DOTA uptake) in the pancreatic head lesion, thus confirming the diagnosis of insulinoma. Biopsy—well-differentiated grade 1 NET with MIB of 1%. The patient was managed by a pancreaticoduodenectomy (Whipple's procedure). (Ga: gallium; CT: computed tomography; NET: neuroendocrine tumor; PET: positron emission tomography)

despite pancreas protocol CT scan, MRI, nuclear imaging, and EUS, further attempt at localization can be done with selective arterial calcium stimulation test.

Regardless of their size, all insulinomas must be managed by surgical resection because of the presence of disabling hypoglycemic symptoms. Enucleation is the surgical procedure of choice for exophytic or peripherally located tumors as they are primarily benign. If enucleation is not feasible either due to local invasion or intrapancreatic location, then pancreatoduodenectomy for tumors in the pancreatic head, central/median pancreatectomy for small body tumors or distal pancreatectomy with or without splenectomy for tumors in the tail is to be considered. Distal pancreatectomy can be performed laparoscopically. In experienced high-volume centers, laparoscopic procedures are safe for patients with insulinomas and may be associated with shorter hospital stays.[30] Radiofrequency ablation remains a viable option in patients who are at high risk for surgery.

Gastrinoma

Gastrinomas are the most common functional NETs of the duodenum, which are located within the Passaro's (gastrinoma) triangle formed by the junction of (1) the cystic duct and the common hepatic duct (superiorly), (2) the junction of the second and third portions of the duodenum (inferiorly), and (3) the head and neck of the pancreas (medially). Peptic ulcer disease (PUD) is present in majority of patients (90%) with gastrinoma. This occurs secondary to the high acid output caused due to the elevation in serum gastrin levels and typically manifests as anemia, dyspepsia, or complications of PUD (perforation, gastric outlet obstruction, or hematemesis/melena). Other symptoms of gastrinoma include diarrhea, heartburn, nausea/vomiting, and weight loss. The classic "ZES" from gastrinomas was described first in 1955, consisting of gastric acid hypersecretion, PUD, and diarrhea. Raised serum gastrin levels with high acid output are essential to diagnose ZES. Measurements should be done after stopping PPIs for at least 5 days and H_2 receptor blockers for a minimum of 2 days. Causes of secondary hypergastrinemia (*Helicobacter pylori* infection, kidney failure, previous vagotomy) and other causes of gastric acid hypersecretion should be ruled out. Serum gastrin levels >1,000 pg/mL and a gastric pH <2 are confirmatory of diagnosis. Gastrin levels between 100 and 1,000 pg/mL and gastric pH >2 require further evaluation in the form of basal gastric acid output measurement and secretin stimulation test. The basal acid output of >15 mEq/h and an increase of serum gastrin by >110–200 pg/mL on secretin stimulation are diagnostic of the syndrome. CECT is the primary modality for localization, assessment of tumor extent, and operability. It detects up to two-thirds of the lesions. ^{68}Ga DOTA-PET has a higher sensitivity compared with both CT and somatostatin receptor scintigraphy. EUS is useful for the detection of small primary tumors. Careful search for additional small lesions is necessary to detect multifocal tumors, particularly in patients with associated MEN1 syndrome.

The treatment of gastrinomas usually depends on the location of the tumor and also on the findings during exploratory laparotomy. If the lesion is not identified in the pancreas on exploration, the entire area included in the "gastrinoma triangle" must be carefully examined. If the lesion still cannot be isolated, a duodenotomy must be performed to rule out duodenal gastrinomas. An intraoperative ultrasound with local resection or enucleation of tumors and periduodenal node dissection must be performed. Gastrinomas in the distal pancreas are treated with a distal pancreatectomy with or without splenectomy. The role of routine splenectomy in such cases is a matter of debate. However, since gastrinomas are known to potentially involve regional lymph nodes, splenectomy may be required to enable a complete lymphadenectomy.

Glucagonomas

Glucagonomas are rare tumors. They are almost always found within the pancreas and commonly in the body and tail region of the organ. Tumor has equal gender distribution and patients are typically seen in the fifth decade of life. About 60–70% of glucagonomas are malignant. Most are sporadic and are rarely associated with MEN1 syndrome. The clinical manifestations of a glucagonoma are classically referred to as the "four-D syndrome." It includes type 2 diabetes mellitus, dermatitis (necrolytic migratory erythema), deep vein thrombosis, and depression. Patients may also have associated anemia, weakness, weight loss, and mental changes. Necrolytic migratory erythema is a characteristic rash of glucagonoma present in about 70% of patients. Fasting serum glucagon levels >1,000 pg/mL are diagnostic. Most tumors are large, usually >4 cm, and easily localized and assessed with a CECT. SSTR-PET scan can be useful for long-term follow-up. SSAs control circulating levels of glucagon and induce anabolism. R_0 resection should be the goal for good symptom control and possible cure. Resection/debulking of the primary and metastatic disease can offer meaningful palliation. For nonresectable lesions, SSAs can provide good symptom control. Dacarbazine and streptozotocin have been used to treat metastatic glucagonomas.

VIPomas

VIPomas are rare functional Pan-NETs, and majority of them are benign. Similar to glucagonomas, >90% of VIPomas are located in the pancreas, commonly in the body and tail of the pancreas. In 1958, Verner and Morrison first described this as WDHA or Verner–Morrison syndrome. Flushing and weight loss are also notable features. Diarrhea in VIPomas is classically described as being painless, odorless, large volume, and secretory diarrhea (6–8 L/day), which persists on fasting. Fasting serum VIP level should be >200 pg/mL and average levels are often close to 1,000 pg/mL. CECT scan usually suffices for localization and assessment owing to frequent large size and distal pancreatic location. Hypokalemia and acidosis can be very severe and need to be corrected as a first step in the management of these tumors. SSAs and glucocorticoids can help in the symptomatic control of diarrhea. When radical resection is not possible, palliation can usually be achieved by debulking of the metastatic tumor in combination with the use of SSAs. Streptozocin-based chemotherapy (with 5-FU) has been combined with SSAs with some success. Dacarbazine and interferon have also been used.

Somatostatinomas

Somatostatinomas are the most uncommon tumors. They represent around 1% of all functional Pan-NETs. Somatostatinoma syndrome includes hyperglycemia, cholelithiasis, steatorrhea, and diarrhea. The mean age of patients at diagnosis is 50 years, with an equal distribution between men and women. They may be located in the pancreas or duodenum and sometimes in the biliary tract or even in the small bowel. In most patients (>90%), the lesions are solitary and large (5–6 cm). Localization is easily achieved by a CECT scan. Size of the lesion is the predictor of liver metastasis and prognosis. Surgical resection is the treatment of choice. As with most other Pan-NETs, many patients have metastasis on presentation, and curative surgery is often not possible. Debulking can give good symptom control and survival. In unresectable disease, octreotide and interferon-alpha may improve symptoms.

Small Intestinal Neuroendocrine Tumors

Small intestinal neuroendocrine tumors account for approximately 25-30% of GEP-NETs, with the most common site being the distal ileum. Primary tumors are generally small (1-2 cm) and may be multiple. At the time of diagnosis, approximately 60% have metastatic disease in the mesenteric lymph nodes, para-aortic lymph nodes, and/or the liver. The primary tumor or the mesenteric lymph node metastasis predisposes to tumor-induced fibrosis, which results in bowel obstruction and vascular encasement. Less than 20% of the patients at diagnosis present with flushing and diarrhea due to carcinoid syndrome. CT/MRI and SSTR-PET are the imaging modalities indicated for the diagnosis and staging. Echocardiography and NT-proBNP should be done to evaluate possible carcinoid heart disease in patients with metastatic disease and/or when symptoms of carcinoid syndrome appear. Patients with SI-NETs must be considered for curative resection, independent of tumor stage, if R0/R1 resection is feasible. In case of emergency surgery, extensive central mesenteric dissection should be avoided as this may result in damage to the mesenteric vessels causing short bowel syndrome. In patients with stage IV disease, which is not amenable to a complete R_0 resection, surgery is to be considered only in an acute emergency situation (bowel obstruction or ischemia). However, surgery should be attempted in patients with liver metastasis when R_0 resection is possible or when the aim is to reduce the endocrine symptoms. SSA is the treatment of choice for patients with disseminated metastatic disease not amenable to surgery and requiring control of symptoms. For SSA refractory serotonin-induced diarrhea, telotristat ethyl can be used, and for those who have progressed on SSA therapy, PRRT is recommended.

Appendiceal Neuroendocrine Tumors

Most appendiceal NETs are present on a clinical background of "appendicitis," and the NET is identified incidentally on final histopathology after appendicectomy (incidence 1-2%). Appendectomy alone is recommended in patients with tumor size <1 cm. Larger tumors of size >2 cm are considered as candidates for a completion right hemicolectomy. However, the role of additional hemicolectomy for lesions between 1 and 2 cm in size is debatable. Most of the incidental findings occur in a relatively young age population on a background of clinical appendicitis. Further resection by a right hemicolectomy may indeed be a considerable undertaking in these groups of patients.

Colorectal Neuroendocrine Tumors

Incidentally detected colorectal NETs have increased because of the widespread use of colonoscopy and adoption of screening programs for colorectal cancer. This has resulted in the early detection of sporadic lesions having a favorable prognosis. Metastasis is rare in smaller tumors <2 cm, but the risk of metastasis significantly increases with the increase in size of the tumor >2 cm.[31] Colonic NETs are uncommon (<1% of all GEP-NETs). Grades 1 and 2 tumors are treated by conventional oncological resection with standard lymphadenectomy. Rectal NETs are often encountered as incidental finding, and those with size <1-2 cm can be managed by endoscopic resection. A recent randomized trial found no statistical difference between the type of endoscopic resection (endoscopic mucosal resection vs. endoscopic submucosal dissection) for small (<10 mm) rectal NETs.[32] For tumors <2 cm, it is recommended to perform transanal EUS for the assessment of tumor depth. Endoscopic removal is contraindicated for tumors invading the muscular propria, and oncological rectal surgery (anterior resection/abdominoperineal resection) is recommended depending on the tumor location in rectum and local invasion. Although high-grade (grade 3) NETs or NECs of the rectum carry an overall poor prognosis, surgical management as per oncological principles is recommended for localized nonmetastatic disease.

Neuroendocrine Liver Metastasis

Surgery is the first choice for patients with resectable metastatic liver disease. Transarterial chemoembolization (TACE), transarterial radioembolization (TARE), and thermal ablation (radiofrequency and microwave) are other techniques used for the treatment of liver lesions. Frilling et al. have described three major morphological categories of NELM:[33]

1. *Type I*: Single metastasis of any size
2. *Type II*: Metastasis predominantly involving one lobe with smaller lesions in the other
3. *Type III*: Disseminated bilobar metastasis

Neuroendocrine liver metastases are typically hypervascular in the hepatic arterial phase of CECT scan. MRI is superior for lesion detection, particularly in the hepatic arterial phase or fat-suppressed T2-weighted imaging. The only modality conferring the possibility of cure is hepatectomy with negative margins, which should be the first choice for grade 1 or 2 GEP-NETs (Ki-67 <20%) with type I NELM with no or limited extrahepatic disease burden. R_2 liver resections with the intent to "debulk" the NELM may be an option for hormonally hypersecreting tumors with poorly controlled symptoms refractory to other systemic therapies. The target, traditionally, was to debulk 90% of the liver tumor burden. However, this cutoff was based on older studies. With the advent of SSAs, transarterial liver-directed therapies, and PRRT, these traditional cutoffs should be viewed with caution, and the role of liver debulking surgery should be continuously reevaluated.

Liver transplantation for NELM is another feasible option having favorable long-term outcomes after following strict selection criteria as follows:[34]
- Low-grade NETs (clinical syndrome irrelevant)
- Primary tumor drained by portal venous system
- Age ≤55 years
- Liver involvement ≤50%
- Complete resection of the primary tumor and any extrahepatic disease
- At least 6 months of stable disease/response to treatment prior to transplantation

■ CONCLUSION

Our improved understanding of the tumor biology of GEP-NETs has led to the development of a variety of treatment modalities in the recent past. With the advent of these new therapies, the correct sequencing of these modalities assumes great importance. Although improvement in the long-term survival outcomes of patients with GEP-NETs remains the ultimate goal, due consideration to optimize the quality of life cannot be overlooked.

■ ACKNOWLEDGMENTS

We acknowledge Dr Subhash Yadav, Professor and Pathologist, Division of GI and HPB Pathology, Department of Surgical Pathology, Tata Memorial Hospital, Mumbai, Maharashtra, India, for contributing to the histopathology images of GEP-NETs; Dr Ameya Puranik, Department of Nuclear Medicine, Tata Memorial Hospital and Homi Bhabha National Institute, Mumbai, for providing the radiological/PET-CT images of GEP-NETs; and Dr Sridhar Sundaram, Associate Professor, Department of Digestive Diseases and Clinical Nutrition, Tata Memorial Hospital, Mumbai, for providing the endoscopic images of gastric/duodenal NETs.

■ REFERENCES

1. Pavel M, Öberg K, Falconi M, Krenning EP, Sundin A, Perren A, et al. Gastroenteropancreatic neuroendocrine neoplasms: ESMO Clinical Practice Guidelines for diagnosis, treatment and follow-up. Ann Oncol. 2020;31(7):844-60.
2. Nagtegaal ID, Odze RD, Klimstra D, Paradis V, Rugge M, Schirmacher P, et al. The 2019 WHO classification of tumours of the digestive system. Histopathology. 2020;76(2):182-8.
3. Xu Z, Wang L, Dai S, Chen M, Li F, Sun J, et al. Epidemiologic trends of and factors associated with overall survival for patients with gastroenteropancreatic neuroendocrine tumors in the United States. JAMA Netw Open. 2021;4(9): e2124750.
4. Palepu J, Shrikhande SV, Bhaduri D, Shah RC, Sirohi B, Chhabra V, et al. Trends in diagnosis of gastroenteropancreatic neuroendocrine tumors (GEP-NETs) in India: a report of multicenter data from a web-based registry. Indian J Gastroenterol. 2017;36(6):445-51.

5. Brierley JD, Gospodarowicz MK, Wittekind C (Eds). TNM Classification of Malignant Tumours, 8th edition. Hoboken: Wiley; 2017.
6. Halperin DM, Shen C, Dasari A, Xu Y, Chu Y, Zhou S, et al. Frequency of carcinoid syndrome at neuroendocrine tumour diagnosis: a population-based study. Lancet Oncol. 2017;18(4):525-34.
7. Feldman JM, O'Dorisio TM. Role of neuropeptides and serotonin in the diagnosis of carcinoid tumors. Am J Med. 1986;81(6B):41-8.
8. van Adrichem RCS, Kamp K, Vandamme T, Peeters M, Feelders RA, de Herder WW. Serum neuron-specific enolase level is an independent predictor of overall survival in patients with gastroenteropancreatic neuroendocrine tumors. Ann Oncol. 2016;27(4):746-7.
9. Tan EH, Tan CH. Imaging of gastroenteropancreatic neuroendocrine tumors. World J Clin Oncol. 2011;2(1):28-43.
10. Rockall AG, Reznek RH. Imaging of neuroendocrine tumours (CT/MR/US). Best Pract Res Clin Endocrinol Metab. 2007;21(1):43-68.
11. Rösch T, Lightdale CJ, Botet JF, Boyce GA, Sivak MV, Yasuda K, et al. Localization of pancreatic endocrine tumors by endoscopic ultrasonography. N Engl J Med. 1992;326(26):1721-6.
12. Brabander T, Kwekkeboom DJ, Feelders RA, Brouwers AH, Teunissen JJM. Nuclear medicine imaging of neuroendocrine tumors. Front Horm Res. 2015;44:73-87.
13. Gabriel M, Decristoforo C, Donnemiller E, Ulmer H, Watfah Rychlinski C, Mather SJ, et al. An intrapatient comparison of 99mTc-EDDA/HYNIC-TOC with 111In-DTPA-octreotide for diagnosis of somatostatin receptor-expressing tumors. J Nucl Med. 2003;44(5):708-16.
14. Geijer H, Breimer LH. Somatostatin receptor PET/CT in neuroendocrine tumours: update on systematic review and meta-analysis. Eur J Nucl Med Mol Imaging. 2013;40(11):1770-80.
15. Chan DL, Ulaner GA, Pattison D, Wyld D, Ladwa R, Kirchner J, et al. Dual PET imaging in bronchial neuroendocrine neoplasms: the NETPET score as a prognostic biomarker. J Nucl Med. 2021;62(9):1278-84.
16. Capurso G, Bettini R, Rinzivillo M, Boninsegna L, Delle Fave G, Falconi M. Role of resection of the primary pancreatic neuroendocrine tumour only in patients with unresectable metastatic liver disease: a systematic review. Neuroendocrinology. 2011;93(4):223-9.
17. Rinke A, Müller HH, Schade-Brittinger C, Klose KJ, Barth P, Wied M, et al. Placebo-controlled, double-blind, prospective, randomized study on the effect of octreotide LAR in the control of tumor growth in patients with metastatic neuroendocrine midgut tumors: a report from the PROMID Study Group. J Clin Oncol. 2009;27(28):4656-63.
18. Caplin ME, Pavel M, Ćwikła JB, Phan AT, Raderer M, Sedláčková E, et al. Lanreotide in metastatic enteropancreatic neuroendocrine tumors. N Engl J Med. 2014;371(3):224-33.
19. Caplin ME, Pavel M, Ćwikła JB, Phan AT, Raderer M, Sedláčková E, et al. Anti-tumour effects of lanreotide for pancreatic and intestinal neuroendocrine tumours: the CLARINET open-label extension study. Endocr Relat Cancer. 2016;23(3):191-9.
20. Strosberg J, El-Haddad G, Wolin E, Hendifar A, Yao J, Chasen B, et al. Phase 3 trial of ^{177}Lu-DOTATATE for midgut neuroendocrine tumors. N Engl J Med. 2017;376(2):125-35.

21. Clewemar Antonodimitrakis P, Sundin A, Wassberg C, Granberg D, Skogseid B, Eriksson B. Streptozocin and 5-fluorouracil for the treatment of pancreatic neuroendocrine tumors: efficacy, prognostic factors and toxicity. Neuroendocrinology. 2016;103(3-4):345-53.
22. Bongiovanni A, Liverani C, Foca F, Fausti V, Di Menna G, Mercatali L, et al. Temozolomide alone or combined with capecitabine for the treatment of metastatic neuroendocrine neoplasia: a "real-world" data analysis. Neuroendocrinology. 2021;111(9):895-906.
23. Yao JC, Shah MH, Ito T, Bohas CL, Wolin EM, Van Cutsem E, et al. Everolimus for advanced pancreatic neuroendocrine tumors. N Engl J Med. 2011;364(6):514-23.
24. Pavel ME, Baudin E, Öberg KE, Hainsworth JD, Voi M, Rouyrre N, et al. Efficacy of everolimus plus octreotide LAR in patients with advanced neuroendocrine tumor and carcinoid syndrome: final overall survival from the randomized, placebo-controlled phase 3 RADIANT-2 study. Ann Oncol. 2017;28(7):1569-75.
25. Yao JC, Fazio N, Singh S, Buzzoni R, Carnaghi C, Wolin E, et al. Everolimus for the treatment of advanced, non-functional neuroendocrine tumours of the lung or gastrointestinal tract (RADIANT-4): a randomised, placebo-controlled, phase 3 study. Lancet Lond Engl. 2016;387(10022):968-77.
26. Delle Fave G, O'Toole D, Sundin A, Taal B, Ferolla P, Ramage JK, et al. ENETS consensus guidelines update for gastroduodenal neuroendocrine neoplasms. Neuroendocrinology. 2016;103(2):119-24.
27. Massironi S, Campana D, Partelli S, Panzuto F, Rossi RE, Faggiano A, et al. Heterogeneity of duodenal neuroendocrine tumors: an Italian multi-center experience. Ann Surg Oncol. 2018;25(11):3200-6.
28. Partelli S, Javed AA, Andreasi V, He J, Muffatti F, Weiss MJ, et al. The number of positive nodes accurately predicts recurrence after pancreaticoduodenectomy for nonfunctioning neuroendocrine neoplasms. Eur J Surg Oncol. 2018;44(6):778-83.
29. Sharma P, Arora S, Karunanithi S, Khadgawat R, Durgapal P, Sharma R, et al. Somatostatin receptor based PET/CT imaging with 68Ga-DOTA-Nal3-octreotide for localization of clinically and biochemically suspected insulinoma. QJ Nucl Med Mol Imaging. 2016;60(1):69-76.
30. Su AP, Ke NW, Zhang Y, Liu XB, Hu WM, Tian BL, et al. Is laparoscopic approach for pancreatic insulinomas safe? Results of a systematic review and meta-analysis. J Surg Res. 2014;186(1):126-34.
31. Anthony LB, Strosberg JR, Klimstra DS, Maples WJ, O'Dorisio TM, Warner RRP, et al. The NANETS consensus guidelines for the diagnosis and management of gastrointestinal neuroendocrine tumors (nets): well-differentiated nets of the distal colon and rectum. Pancreas. 2010;39(6):767-74.
32. Gao X, Huang S, Wang Y, Peng Q, Li W, Zou Y, et al. Modified cap-assisted endoscopic mucosal resection versus endoscopic submucosal dissection for the treatment of rectal neuroendocrine tumors ≤10 mm: a randomized noninferiority trial. Am J Gastroenterol. 2022;117(12):1982-9.
33. Frilling A, Li J, Malamutmann E, Schmid KW, Bockisch A, Broelsch CE. Treatment of liver metastases from neuroendocrine tumours in relation to the extent of hepatic disease. Br J Surg. 2009;96(2):175-84.
34. Mazzaferro V, Sposito C, Coppa J, Miceli R, Bhoori S, Bongini M, et al. The Long-term benefit of liver transplantation for hepatic metastases from neuroendocrine tumors. Am J Transplant. 2016;16(10):2892-902.

CHAPTER 6

Newer Terminology in Ventral Hernia Repair

Sanjeet Kumar Rai, Aditya Baksi, Asuri Krishna, Virinder Kumar Bansal

■ INTRODUCTION

In the 19th and first half of the 20th century, herniorrhaphy was the standard of care for ventral hernias—both primary and incisional. In 1963, Francis Usher reported the use of polypropylene mesh in hernia repair.[1] But it took a few more decades before mesh repair became the standard of care globally for ventral hernias. Surgeons experimented with various types of mesh materials and various layers of the abdominal wall for placing the mesh. Four main positions were described: *Onlay*, where the mesh is placed above the anterior rectus sheath; *inlay*, where the mesh is stitched to the margins of the defect; *sublay*, where the mesh is placed either on the posterior rectus sheath (PRS), i.e., deep to the rectus abdominis or "retrorectus," or between the PRS and the peritoneum (preperitoneal); and, *underlay*, where the mesh is intraperitoneal, i.e., attached to the parietal peritoneum **(Fig. 1)**. The sublay repair, popularized by Rives and Stoppa in the 1980s, became the gold standard in ventral hernia repair.[2] It had its limitations though. The size of the retrorectus mesh was limited by the bilateral semilunar lines, and open surgery had its share of surgical site infection (SSI). To circumvent these problems, newer approaches to hernia repair were described in the 1990s. Ramirez, et al. described the anterior component separation[3] that enabled repair of larger hernias, and LeBlanc and Booth popularized laparoscopic underlay repair with intraperitoneal mesh placement.[4] Open component separation techniques had a very high rate of seroma and SSI. On the other hand, the laparoscopic technique, which later came to be known as intraperitoneal onlay mesh (IPOM), became the gold standard for laparoscopic ventral hernia repair. However, it had several drawbacks. It required coated or composite mesh to prevent adhesion to bowel. These meshes were almost 10 times more expensive than the polypropylene meshes used in open surgery. That, along with the cost of tackers needed to fix the mesh to the parities, made IPOM a costly operation, not affordable by many, especially in low-middle-income countries. Also, the tacks resulted in severe postoperative pain, increasing hospital stay. With longer follow-up, occasional reports of mesh erosion into bowel started to come up.[5] These concerns led surgeons to look for alternative minimal access approaches to hernia repair, which

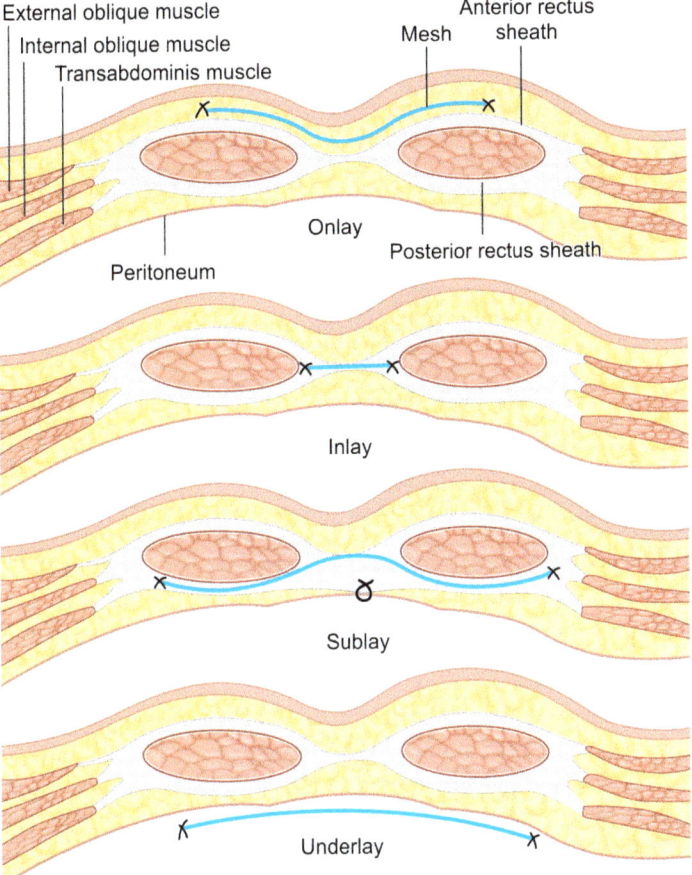

Fig. 1: Schematic diagram showing placement of mesh at different sites.

would be less painful and more cost-effective and avoid intraperitoneal mesh placement. This has led to the development of an array of procedures in the last two decades and the consequent new terminologies in hernia literature.

UNDERLAY REPAIRS

Intraperitoneal Onlay Mesh

The technique of IPOM was first described by Karl LeBlanc in 1993,[4] although they did not use this acronym till much later, when it had gained wider publicity. IPOM is performed using three lateral ports—two 5-mm working ports on either side of a 10-mm camera port. The ports are placed on the left flank for midline and right-sided ventral hernias and on the right flank for left-sided ventral hernias. After the creation of pneumoperitoneum and placement of ports, the contents of the hernia sac are reduced, followed by insertion of a composite mesh, which is fixed to the parities, typically with

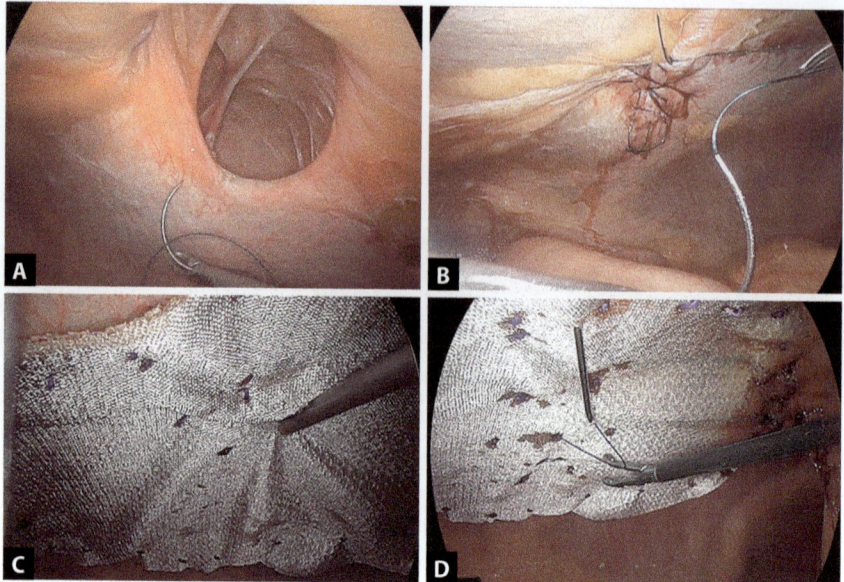

Figs. 2A to D: Intraperitoneal onlay mesh (IPOM) plus repair of ventral hernia: (A) Hernia defect; (B) Defect closure; (C) IPOM implantation; (D) Suture transfixation.

a double crown of tacks and four-corner transfascial sutures. Important technical considerations include large mesh overlap of at least 5 cm all around the defect and placement of outer tacks at intervals of 1.5–2 cm along the periphery of the mesh.

Intraperitoneal Onlay Mesh Plus

The traditional IPOM, described by LeBlanc, was a bridging repair in which the fascial defect was not closed, and a mesh was simply applied as a patch over the defect. Proponents of IPOM argue that closing the defect would result in tension, which is a known cause of postoperative pain and recurrence. However, many surgeons prefer to close the defect with intracorporeal or extracorporeal sutures, as this has been shown to reduce seroma formation **(Figs. 2A to D)**.[6] It is believed to improve abdominal wall dynamics, resulting in postoperative bulging. In in its latest update of guidelines for laparoscopic ventral hernia repair, the International Endohernia Society has recommended closure of the fascial defect.[7]

Hybrid Intraperitoneal Onlay Mesh

Some hernias may not be manageable by a laparoscopic approach. By performing some steps by open technique, a full-fledged conversion to open surgery may be avoided, thus reducing the size of the incision and risk of SSI. A hybrid approach[8] is especially useful in incarcerated hernias not reducible by laparoscopic means or in the presence of dense intrabdominal adhesions not amenable to laparoscopic adhesiolysis.

Transabdominal Partially Extraperitoneal

Transabdominal partially extraperitoneal (TAPE) repair is a variant of IPOM, which has been used in suprapubic (M5) and iliac (L3) hernias, when the distance between the lower margin of the defect and the pubic arch is <5 cm.[9] Raising a peritoneal flap ensures a mesh overlap of 5 cm caudally. The flap is raised, extending from one anterior superior iliac spine to the other, and dissected caudally up to the space of Retzius and spaces of Bogros bilaterally to expose the pubic arch and Cooper's ligaments. The technique has also been described for lumbar (L4) hernias, where the colon is mobilized along the white line of Toldt, and the extraperitoneal space is dissected up to the psoas major to identify the posterior border of the defect. The mesh is then fixed to the psoas with sutures or glue. Tacks are avoided to prevent injury to nerves. The colon may be repositioned and fixed with interrupted sutures to the mesh.[10]

Laparoscopic Intracorporeal Rectus Aponeuroplasty

Laparoscopic intracorporeal rectus aponeuroplasty (LIRA), popularized by Salvador Morales-Conde from Spain,[11] is a modification of IPOM that entails longitudinal release incisions on two sides of a medium-sized (4–10 cm) midline hernia defect. This creates two flaps, which are sutured together in the midline, achieving closure of the fascial defect without any tension, unlike in IPOM plus, which is not tension-free. Morales-Conde found lower rates of bulging and recurrence with LIRA compared to IPOM plus.[12] The use of LIRA has been extended to patients with multiple midline Swiss cheese defects, lateral hernias, and suprapubic hernias.[13,14]

■ SUBLAY REPAIRS

eTEP/eTEP-RS

The enhanced-view totally extraperitoneal (eTEP) technique was first described for inguinal hernia repair by Jorge Daes in 2012.[15] Igor Belyansky applied the eTEP approach to ventral hernia repair and reported the outcomes in a multicentric study in 2018.[16]

The patient is positioned supine with the table flexed to increase the space between the costal margins and the iliac crests. Access to one of the retrorectus spaces is gained by Hasson's technique or via optical trocar entry. The space is dissected, and then crossover to the contralateral retrorectus space is done, typically done near the falciform ligament or below the arcuate ligament. For crossover, the medial aspect of the ipsilateral PRS is incised sharply to enter the preperitoneal space in the midline; then, the medial edge of the contralateral PRS is incised. The contralateral retrorectus space is then dissected craniocaudally. The hernia sac, if possible, is mobilized and reduced into the peritoneal cavity; otherwise, it is transected, and its contents are reduced after necessary adhesiolysis.

The anterior defect is closed along with restoration of linea alba in case of a concomitant rectus diastasis. Any defect in the PRS is also closed to maintain a barrier between the mesh and the bowel. A nonabsorbable mesh of appropriate size is deployed in this space, which does not need fixation with tacks or transfascial sutures, as it is sandwiched between the anterior and PRSs **(Figs. 3A to I)**.

Thus, the eTEP repair achieves all the goals of an ideal hernia repair—large, inexpensive mesh in sublay position without painful penetrating fixation. It also offers a lot of flexibility in port positioning. However, it is technically challenging and has a steep-learning curve.

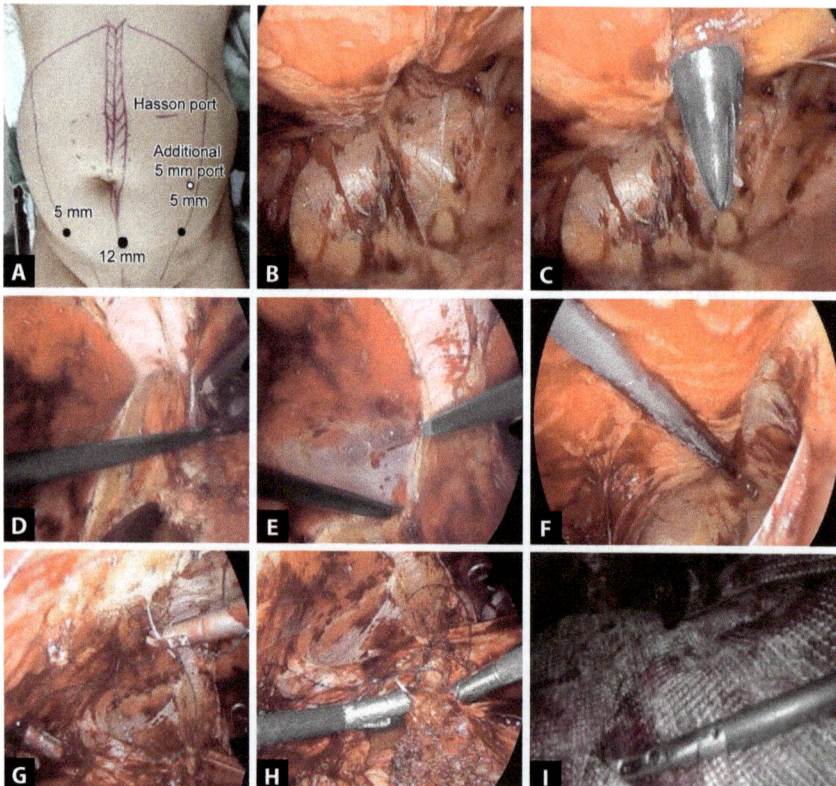

Figs. 3A to I: Enhanced-view totally extraperitoneal (eTEP) repair. (A) Port position; (B) Retrorectus telescopic dissection; (C) Suprapubic port insertion; (D) Left posterior rectus sheath (PRS) division; (E) Right PRS division; (F) Caudal extent of dissection; (G) Anterior defect closure; (H) PRS closure; (I) Mesh placement.

MILOS

MILOS (mini- and less-open sublay) surgery, first described by Wolfgang Reinpold,[17] allows the placement of a large retrorectus mesh through a small (2–6 cm = mini open, 6–12 cm = less open) incision directly over the hernia defect. After skin incision, the hernia sac is dissected out, herniotomy is done to inspect the contents, and the sac is resected. The edges of the defect are defined. Using retractors to lift the abdominal wall, dissection is done in the retrorectus plane, at least 8 cm all around the defect, using standard laparoscopic instruments and an Endotorch™. Polypropylene mesh of appropriate size is placed, usually without any fixation. The fascial defect is closed with nonabsorbable or delayed absorbable sutures. According to Reinpold, this procedure is suitable for most hernias, except for the very small (defect <2 cm) and very large ones.

EMILOS

The Endoscopic MILOS (EMILOS), described by Schwarz and Bittner,[18] is a hybrid technique, most suitable for midline hernias with significant rectus diastasis, which requires large mesh overlap to prevent recurrence. It is basically a reverse totally extraperitoneal (TEP) procedure. The initial steps are just like MILOS, dissecting out the hernia sac. The PRS of one side is incised, and the retrorectus space is developed till the symphysis pubis using a balloon. The opposite PRS is also incised, and the retrorectus space is created. The skin incision is provisionally closed, and endoscopic instruments are used to extend the retrorectus spaces cranially beyond the costal margins and xiphoid. The PRS is closed, and a large polypropylene mesh is placed. The skin is reopened, and the hernia defect is closed as in open surgery, followed by skin closure. The hybrid approach obviates the need for laparoscopic suturing of the linea alba, which is technically challenging.

TAPP

TAPP (transabdominal preperitoneal) repair for ventral hernia was described as early as 2003 by Chowbey et al.[19] In this technique, a nonabsorbable mesh is placed in the preperitoneal space, just like in TAPP repair of groin hernia. However, it is technically more challenging than the inguinal counterpart due to the variability in preperitoneal fat from person to person and at different parts of the abdominal wall. This results in frequent peritoneal tears, which need to be repaired. Ports are placed about 5 cm distant from the planned peritoneal incision, which is made by taking into account the defect location and size, with a minimum of 5 cm overlap all around. Dissection of the hernia sac is done after the peritoneal flap is created on both sides of the defect. The defect is closed with nonabsorbable or delayed absorbable sutures, followed by mesh placement and closure of the peritoneal defect.

Because of the technical difficulty, the procedure had limited acceptance since its conception. However, with rising enthusiasm in robotic surgery in the last decade, there is renewed interest in this procedure, as evident from several reports of robot-assisted TAPP (rTAPP) in recent years.[20-22] Due to the added precision offered by the robotic platform, raising the peritoneal flap is less cumbersome.

TARUP

In 2013, Schroeder et al. described a laparoscopic transabdominal approach to the retrorectus plane using lateral ports.[23] The procedure was similar to TAPP, except that the peritoneal incision was deepened to incise the PRS as well. Five years later, Muysoms et al. performed the procedure robotically and named it rTARUP (robot-assisted transabdominal retromuscular umbilical prosthetic) repair.[24] Being a pilot project, they restricted the procedure to patients having umbilical hernias smaller than 5 cm, so that a 15 cm × 15 cm mesh could be used consistently. Ports were placed on the patient's left flank. Dissection was carried out in the retrorectus space. The composite PRS–peritoneal flap largely eliminates the risk of peritoneal tears that frequently occur in TAPP.

TARM

Described by Ashwin Masurkar,[25] TARM (transabdominal retromuscular) repair is, in principle, the same as TARUP, except for the port position. Three ports are placed in triangulation at least 10 cm cranial or caudal to the center of the defect. The retromuscular space is developed by raising a PRS–peritoneum flap 8 cm beyond the defect, with meticulous dissection, preserving the neurovascular bundles at the linea semilunaris. The hernia defect is closed, followed by mesh placement and closure of the PRS–peritoneum incision. For large or multiple defects, and concomitant divarication of recti, six ports are used—three in the upper abdomen and three in the lower abdomen. Two PRS–peritoneum flaps are raised, one from above and one from below. After creation of the retromuscular space, the initial three ports in the upper abdomen are withdrawn into the retromuscular space, followed by closure of defects and the initial PRS–peritoneum incision. The procedure is completed by closing the anterior defect, mesh placement, and, finally, the second PRS–peritoneum incision (**Figs. 4A to F**).

■ SUPRAFASCIAL (ONLAY) REPAIRS
SCOLA/TESLAR/REPA

SCOLA (subcutaneous onlay laparoscopic approach), first described by Claus et al.[26] in 2018, is a laparoscopic onlay mesh repair, most suitable for patients with ventral hernias and concomitant diastasis recti, who do not want or need

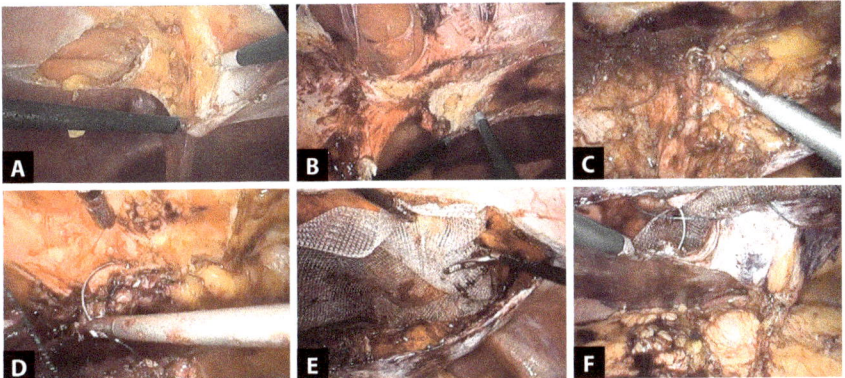

Figs. 4A to F: Transabdominal retromuscular (TARM) repair epigastric hernia. (A and B) Transabdominal retrorectus space dissection; (C) Defect closure in posterior rectus sheath (PRS); (D) Hernia defect closure anteriorly; (E) Mesh placement rectrorectus space; (F) Posterior flap closure using V-Loc.

abdominoplasty. The authors recommend SCOLA for patients with a body mass index of 22–32 kg/m². The procedure is also known by other acronyms such as TESLAR (total endoscopic-assisted linea alba reconstruction) and REPA (preaponeurotic endoscopic repair).[27]

The procedure is done with the patient supine, with hips slightly extended, and legs abducted. The surgeon stands between the legs of the patient. A 2-cm incision is made just above the pubis, and subcutaneous fat is dissected to reach the anterior rectus sheath. Dissection is done cranially and laterally to create space for insertion of a 10-mm port (camera) and two working 5-mm ports in triangulation. Carbon dioxide insufflation pressure is maintained at 8–10 mm Hg. Using a grasper and monopolar hook or scissors, the subcutaneous fat is dissected off the anterior rectus sheath and linea alba. Cranially, dissection is done up to the xiphoid process and laterally for at least 12–15 cm. The hernia defect and the diastasis are approximated using a nonabsorbable or delayed absorbable barbed suture from the xiphoid to at least 2 cm below umbilicus. Mesh is placed to cover the area from xiphoid to at least 3 cm below umbilicus and laterally at least 3 cm. A closed suction drain is placed. The procedure is technically simpler than the sublay repairs but has a high incidence of seroma (27% in the initial series).

ELAR

Like EMILOS, ELAR (endoscopic-assisted linea alba reconstruction) is a hybrid technique described by Köckerling et al., indicated in patients with umbilical or epigastric hernias with concomitant rectus diastasis.[28] The skin incision is a half-loop to the left of the umbilicus, extended 2–3 cm cranially in the midline. The hernia sac is dissected out, opened, and contents repositioned or resected. Further dissection up to the xiphoid is carried out endoscopically between the subcutaneous fat and the anterior rectus sheaths, as in SCOLA. Next, release incisions are made on the two rectus sheaths from xiphoid to just below umbilicus, 2-3 cm from their medial margin. A new linea alba is reconstructed by approximating the two medial parts with nonabsorbable sutures. This is followed by mesh placement, which is sutured to the incised margins bilaterally to replace the medial parts.

COMPONENT SEPARATION TECHNIQUES

In 1990, Ramirez first used the term "component separation" to describe a technique to reconstruct large abdominal wall defects with a functional transfer of abdominal wall components.[3] He described the anterior component separation technique. Later, "posterior component separation (PCS)" was described by Carbonell et al. in 2008 as a modification of the classical Rives-Stoppa retrorectus repair.[29] Novitsky et al. in 2012 described a modification of the PCS, which they named as "transversus abdominis release (TAR)".[30] The PCS–TAR technique, described below, has gained rapid popularity in the last decade and is frequently needed for minimally invasive repair of hernias with defects >6 cm.

Posterior Component Separation–transversus Abdominis Release

The procedure begins with dissection of the retrorectus space after medial division of the PRS (Rives-Stoppa technique). The dissection is continued up to the linea semilunaris, which is marked by large neurovascular bundles and the deep inferior epigastric vessels. For further mobilization, the posterior lamella of the internal oblique muscle is incised, and dissection is continued laterally between the internal oblique and the transversus abdominis muscles (PCS). Next, the transversus abdominis muscle is divided along its entire medial edge, allowing entry into the plane between the fascia transversalis and the transversus abdominis muscle. This plane is continuous with the retroperitoneum and can be extended further laterally up to the psoas major if needed. Inferiorly, dissection is done to develop the space of Retzius (anterior to urinary bladder) and space of Bogros laterally to expose Cooper's ligament and pubic arch. Superiorly, dissection is done up to the subxiphoid space medially and beyond the costal margins laterally **(Figs. 5A to F)**.

Posterior component separation–transversus abdominis release can be done unilaterally or bilaterally as per necessity. It can be combined with any of the sublay repairs (e.g., eTEP-TAR, EMILOS-TAR, or TARM-TAR) to achieve tension-free closure of the PRS and linea alba. The discovery of TAR has revolutionized hernia repair, as it has made possible the gold standard sublay repair in hernias with very large defects.

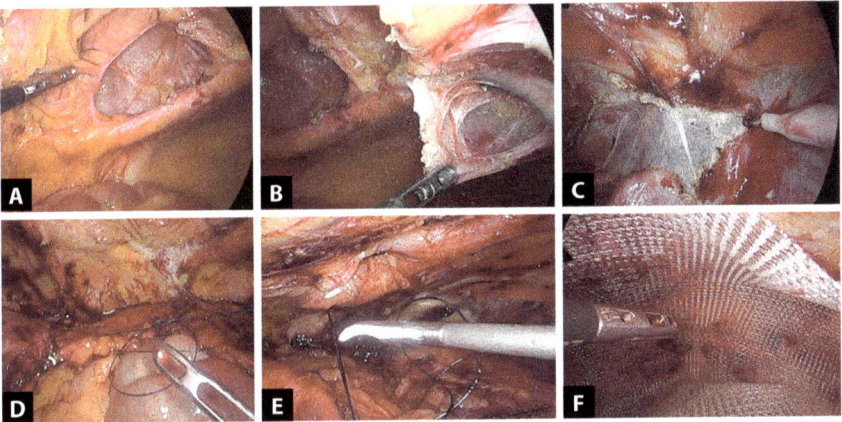

Figs. 5A to F: Transversus abdominis release (TAR). (A) Infraumbilical incisional hernia; (B) Retrorectus space creation; (C) Right TAR with cranial extension; (D) Posterior sheath closure after left-sided dissection; (E) Anterior hernial defect closure; (F) Mesh placement.

TABLE 1: Newer terminology in ventral hernia repair.

Mesh position	Acronym	Procedure name
Underlay	IPOM	Intraperitoneal onlay mesh
	IPOM plus	Intraperitoneal onlay mesh plus
	Hybrid IPOM	Hybrid intraperitoneal onlay mesh
	TAPE	Transabdominal partially extraperitoneal
	LIRA	Laparoscopic intracorporeal rectus aponeuroplasty
Sublay	eTEP-RS	Enhanced-view totally extraperitoneal—Rives-Stoppa
	MILOS	Mini- or less-open sublay
	EMILOS	Endoscopic mini- or less-open sublay
	TAPP	Transabdominal preperitoneal
	TARUP	Transabdominal retromuscular umbilical prosthetic
	TARM	Transabdominal retromuscular
	PCS–TAR	Posterior component separation—transversus abdominis release
Onlay	SCOLA/TESLAR/REPA	Subcutaneous onlay laparoscopic approach/total endoscopic-assisted linea alba reconstruction/preaponeurotic endoscopic repair
	ELAR	Endoscopic-assisted linea alba reconstruction

■ CONCLUSION

A list of newer terminology in ventral hernia repair is given in **Table 1**.

The last two decades have witnessed a multitude of innovations in hernia repair and a tremendous rise in enthusiasm for hernia surgery among general surgeons. However, most of these newer procedures come with one caveat, i.e., a steep-learning curve. A thorough knowledge of the abdominal wall anatomy and expertise in laparoscopic dissection and suturing are paramount to safe performance of these procedures. To this end, there has been a steady increase in hernia workshops and conferences in India as well as globally. Newer procedures come with newer complications, and proper training is required to both avoid and manage these complications. A rise in robot-assisted hernia repairs is also expected in the coming years, as the robotic platform has been found to be beneficial in performing these technically challenging procedures. All said and done, despite these promising innovations, IPOM/IPOM plus continues to be the most commonly performed hernia repair in most centers. Long-term follow-up studies of these procedures and improved training opportunities might, however, lead to a change in hernia practice in the future.

■ REFERENCES

1. Usher FC. Hernia repair with knitted polypropylene mesh. Surg Gynecol Obstet. 1963;117:239-40.
2. Forte A, Zullino A, Manfredelli S, Montalto G, Covotta F, Pastore P, et al. Rives technique is the gold standard for incisional hernioplasty. An institutional experience. Ann Ital Chir. 2011;82(4):313-7.
3. Ramirez OM, Ruas E, Dellon AL. "Components separation" method for closure of abdominal-wall defects: an anatomic and clinical study. Plast Reconstr Surg. 1990;86(3):519-26.
4. LeBlanc KA, Booth WV. Laparoscopic repair of incisional abdominal hernias using expanded polytetrafluoroethylene: preliminary findings. Surg Laparosc Endosc. 1993;3(1):39-41.
5. Soare AM, Cârțu D, Nechita SL, Andronic O, Șurlin V. Complications of intraperitoneal mesh techniques for incisional hernia: a systematic review. Chirurgia (Bucur). 2021;116(6 Suppl):S36-42.
6. He C, Lu J, Ong MW, Lee DJK, Tan KY, Chia CLK. Seroma prevention strategies in laparoscopic ventral hernia repair: a systematic review. Hernia J Hernias Abdom Wall Surg. 2020;24(4):717-31.
7. Bittner R, Bain K, Bansal VK, Berrevoet F, Bingener-Casey J, Chen D, et al. Update of Guidelines for laparoscopic treatment of ventral and incisional abdominal wall hernias (International Endohernia Society (IEHS))—part A. Surg Endosc. 2019;33(10):3069-139.
8. Ahonen-Siirtola M, Rautio T, Biancari F, Ohtonen P, Mäkelä J. Laparoscopic versus hybrid approach for treatment of incisional ventral hernia. Dig Surg. 2017;34(6):502-6.
9. Sharma A, Dey A, Khullar R, Soni V, Baijal M, Chowbey PK. Laparoscopic repair of suprapubic hernias: transabdominal partial extraperitoneal (TAPE) technique. Surg Endosc. 2011;25(7):2147-52.

10. Sun J, Chen X, Li J, Zhang Y, Dong F, Zheng M. Implementation of the transabdominal partial extra-peritoneal (TAPE) technique in laparoscopic lumbar hernia repair. BMC Surg. 2015;15(1):118.
11. Gómez-Menchero J, Guadalajara Jurado JF, Suárez Grau JM, Bellido Luque JA, García Moreno JL, Alarcón Del Agua I, et al. Laparoscopic intracorporeal rectus aponeuroplasty (LIRA technique): a step forward in minimally invasive abdominal wall reconstruction for ventral hernia repair (LVHR). Surg Endosc. 2018;32(8):3502-8.
12. Gómez-Menchero J, Balla A, García Moreno JL, Gila Bohorquez A, Bellido-Luque JA, Morales-Conde S. Laparoscopic intracorporeal rectus aponeuroplasty (LIRA) technique versus intraperitoneal onlay mesh (IPOM plus) for ventral hernia repair: a comparative analysis. Hernia. 2023.
13. Gómez-Valles P, Jeri-McFarlane S, Gomez-Menchero J, Morales-Conde S. Moving the concept associated to laparoscopic intracorporeal rectus aponeuroplasty (LIRA) to lateral hernia. Cir Esp. 2022;100(12):780-2.
14. Jeri-McFarlane S, Gómez-Valles P, Gomez-Menchero J, Sánchez-Ramírez M, Morales-Conde S. Expanding indication of laparoscopic intracorporeal rectus aponeuroplasty (LIRA) to suprapubic area: LIRA & TAPE. Cir Esp. 2022;100(10):641-3.
15. Daes J. The enhanced view-totally extraperitoneal technique for repair of inguinal hernia. Surg Endosc. 2012;26(4):1187-9.
16. Belyansky I, Daes J, Radu VG, Balasubramanian R, Reza Zahiri H, Weltz AS, et al. A novel approach using the enhanced-view totally extraperitoneal (eTEP) technique for laparoscopic retromuscular hernia repair. Surg Endosc. 2018;32(3):1525-32.
17. Reinpold W, Schröder M, Berger C, Nehls J, Schröder A, Hukauf M, et al. Mini- or less-open sublay operation (MILOS): a new minimally invasive technique for the extraperitoneal mesh repair of incisional hernias. Ann Surg. 2019;269(4):748-55.
18. Schwarz J, Reinpold W, Bittner R. Endoscopic mini/less open sublay technique (EMILOS): a new technique for ventral hernia repair. Langenbecks Arch Surg. 2017;402(1):173-80.
19. Chowbey PK, Sharma A, Khullar R, Soni V, Baijal M. Laparoscopic ventral hernia repair with extraperitoneal mesh: surgical technique and early results. Surg Laparosc Endosc Percutan Tech. 2003;13(2):101-5.
20. Kennedy M, Barrera K, Akcelik A, Constable Y, Smith M, Chung P, et al. Robotic TAPP ventral hernia repair: early lessons learned at an inner-city safety net hospital. JSLS. 2018;22(1):e2017.00070.
21. Cabrera ATG, Lima DL, Pereira X, Cavazzola LT, Malcher F. Robotic transabdominal preperitoneal approach (TAPP) approach for lateral incisional hernias. Arq Bras Cir Dig. 2021;34(2):e1599.
22. Kudsi OY, Gokcal F, Bou-Ayash N, Crawford AS, Chung SK, Chang K, et al. Learning curve in robotic transabdominal preperitoneal (rTAPP) ventral hernia repair: a cumulative sum (CUSUM) analysis. Hernia. 2021;(3):755-64.
23. Schroeder AD, Debus ES, Schroeder M, Reinpold WMJ. Laparoscopic transperitoneal sublay mesh repair: a new technique for the cure of ventral and incisional hernias. Surg Endosc. 2013;27(2):648-54.
24. Muysoms F, Van Cleven S, Pletinckx P, Ballecer C, Ramaswamy A. Robotic transabdominal retromuscular umbilical prosthetic hernia repair (TARUP):

observational study on the operative time during the learning curve. Hernia J Hernias Abdom Wall Surg. 2018;22(6):1101-11.
25. Masurkar AA. Laparoscopic trans-abdominal retromuscular (TARM) repair for ventral hernia: a novel, low-cost technique for sublay and posterior component separation. World J Surg. 2020;44(4):1081-5.
26. Claus CMP, Malcher F, Cavazzola LT, Furtado M, Morrell A, Azevedo M, et al. Subcutaneous onlay laparoscopic approach (SCOLA) for ventral hernia and rectus abdominis diastasis repair: technical description and initial results. Arq Bras Cir. 2018;31(4):e1399.
27. Juárez Muas DM. Preaponeurotic endoscopic repair (REPA) of diastasis recti associated or not to midline hernias. Surg Endosc. 2019;33(6):1777-82.
28. Köckerling F, Botsinis MD, Rohde C, Reinpold W. Endoscopic-assisted linea alba reconstruction plus mesh augmentation for treatment of umbilical and/or epigastric hernias and rectus abdominis diastasis—early results. Front Surg. 2016;3:27.
29. Carbonell AM, Cobb WS, Chen SM. Posterior components separation during retromuscular hernia repair. Hernia. 2008; 12(4):359-62.
30. Novitsky YW, Elliott HL, Orenstein SB, Rosen MJ. Transversus abdominis muscle release: a novel approach to posterior component separation during complex abdominal wall reconstruction. Am J Surg. 2012;204(5):709-16.

CHAPTER 7

Management of Benign Biliary Stricture

Mahesh Thombare, Magnus Jayaraj Mansard, VK Kapoor

■ INTRODUCTION

Benign biliary stricture (BBS) is caused by varied etiology, the most common being post-cholecystectomy bile duct injury (BDI) and following liver transplantation. Other causes commonly include chronic pancreatitis and inflammatory cholangiopathy **(Table 1)**.[1] Cholecystectomy is now one of the most common surgeries done in India. There are no records of the total number of cholecystectomies done in a year. Approximately 750,000 cholecystectomies are done yearly in the United States. Most of the cholecystectomies go well. About 0.4–0.6% of open and laparoscopic cholecystectomies develop the most feared complication, iatrogenic BDI.[2]

TABLE 1: Cause of benign biliary strictures.[1]

Categories	Etiologies
Iatrogenic	• Cholecystectomy (open or laparoscopic) • Liver transplantation • Partial hepatectomy • Bilioenteric anastomosis • Sphincterotomy • Transarterial chemoembolization (TACE) • Radiation therapy
Inflammatory cholangiopathy	• Acute or chronic pancreatitis of any etiology • Primary or secondary sclerosing cholangitis • Immunoglobulin G4 (IgG4)-related cholangiopathy • Eosinophilic cholangiopathy • Primary or secondary sclerosing cholangitis
Ischemia	• Hypotension • Hepatic artery thrombosis
Others	• Papillary stenosis • Mirizzi syndrome • Portal biliopathy • Parasitic infestation • Trauma

More recently, the reported incidence of major BDI is between 0.08 and 0.3%. Surgery in the right upper quadrant, such as gastric resection, hepatectomy, pancreatic resection, hepatectomy, lymphadenectomy, and other surgical procedures in proximity to the hepatoduodenal ligament, can also cause BDI.

The initial two to three times higher incidence of BDI after laparoscopic cholecystectomy was ascribed to the initial learning curve of laparoscopy. These rates have remained almost constant in the last three decades. The recent reports suggest that the incidence of postlaparoscopic cholecystectomy BDI is decreasing. Post-cholecystectomy BDI results in high morbidity, mortality, cost of treatment, and all-cause mortality in the long term. The all-cause mortality is between 7.2 and 14.5%.[3] BDI occurs when the surgeon fails to avoid the bile duct during dissection. The bile duct is also at risk for injury in any surgery in the right upper quadrant, such as hepatectomy and gastrectomy.

Factors that Result in Bile Duct Injury

Failure to identify cystic duct before clipping or dividing it is an independent risk factor for BDI. The critical view of safety (CVS) is also an important factor in the pathogenesis of BDI. The risk of injury doubles in surgery for acute cholecystitis and quadruples in severe cholecystitis due to obscure anatomy due to inflammation. Other factors include variation in biliovascular anatomy, choledocholithiasis, urgent surgery, the experience of the operating surgeon, and volume of surgery. Recent studies do not show a relation between low-volume centers and high-volume centers, and the incidence is low when the residency training involves laparoscopic techniques.

Diagnosis

Clinical Presentation

Most of the bile duct injuries (BDI) are not diagnosed intraoperatively. The majority of the undiagnosed bile duct injuries are cystic duct leaks and leaks from the duct of Luschka, which is in continuity with the common bile duct (CBD) where internal drainage with endoscopic treatment is usually successful.

True bile duct injuries, such as partial injury or transection, are diagnosed intraoperatively in 70–80% of the cases. An unexplained source of bile or bile staining during cholecystectomy, whether open or laparoscopic, should raise the suspicion of BDI, either due to complete severance or partial injury or incompletely clipped cystic duct.

When BDI is suspected, intraoperative cholangiography is useful in delineating the biliary tree anatomy and site of injury. Intraoperative cholangiography will not be able to raise suspicion in patients with complete occlusion of the extrahepatic biliary tree.

Any patient who is unwell in the postoperative period should be carefully examined, and suspicion of bile leak or bile stasis should be kept in mind and investigated. Abdominal pain, tenderness, nausea, vomiting, hiccups, fever, ileus, or bile in the drain (if placed) or in the wound will lead to the diagnosis of BDI with further investigation.

The level of suspicion should be high in a patient who is unwell in the postoperative period, with prompt specialist consultation or referral to a tertiary referral biliary center. Patients have leukocytosis, with a shift to the left. Patients with neglect may develop hypotension due to sepsis as a result of bilioma, biliary peritonitis, and cholangitis.

Investigations

Intraoperatively Strasberg A–D type injuries are identified in up to 30% of patients, while Strasberg type E injuries are detected in about 70-80% of patients. Identifying BDI, both intraoperatively and postoperatively, is a challenge to a surgeon. Intraoperatively, the surgeon should get cautioned if he/she sees more than two ducts joining the gallbladder and should refrain from clipping any structure and dividing it. Such a situation warrants cholangiography intraoperatively to identify CBD anatomy.

A continuous flow of bile from the hepatoduodenal ligament area should be considered to be coming from BDI unless proven otherwise. It is also a good idea to review the recording of the procedure and call for help and fresh input for an unbiased opinion. A CBD injury should be considered if at any time more than a single duct is ligated or divided. Hyperbilirubinemia with elevated alkaline phosphate and clinical jaundice is seen in 30-50% of patients. Jaundice also occurs due to the reabsorption of bile from the peritoneal cavity.

The most commonly available investigation is ultrasonography (US) of the abdomen, which may show extrahepatic fluid collections, dilated intrahepatic biliary radicles (IHBR)/CBD in case of distal obstructions, and free fluid in the abdomen. Concomitant use of color Doppler can identify vascular injury if any. If sonography is suspicious of BDI, or when peritonism or peritonitis, diffuse abdominal pain, and tenderness is present, a contrast-enhanced computed tomography (CT) scan should be ordered which will highlight bilioma, abscess, ascites, proximal biliary dilation, and inflammation as well as hepatic arterial perfusion and liver atrophy. As these findings are nonspecific, they should be interpreted in the clinical context. Up to 20% of patients with BDI have an injury to the right hepatic artery. The US and CT scans cannot determine the nature of the fluid collection or its source.

Confirmation of bile leak is possible with the use of magnetic resonance cholangiopancreatography (MRCP) or hepatobiliary iminodiacetic acid (HIDA) scan. HIDA scan is more sensitive and specific than MRCP, US, or CT scan in detecting the source of bile leak and fluid collections, but the exact site of the leak is not demonstrated due to poor spatial resolution. A HIDA scan can be repeated to know about the stoppage of the leak after draining the CBD.

Endoscopic retrograde cholangiopancreaticography (ERCP) is an invasive investigation that will demonstrate the anatomy of the bile duct usually below the site of the block only, but at the same time it has therapeutic potential. Drainage of a biliary tree, dilatation of the stricturing biliary tree, and placement of stents have a definitive role in the management of biliary injury. The success rate of ERCP is increased if the injury is to the extrahepatic biliary tree, 5 mm or less in diameter, and without concomitant abscess. ERCP may be wrongly interpreted as normal due to no contrast leak, despite bile in the drain, in isolated right hepatic duct or the right segmental biliary duct draining into the cystic duct. Comparing preoperative MRCP with ERCP may be able to suggest this type of injury. Fistulography done through the percutaneous catheter may be able to delineate the anatomy, especially when the tract of the catheter is formed.

Patients presenting with suspected complete block and cholangitis should undergo urgent percutaneous transhepatic cholangiography (PTC) and percutaneous transhepatic biliary drainage (PTBD). PTC is also indicated when ERCP fails. PTC is a technically challenging procedure in patients with BDI due to lack of dilation of IHBR. A combination of PTC and ERCP, known as a rendezvous technique, is also described in complex biliary injuries as a safe definitive procedure or as a bridge to surgical repair, with a success rate of 55%.

Endoscopic retrograde cholangiopancreatography and percutaneous transhepatic cholangiography are also associated with a small but definitive risk of acute pancreatitis, bleeding, perforation, and cholangitis, especially after PTC. The diagnostic abilities of ERCP and PTC are almost completely replaced by noninvasive MRCP. MRCP delineates the anatomy above and below the injury, detects vascular injury, and is thus important before treatment planning **(Figs. 1 and 2)**.

Contrast-enhanced MRCP with specific liver-excreted contrast agents detects a leak and localizes it accurately with an accuracy of 100%. Complete cholangiography is key to good surgical success; incomplete cholangiography or no cholangiography is associated with a significantly reduced success rate after repair of BDI.[4]

Investigations in Patients without Prior History of Surgery

Ultrasonography has a high sensitivity for the detection of biliary obstruction but has low accuracy in showing the extent of the obstruction.

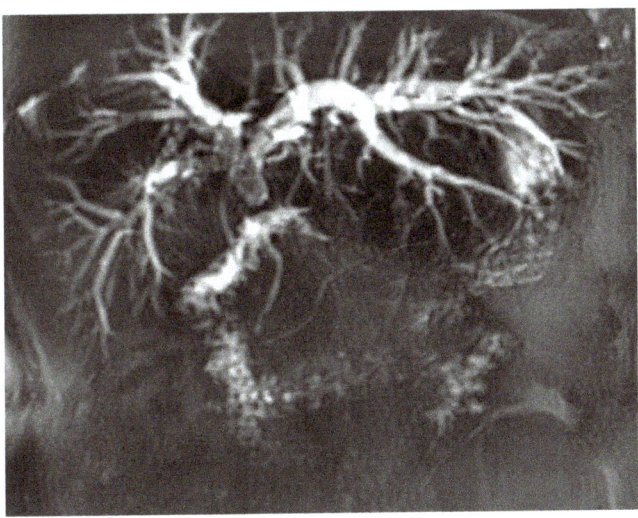

Fig. 1: MRCP showing postcholecystectomy Bismuth type 2 benign biliary stricture.

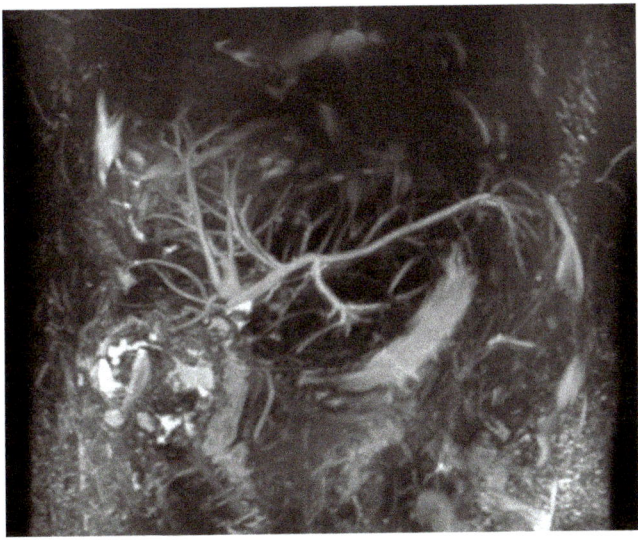

Fig. 2: MRCP representing postcholecystectomy stricture of right hepatic duct with common hepatic duct (Bismuth type-5)

Differentiation of benign strictures from malignant strictures is difficult, with a specificity of 30–70%. CT scan is the next logical investigation to detect the biliary obstruction and the extent of the biliary obstruction and differentiate between benign and malignant obstruction. MRCP is increasingly used as it is non-invasive investigation that can differentiate between benign and malignant strictures and is important to plan endoscopic therapy. Endoscopic US (EUS) provides morphology and

TABLE 2: Diagnostic tools for benign biliary strictures.[5]

Investigation	Sensitivity (%)	Specificity (%)	Positive predictive value (PPV) (%)	Negative predictive value (NPV) (%)
CT	79	79	73	84
MRCP	88	85	80.8	91
EUS-FNA	47	100	100	50

(CT: computed tomography; EUS-FNA: endoscopic ultrasound-fine-needle aspiration; MRCP: magnetic resonance cholangiopancreatography)

TABLE 3: Endoscopic retrograde cholangiopancreatography (ERCP) and cholangioscopy-directed investigations for undiagnosed benign biliary stricture.[6]

	Sensitivity (%)	Specificity	Accuracy
ERCP	88	46	52–83
IDUS	98	98	92
POCS	100	77	74–97
pCLE	94	92	93
Tissue sampling under POCS	82	100	90

(IDUS: intraductal ultrasound; pCLE: probe-based confocal laser endomicroscopy; POCS: peroral cholangioscopy)

evaluation, allows fine needle aspiration cytology (FNAC) of the stricture[5] **(Table 2)**.

Intraductal US (IDUS) and confocal laser endomicroscopy are recent additions to the armamentarium to differentiate benign strictures from malignant. It is less invasive than direct cholangioscopy and direct biopsy. IDUS is more accurate than EUS in determining the nature of the biliary stricture—89 versus 76%—and deciding the T stage and operability. Bile duct wall destruction, raised tumor, and polypoid mass size >8 mm are suggestive of malignancy.

For undiagnosed biliary strictures, per-oral cholangioscopy (POCS) can be performed along with probe-based confocal laser endomicroscopy (pCLE), and POCS-guided biopsy can visualize the stricture and characterize it.[7] Cholangioscopy-guided pCLE is better than fluoroscopy-guided pCLE **(Table 3)**. pCLE can be done either by intravenous injection of fluorescein or by drip method via catheter directly onto the bile duct mucosa.

Percutaneous transhepatic cholangioscopy (PTCS) is another investigation that is not frequently utilized by radiologists.[7] An afferent loop of the Roux-en-Y hepaticojejunostomy anchored to the anterior abdominal wall called a modified Hutson loop can be used in patients undergoing liver transplant for primary sclerosing cholangitis or those undergoing redo HJ for stricture.

Retrograde biliary interventions using percutaneous transjejunal access (PTJA) are successful in 88–95% with a low complication rate.[8] This access can be used repeatedly when required, without a need for a biliary drain. PTCS can also be done through the PTBD tract after maturation with a flexible small-diameter endoscope. The right-side approach is more frequently used than the left side approach.

Management Options

The management aims to control the sepsis and establish biliary-enteric communication with durability. It is also important to rule out vascular injury as it will affect the outcome of the biliary repair. The benefit of arterial reconstruction is still not clear.

Need for Referral and Timing of Repair

When BDI is suspected, it is in the patient's best interest not to do further dissection, place a drain in the subhepatic space, and refer the patient to a tertiary referral biliary center. If the injury is suspected in laparoscopic cholecystectomy, do not convert to open surgery just to put a drain. Management of BDI involves multiple specialties—radiologist, endoscopist, and hepatobiliary surgeon; thus, referral to a tertiary biliary center is the standard of care.

Late referral after more than 72 hours is associated with more morbidity and longer intensive care unit (ICU) stays. When the BDI is identified during the cholecystectomy, the help of a hepatobiliary surgeon should be sought and primary repair should be attempted. Previously attempted inadequate repair of intraoperatively detected BDI is a risk factor for postoperative morbidity and poor long-term outcome.

Repair of BDI done by primary nonhepatobiliary surgeons is associated with a higher incidence of stricture, reoperation, and morbidity. Stewart and Way showed that only 13% of hepaticojejunostomy done by index surgeons were successful in patients referred to tertiary biliary centers after doing hepaticojejunostomy.[9] For bile duct injuries diagnosed post-operatively, early referral should be sought to a tertiary referral biliary center. If the injury occurs in a tertiary biliary center, the help of another colleague should be sought. The repair of BDI done by the primary surgeon is associated with an 11% increase in mortality with poor long-term success rate of 17–24%. When the repair is done early (within 14 or 21 days) or late (after 14 or 21 days) by the hepatobiliary surgeon, the results are similar in terms of overall morbidity, recurrent cholangitis, stricture formation, and reoperation by a hepatobiliary surgeon.

Arterial and portal vein injury repairs are complex reconstructions and usually should be investigated by CT scan to know the extent of the injury. Usually, the right hepatic artery is the most commonly injured in up to 47% of patients with BDI.

As the majority of the blood supply to the liver comes from the portal vein, ligation of the right hepatic artery is usually well tolerated. The ischemic insult from an injury to the right hepatic artery is also influenced by the presence of biliary obstruction, hemodynamic stability, location of the injury, and comorbidities.

In combined biliary and vascular injuries, a cumulative 10% actual incidence of clinically significant liver ischemia should be anticipated. The high level of technical expertise required for attempting a repair, low rates of early diagnosis, and the favorable clinical course; immediate repair upon recognition during the index operation is not advocated, even in tertiary biliary centers.

The timing of surgery is a controversial topic. Proponents of delayed repair, typically 6 weeks after the BDI, state control of sepsis, bile leak, and reduced inflammation in the subhepatic area as factors that make repair easier than early repair. Early repair done within 6 weeks after the BDI has reported more leaks, restricture rate, and mortality in the past. Recent studies have challenged this time frame. In a retrospective study, Sahajpal et al., showed that early repair within 72 hours and late repair after 6 weeks of BDI have fewer stricture rates compared to intermediate repair done between 72 hours and <6 weeks.[10]

Classification of Biliary Stricture and Bile Duct Injury

The Bismuth classification of biliary stricture and the Strasberg classification **(Table 4)** of acute BDI are anatomically oriented, classifying patients according to the location of the injury in the biliary tree. McMahon, Bergman, Neuhaus, and Csendes classifications are other anatomically oriented classifications.

The Bismuth and Strasberg classification did not incorporate vascular injury, another important factor in the outcome of BDI and post-cholecystectomy BBS. Recent systems, such as the Stewart-Way classification, the Hannover classification, and the ATOM (anatomic, time of detection, mechanism) classification, have incorporated information regarding the possible presence of a concomitant vascular injury.[12]

Endoscopic Management

Endoscopy can be used as a temporizing procedure to control bile leak before definitive repair or as definitive management. In patients with incomplete transection with some continuity being maintained, ERCP can be used as

TABLE 4: Strasberg classification expands the Bismuth classification to include bile duct injuries of the laparoscopic era.[11]

A	Leakage from the cystic duct or minor duct in the gall bladder fossa
B	Occlusion of aberrant right hepatic duct
C	Transection of aberrant hepatic duct (without concomitant occlusion)
D	Injury to the common hepatic or CBD lateral wall without transection
E1	Transection >2 cm from the confluence of the hepatic ducts
E2	Transection <2 cm from the confluence of the hepatic ducts **(Fig. 1)**
E3	Transection involving the confluence of the hepatic ducts with continued right and left ductal communication
E4	Transection resulting in the destruction of the hepatic confluence (disruption of the confluence ceiling)
E5	Aberrant right hepatic duct stricture ± CHD stricture **(Fig. 2)**

(CBD: common bile duct; CHD: common hepatic duct)

a definitive tool. ERCP with sphincterotomy with CBD stenting is the most commonly used procedure in patients with type A Strasberg injuries.

The success rate of ERCP to control bile leak is 83%. The majority of the patients would require only a single ERCP intervention; only a minority (7.5%) required repeat ERCP and only 1.5% required surgical intervention. Some studies debate the need for stenting and reported equally good results as that of sphincterotomy with stenting. The majority of patients (82–89%) with CBD injury but without complete transection required only ERCP, sphincterotomy, and stenting.

Eighty percent of the patients with post-cholecystectomy biliary stricture can be definitively managed by ERCP, sphincterotomy with stricture dilation, and stent placement. Balloon dilatation of an anastomotic stricture after hepaticojejunostomy should be done cautiously in the early postoperative period (<30 days) to avoid anastomotic dehiscence and bile leak.

A recent study by Costamagna et al., demonstrated the long-term efficacy of multiple plastic stents (MPS) for post-cholecystectomy biliary strictures with a stricture resolution rate of 97%, a mean treatment duration of 11.8 ± 6.4 months, a mean number of 4.3 stents, and 4.2 ERCPs per patient at long-term follow-up of 11 years.[13] The success rate of MPS is better with distal strictures (≥80%) than with proximal strictures (≤25%). There is no optimal treatment identified regarding the number of stents, type of stents, and frequency of stent exchanges.

For uncomplicated bile duct injuries with leaks from the cystic duct and duct of Luschka, follow-up ERCP may not be required and the stent may be removed by standard gastroscopy. The use of rendezvous techniques in patients with complete CBD transections without tissue loss who are at high risk for surgery is reported. Such techniques use a percutaneous transhepatic approach along with the endoscopic approach to open the obstructing clips and stent the CBD. In a series of 47 patients, Schreuder et al., reported a long-term success rate of 55% for the rendezvous technique, while for another 30% of patients, it provided a bridge to definitive treatment by providing internal biliary drainage. A recent series of 60 consecutive patients with main bile duct transections, with a mean tissue length loss of 17 mm, reported a long-term success rate of 67% with a combined endoscopic and radiologic approach (CERA) and restricture rate of 8.3% at 41 months follow-up.[14] The mean duration of treatment was 526 [standard deviation (SD) ± 415] days, with a median number of eight endoscopies (range 1–33).

A minority of biliary leaks do not respond to either sphincterotomy or plastic stent placement and need either placement of MPS or fully covered self-expanding metal stents (FCSEMS). Due to the large diameter of the stent and its covered nature, FCSEMS diverts bile from the site of the leak more efficiently. In uncontrolled case series, the success rate of FCSEMS is ranging from 90 to 100%.[15] FCSEMS are not usually used for refractory leaks from the common hepatic duct near confluence. Stent migration, blockage, and stricture formation at proximal and distal ends due to the use of oversized stents are complications of FCSEMS. Short duration of stent use might decrease complications. FCSEMS is superior to MPS in the management of refractory bile leak. Single-operator cholangioscopy is used to place guidewire placement in complex strictures that are difficult to intubate by conventional ERCP.

Use of a biodegradable biliary stent made of polyglactic acid and polydioxanone had a satisfactory result in 83% in 21 months' follow-up. In a meta-analysis of covered self-expanding metal stents versus MPS for BBS by Giri et al., the covered self-expanding metal stents (SEMS) were comparable to MPS for stricture resolution, recurrence rate, and complications.[16] Use of modified FCSEMS, in the form of either antimigration waist or conical shape, is better than conventional FCSEMS or MPS in BBS secondary to surgical injuries or anastomoses, with lower stricture recurrence rate of 7% and migration rate of 3% versus 19% and 25% for conventional FCSEMS and 19% and 4% for MPS.

Magnetic compression anastomosis (MCA) can be used in patients with bile duct stricture that does not allow guidewire cannulation.[17] The magnets are kept on both sides of obstruction, delivered via PTC proximally and by ERCP distally. Gradual ischemia and establishment of fistula between biliobiliary and bilioenteric strictures lend themselves to further endotherapy. The success rate of MCA is 87%, with a restructure rate of 7.1%. Use of thermal energy in the form of bipolar radiofrequency ablation (RFA) in various etiologies of BBS has been reported in a small prospective study of nine patients. It could prove to be important adjuvant treatment in patients with refractory strictures.

Use of holmium laser has been reported for patients with hepatolithiasis with intrahepatic stricture, with a recurrence-free rate of 67% at 5 years in a small series of 15 patients. Similarly, in a study of 12 patients with intrahepatic strictures, thulium laser vaporization has reported 100% technical success rate.[18]

Surgical Management

Surgical treatment of BDI is a gold standard treatment for repair and is usually required when ERCP is not therapeutic. Complete transection of the CBD almost always requires operative repair, with occasional use of rendezvous techniques. The operative techniques depend on the injury pattern.

Ligation or Clipping of Cystic Duct

Ligation or clipping of the cystic duct is usually not required due to the effective use of ERCP and sphincterotomy, with or without CBD stenting. When endoscopic support is not available, ligation or clipping of the cystic duct is an effective treatment to stop leaks in Strasberg type A injuries. Transection of small ducts <3 mm in diameter draining a single segment of the liver (Strasberg type C) can also be safely ligated.

Surgery—Simple Repair

Strasberg type D injuries, which are typically lateral injuries to the common hepatic duct or CBD without transection, are repaired with T-tube drainage of CBD. The T-tube can be placed either transcystically or through the choledochotomy. When expertise is available, the injury can be repaired and a T-tube can be inserted laparoscopically.

Timing (Early vs. Delayed) of Repair

A meta-analysis and systemic review by Wang et al., showed that early repair is associated with a higher failure rate compared with delayed repair, and early referral has a better repair rate than delayed referral. Delayed referral is associated with a higher incidence of complications, the requirement for more invasive procedures, and a prolonged period of recovery.[19]

Immediate repair by nonexpert surgeons is associated with poor outcomes. When a hepatobiliary expert is available, the optimal timing of repair is controversial. A recent multicenter, multiarm, parallel-group, randomized controlled trial (RCT) from 10 centers in Egypt reported that avoiding conversion to open surgery, avoiding prereferral repair attempts, controlling abdominal sepsis, repairing by a hepatopancreatobiliary (HBP) surgeon with a wide stoma and transanastomotic stents are associated with successful reconstruction with Roux-En-Y hepaticojejunostomy.[20] When all these variables are reached, the timing of repair does not affect the success. Early reconstruction after abdominal sepsis control can be done at any time with comparable results to those of delayed repair.

The European-African Hepato-Pancreato-Biliary Association (E-AHPBA) Research Collaborative Study management group reported a total of 913 patients by its members over a period of 16 years and found that the timing of hepaticojejunostomy, either early (<7 days), intermediate (1-6 weeks), or late (6 weeks–6 months), did not have any impact on severe postoperative complications, need for reintervention, or liver-related mortality.[21]

Whenever septic complications due to bile leak need to be addressed first, late repair gives the optimum results. Late repair also allows the level of stricture to stabilize by allowing ischemia to reach its final level and to do anastomosis at an adequately safe level. An experienced hepatobiliary team, complete cholangiogram, no sepsis or severe biliary peritonitis, no significant comorbidities, and no vascular injury are the requirements of immediate or early reconstruction with hepaticojejunostomy.

End-to-end Bile Duct Anastomosis

Sharp transection of the bile duct without much tissue loss, no involvement of hilar confluence, and those without vascular injury can be repaired by end-to-end anastomosis. Its advantage is that the bile flow is restored physiologically than bilioenteric anastomosis. There is a larger experience with this technique due to its widespread use in liver transplantation.

The repair is technically demanding due to the bile duct's small diameter. There is a trend toward a higher stricture rate but fewer postoperative complications. The use of T-tube in such anastomosis is controversial.

If the patient develops bile duct stricture, it is still amenable for endoscopic management as well as surgery in about two-thirds of patients, with good results in 80% of patients. In Bismuth type II stricture or Strasberg type E2 injury, Kohneh Shahri et al., achieved better results with end-to-end ductal anastomosis (100%) than with hepaticojejunostomy (71%) during early repair procedures (<30 days after the initial trauma). The recurrent stricture rate of 9.6% was observed for end-to-end repair and 5.3% for hepaticojejunostomy.[22]

Hepaticojejunostomy

Hepaticojejunostomy is the universal gold standard for surgery required for BDI Strasberg type B and sometimes in type D and BBS E1–E5, where there is tissue loss. The anastomosis should be done in an area of the bile duct that is well vascularized and not fibrosed. The anastomosis (stoma) should be made as large as possible; this can be achieved by placing the hepaticotomy (ductotomy) at the biliary ductal confluence (hilum), called hilojejunostomy,[23] and extending it on the extrahepatic portion of the left hepatic duct, called the Hepp–Couinaud technique. Priorly placed PTC stents or new stents can be used in view to prevent anastomotic stricture.

The anastomotic stricture rate of hepaticojejunostomy is in the range of 4–69%. Due to altered anatomy, strictures after hepaticojejunostomy are managed by percutaneous transhepatic balloon stricture dilatation (PTBSD). The overall success rate of PTBD is 66–76% with a morbidity of 11–13%, or by ERCP by long route. Up to 20–25% of patients with hepaticojejunostomy need revision of the anastomosis[24] with a long-term success rate of approximately 90% with a slightly higher morbidity.

Laparoscopic repair of BDI is sparse due to fear of encountering adhesions in the subhepatic area from previous surgery, bile leak, or prior repair, lack of tactile perception, experience, and long-term follow-up. The laparoscopic repair has its predicted advantages of reduced operative time, morbidity, and early discharge. The majority of studies of laparoscopic or robotic biliary-enteric reconstruction are of early repair within 7–11 days, except a study from India, which favored delayed laparoscopic repair after a period of 6 weeks.[25]

Hepaticoduodenostomy is another, less commonly used alternative. Its theoretical advantages, as compared to hepaticojejunostomy, are shorter operative time, decreased bleeding, and a lower incidence of adhesive intestinal obstruction. However, technical parameters limit the feasibility of hepaticoduodenostomy.[26] In type E1–E3 strictures, it is possible to do hepaticoduodenostomy with or without duodenal mobilization. For higher strictures, hepaticojejunostomy is preferred for tension-free repair. The added advantage of HD is its accessibility to endoscopy for any future interventions.

Hepatectomy

A small percentage of patients, up to 1.4%, with BDI require liver resection. Patients in whom several treatment options have failed and resulted in nonfunctional liver segment or lobe with high biliovascular injury resulting in liver atrophy, abscess, recurrent cholangitis, and sepsis, which is refractory to management, are an indication for partial hepatectomy. Patients with Strasberg type B BDI may develop segmental cholestasis of a part of the right lobe of the liver, which may lead to atrophy over a long period of time and need segmental hepatic resection. The BDI proximal to the hepatic confluence, with associated right hepatic artery injuries, is at more risk for hepatectomy.

In the acute setting, hepatectomy cannot be avoided in patients with peritonitis and sepsis in patients with liver necrosis, bile duct necrosis, liver abscess, or persistent segmental bile duct leaks that are not amenable to reconstruction.

A recent review by Furtado et al., identified 8 articles with 2,110 patient cohorts, with 84 patients requiring hepatectomy.[27] Complex vasculobiliary injury was the most common reason. The mean time of the hepatectomy was between 26 and 224 months after the BDI, 67–89% of patients underwent right hepatectomy with variable postoperative morbidity and mortality of 4.7%. Recurrent symptoms were seen in 19% of patients.

Liver Transplantation

Patients with BBS after multiple failed treatment options, BDI with vascular injury, and delayed diagnosis of a BDI leading to permanent impairment of liver function are candidates for liver transplantation. Secondary biliary cirrhosis (SBC) with liver failure is one of the indications for liver transplantation. Rarely, patients may present with acute liver failure requiring urgent transplantation.

A recent retrospective study found 12 patients over 12 years who underwent liver transplants for SBC due to BDI. The time to SBC from injury was 2.4–14 years. Postoperative complications, largely infective (75%) and renal (33%), were observed in 92% of patients. The 5-year survival was 83%.[28]

BENIGN BILIARY STRICTURE DUE TO STRICTURED BILIARY ENTERIC ANASTOMOSIS

Endoscopic management of strictured hepaticojejunostomy **(Fig. 3)** is a technically demanding procedure due to altered anatomy. Balloon enteroscopy-guided ERC is now being commonly reported. In a meta-analysis

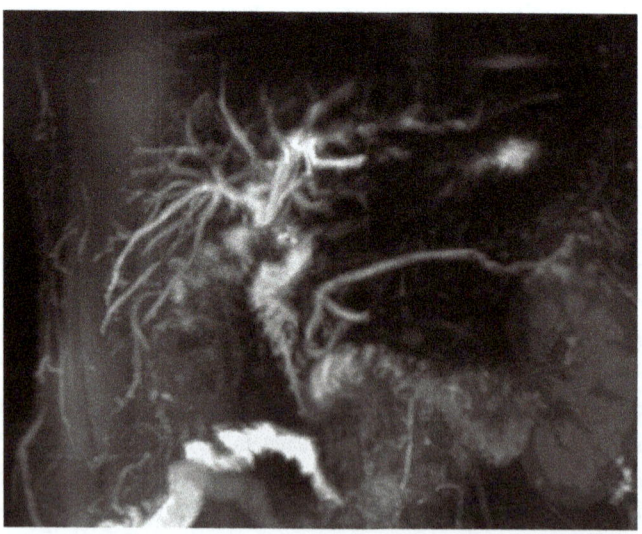

Fig. 3: MRCP showing strictured hepaticojejunostomy done for prior benign biliary stricture.

of 15 studies, Inamdar S et al., showed an 81% success rate for single balloon enteroscopy to reach the papilla, 69% for cholangiogram, and 62% for successful intervention.[29] The use of biodegradable stents in patients with surgically altered anatomy placed by enteroscopy obviates the need for a second procedure to remove the stents.[30]

For most patients with surgically altered anatomy, the other convenient option is EUS-guided hepatico-gastrostomy. The right system is approached either through the hepaticogastrostomy or EUS-guided hepatico-jejunostomy if choledochoduodenostomy is present.

Endoscopic treatment is not always technically successful. Such patients have the option of PTBSD or surgical revision. Patients who have PTBSD followed by long-term internal-external biliary catheter placement, can have stent removal after judging the biliary pressure, typically less than 15 mm Hg.[31]

POST-LIVER TRANSPLANTATION BENIGN BILIARY STRICTURE

Up to 10-15% of patients with liver transplantation will develop biliary stricture, usually within a year after the surgery, and it is the second most common cause of BBS. Biliary strictures after transplantation are both anastomotic and nonanastomotic in nature. Anastomotic stricture is at the anastomotic site and is usually short. Anastomotic and non-anastomotic biliary stricture (NABS) are usually multifactorial such as biliary anomalies, bile leaks, long warm or cold ischemia time, elderly donors, prolonged operative time, size mismatch, anastomotic tension, hepatic artery thrombosis or stenosis, significant reperfusion injury, chronic rejection, immunologically induced injuries such a transplant done for primary sclerosing cholangitis and autoimmune hepatitis. Up to 10-15% of patients will develop biliary stricture after deceased donor liver transplantation and up to 40% in living donor liver transplant. Anastomotic strictures are more common in living donor transplants than in deceased donor transplants and are called Achilles heel of liver transplant. The majority of the patients are asymptomatic and have only graft dysfunction.

Endoscopic management is the most favored treatment modality. Endoscopic treatment consists of ERCP, sphincterotomy, and balloon dilation with stent placement, either plastic or metal stents. Strictures presenting after 6 months are more resistant to endoscopic treatment than those presenting earlier.

Stents are used in three ways: Single plastic stent with periodic exchange every 3 months, MPS usually sequential stent addition, or use of FCSEMS. The technical success reported is 95-100% with a stricture resolution rate of 80-95% with a recurrence rate of 3-37%.[32]

Fully covered self-expanding metal stents are largely used as a secondary intervention with a good stricture resolution rate. Recently, their use as the primary modality of treatment has shown that they can reduce the treatment cost by reducing the number of ERCPs required for stricture resolution. The rate of stent migration, both proximally and distally, is higher with FCSEMs. The use of metal stents with an antimigration design has reduced the rate of migration. In a study by Sung et al., the success rate, recurrence rate, and safety were comparable in patients with FCSEMS, plastic stent, and PTBD, but FCSEMS were associated with shorter resolution time and a smaller number of ERC procedures.[33] The use of MCA was successful in 89% of patients in a study of 75% of post-liver transplant BBS.[34]

Surgical and percutaneous treatments are reserved for patients who have prior hepaticojejunostomy and refractory strictures not responding to endoscopic or percutaneous treatment. Surgery involves either repair or conversion to bilioenteric anastomosis or retransplantation. Early surgery is reserved for only patients with an uncontrolled leak and evidence of biliary peritonitis. Living donor liver transplantation and ex situ liver transplantation biliary strictures have lower success rates (58–76% vs. 80–93%) due to smaller duct size and the need for complex anastomoses. With combined procedures with interventional radiology or implementation of enteroscopy-assisted ERCP and EUS-guided approaches, very few patients ultimately require surgical revision.

Endoscopic management of NABS is more demanding as it involves hilum as well as intrahepatic ducts. NABS, presenting after a year, are more resistant to responding to endoscopic treatment, with a higher number of stricture dilatations, longer duration of stenting, and higher recurrence rate. About 40–82% of patients with NABS will respond to endoscopic therapy.[35]

BENIGN BILIARY STRICTURE DUE TO CHRONIC PANCREATITIS

The most common cause of nonsurgical biliary stricture is chronic pancreatitis (CP) **(Fig. 4)**. They occur in about 13–21% of chronic pancreatitis patients. These strictures typically involve lower CBD and are difficult to treat endoscopically due to pancreatic fibrosis, pancreatic calcifications, CBD wall calcification, and scarring. Occasionally, the CBD obstruction is caused by pancreatic stones in the ampulla rather than stricture. Cross-sectional imaging, such as CT or MRI is necessary to rule out malignancy in the head of the pancreas. The presence of pancreatic head calcifications increases the risk of endoscopic treatment failure by 17-fold. Symptomatic patients, those with raised alkaline phosphatase and/or bilirubin for >6 weeks, should be treated.

Siiki et al., in a review of 25 studies, showed the success rate of covered SEMS to be 77% compared to 33% with plastic stents at 1-year follow-up.[36]

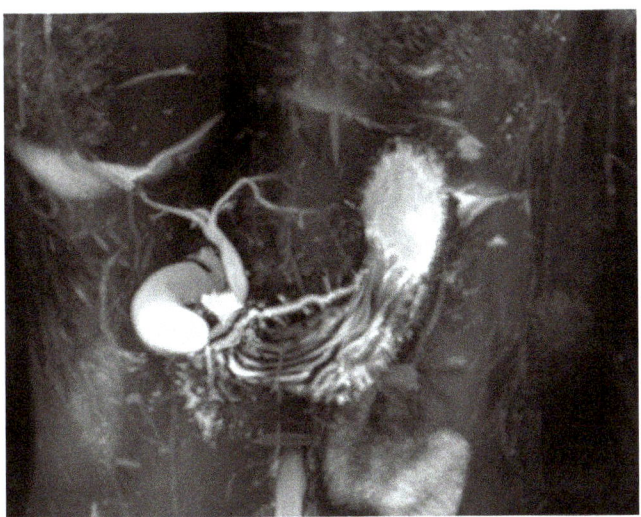

Fig. 4: MRCP in chronic pancreatitis with lower CBD stricture and dilated main PD with side branches.

The median number of ERCP procedures required was 3.9 for plastic stents versus 1.5 for SEMS in chronic pancreatitis. Uncovered SEMS are strongly discouraged due to difficulty in stent removal due to tissue ingrowth. An RCT by Ramchandani et al., used MPS and covered SEMS for a period of 12 months and showed a similar stricture resolution rate of 77.1 versus 75.8% for both procedures at 24 months with a stent migration rate of 20%.[37] A small percentage of patients would not respond to endoscopic treatment and will require surgical treatment. Also, patients who have associated intractable pain or other complications requiring surgical treatment are best served by Frey's procedure with biliojejunal anastomosis. Regimbeau et al., reported 52% incomplete stricture resolution in the endoscopic treatment group of 33 patients (extractible metallic stents in 35% and MPS in 65%) who required secondary surgical treatment.[38] Choledochojejunostomy is better than reinsertion of CBD in the resection cavity which is associated with high stricture recurrence.

BENIGN BILIARY STRICTURE DUE TO PRIMARY SCLEROSING CHOLANGITIS

During the disease course, 50% of the patients with PSC develop dominant biliary stricture. The biliary stricture in PSC can be benign or malignant (10–15%). It can also be multifocal and both intrahepatic and extrahepatic **(Fig. 5)**. Differentiating the nature of the stricture, whether benign or malignant, is an important but difficult task. Fluctuating cholestasis on LFTs and jaundice, irrespective of dominant stricture or endoscopic treatment,

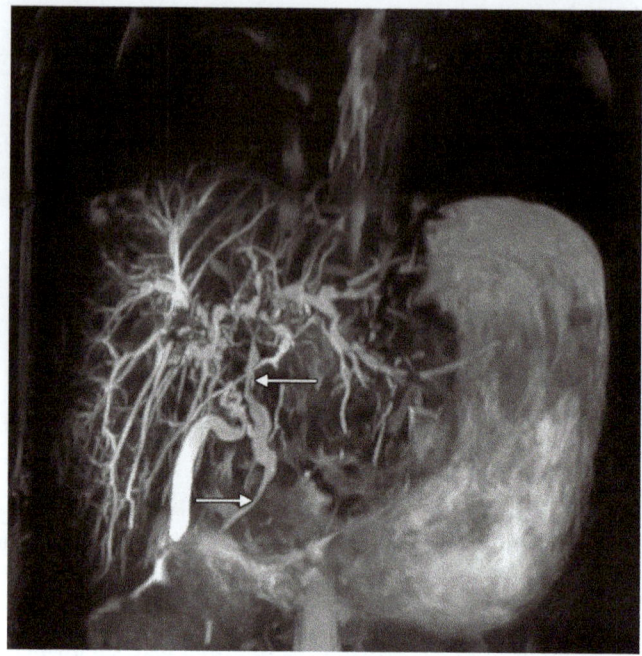

Fig. 5: MRCP—a case of sclerosing cholangitis with multiple extrahepatic and intrahepatic strictures.

is a feature of PSC, and a multidisciplinary team should be involved in the decision-making of PSC treatment.

It is indicated to do MRCP first to locate the dominant stricture prior to ERCP. Extrahepatic bile duct severe stricture with proximal dilatation is more likely to respond to endoscopic treatment than those with multiple intrahepatic strictures without dilatation. Brush cytology obtained during ERCP has a sensitivity of 43% but has a high specificity of 97% for cholangiocarcinoma. In a meta-analysis by Navaneethan et al., fluorescent in situ hybridization (FISH) in PSC had a sensitivity of 68% and specificity of 70% for diagnosing cholangiocarcinoma.[39] The endoscopic therapy for BBS in PSC is a balloon or bougie dilatation with or without stent placement of dominant biliary stricture. The complications, such as cholangitis and pancreatitis, were significantly less with balloon dilatation than with stenting. Balloon dilatation is repeated at intervals of 1–4 weeks till technical success is obtained, and on average, it requires 2–3 sessions to achieve this. Stent placement, compared to balloon dilatation, has more complication rate without significant differences. If balloon dilatation fails, another option is to place a plastic stent for a short duration of 1–2 weeks to avoid the risk of stent occlusion.

For dominant stricture below the hilar confluence, FCSEMS are used. In PSC, endoscopic resolution of strictures is rare, and repeated treatments are required due to the relapse or the development of new strictures.[40] Liver transplantation is the only proven treatment that modifies the natural history of PSC. Surveillance for ulcerative colitis and colorectal cancer, cholangiocarcinoma, and gall bladder cancer should be provided lifelong.

■ IMMUNOGLOBULIN G4 SCLEROSING CHOLANGITIS

Immunoglobulin G4 (IgG4) cholangiopathy is an autoimmune inflammatory disease associated with other autoimmune disorders, such as autoimmune pancreatitis. The patients can have extra or intrahepatic bile duct stricture. BBS can involve any part of the biliary tree and is associated with inflammation of the biliary wall or external compression from inflammatory or malignant mass in the head of the pancreas. The first-line treatment is usually corticosteroids with a high rate of resolution. Prednisone is used in a dose of 20–40 mg/day, tapered by 2–10 mg every 1–4 weeks.

Rituximab is used either at onset for patients with glucocorticoid intolerance or those with disease flare on glucocorticoids. It is associated with a high remission rate but high relapse rate if there is involvement of multiple organs with limited adverse events.[41] Biliary stenting is required if the patient has cholangitis or significant biliary obstruction, in those for whom steroids are contraindicated, or when the diagnosis is not confirmed and requires biliary brush cytology or biopsy. If the stent is placed before starting corticosteroids, the stent needs to be removed within 2 weeks of improvement after starting corticosteroids to prevent stent dislodgment.[42] Obstructive jaundice patients with IgG4 cholangiopathy can be treated with corticosteroids alone without biliary tract infection. In Japan, patients with IgG4 sclerosing cholangitis receive long-term low-dose (5 mg/day) prednisone to prevent relapse.[43]

■ CONCLUSION

The gold standard for the management of post cholecystectomy BBS is a Roux-en-Y hepaticojejunostomy. Surgery is a one-time treatment in the majority of patients with good long-term patency. It is preferred in patients with high strictures, those with complete transection of the bile duct, i.e., no biliary ductal continuity, or segmental loss of the bile duct, or after failed endoscopic treatment. Surgery is also a one-time treatment for patients with chronic pancreatitis with biliary stricture who require concomitant pancreatic surgery. For strictures that are low, short segment, and incomplete, i.e., with biliary ductal continuity, as seen in some patients of post-cholecystectomy BBS, dominant stricture in PSC, biliary stricture in chronic pancreatitis, and anastomotic stricture after liver transplant, endoscopic management is also an effective treatment with results equal to that of surgery. Advances in therapeutic endoscopy, such as the use of MPS and FCSEMS, have improved the results of endoscopy. The drawback of endoscopic treatment is the need for prolonged treatment, repeated intervention, repeated hospitalizations, and higher costs.

REFERENCES

1. Ma MX, Jayasekeran V, Chong AK. Benign biliary strictures: prevalence, impact, and management strategies. Clin Exp Gastroenterol. 2019;12:83-92.
2. Halbert C, Pagkratis S, Yang J, Meng Z, Altieri MS, Parikh P, et al. Beyond the learning curve: incidence of bile duct injuries following laparoscopic cholecystectomy normalize to open in the modern era. Surg Endosc. 2016;30(6):2239-43.
3. Fong ZV, Pitt HA, Strasberg SM, Loehrer AP, Sicklick JK, Talamini MA, et al. Diminished survival in patients with bile leak and ductal injury: management strategy and outcomes. J Am Coll Surg. 2018;226(4):568-76.e1.
4. Stewart L, Way LW. Bile duct injuries during laparoscopic cholecystectomy. Factors that influence the results of treatment. Arch Surg. 1995;130(10):1123-8; discussion 1129.
5. Schepis T, Boškoski I, Tringali A, Costamagna G. Role of ERCP in benign biliary strictures. Gastrointest Endosc Clin N Am. 2022;32(3):455-75.
6. Tanisaka Y, Ryozawa S, Nonaka K, Yasuda M, Fujita A, Ogawa T, et al. Diagnosis of biliary strictures using probe-based confocal laser endomicroscopy under the direct view of peroral cholangioscopy: results of a prospective study (with video). Gastroenterol Res Pract. 2020;2020:6342439.
7. Riaz A, Entezari P, Ganger D, Gabr A, Thornburg B, Russell E, et al. Percutaneous access of the modified Hutson loop for retrograde cholangiography, endoscopy, and biliary interventions. J Vasc Interv Radiol. 2020;31(12):2113-20.e1.
8. Sj M, Rn G, Na C, Tg S, Nd S. Percutaneous transjejunal biliary intervention: 10-year experience with access via Roux-en-Y loops. Radiology. 1998;206(3):665-72.
9. Stewart L, Way LW. Laparoscopic bile duct injuries: timing of surgical repair does not influence success rate. A multivariate analysis of factors influencing surgical outcomes. HPB. 2009;11(6):516-22.
10. Sahajpal AK, Chow SC, Dixon E, Greig PD, Gallinger S, Wei AC. Bile duct injuries associated with laparoscopic cholecystectomy: timing of repair and long-term outcomes. Arch Surg Chic. 2010;145(8):757-63.
11. Strasberg SM, Hertl M, Soper NJ. An analysis of the problem of biliary injury during laparoscopic cholecystectomy. J Am Coll Surg. 1995;180(1):101-25.
12. Chun K. Recent classifications of the common bile duct injury. Korean J Hepatobiliary Pancreat Surg. 2014;18(3):69-72.
13. Costamagna G, Tringali A, Perri V, Familiari P, Boškoski I, Barbaro F, et al. Endotherapy of postcholecystectomy biliary strictures with multiple plastic stents: long-term results in a large cohort of patients. Gastrointest Endosc. 2020;91(1):81-9.
14. Schreuder AM, Booij KAC, de Reuver PR, van Delden OM, van Lienden KP, Besselink MG, et al. Percutaneous-endoscopic rendezvous procedure for the management of bile duct injuries after cholecystectomy: short- and long-term outcomes. Endoscopy. 2018;50(6):577-87.

15. Wang AY, Ellen K, Berg CL, Schmitt TM, Kahaleh M. Fully covered self-expandable metallic stents in the management of complex biliary leaks: preliminary data: a case series. Endoscopy. 2009;41(9):781-6.
16. Giri S, Jearth V, Sundaram S. Covered self-expanding metal stents versus multiple plastic stents for benign biliary strictures: an updated meta-analysis of randomized controlled trials. Cureus. 2022;14(4):e24588.
17. Jang SI, Cho JH, Lee DK. Magnetic compression anastomosis for the treatment of post-transplant biliary stricture. Clin Endosc. 2020;53(3):266-75.
18. Thai Binh N, Tra My TT, Lan Oanh DT, Minh Duc N. Percutaneous transhepatic endoscopic thulium laser vaporesection for management of severe and focal benign biliary strictures. Clin Ter. 2023;174(4):360-4.
19. Wang X, Yu WL, Fu XH, Zhu B, Zhao T, Zhang YJ. Early versus delayed surgical repair and referral for patients with bile duct injury: a systematic review and meta-analysis. Ann Surg. 2020;271(3):449-59.
20. Omar MA, Kamal A, Redwan AA, Alansary MN, Ahmed EA. Post-cholecystectomy major bile duct injury: ideal time to repair based on a multicentre randomized controlled trial with promising results. Int J Surg Lond Engl. 2023;109(5):1208-21.
21. A European-African HepatoPancreatoBiliary Association (E-AHPBA) Research Collaborative Study Management Group, Other members of the European-African HepatoPancreatoBiliary Association Research Collaborative. Post cholecystectomy bile duct injury: early, intermediate or late repair with hepaticojejunostomy—an E-AHPBA multi-center study. HPB. 2019;21(12):1641-7.
22. Kohneh Shahri N, Lasnier C, Paineau J. Bile duct injuries at laparoscopic cholecystectomy: early repair results. Ann Chir. 2005;130(4):218-23.
23. Kapoor VK. What's in a name? Hilo-jejunostomy, not hepaticojejunostomy, for post cholecystectomy iatrogenic benign biliary stricture. SOJ Surg. 2016;3:1-3.
24. Booij KAC, Coelen RJ, de Reuver PR, Besselink MG, van Delden OM, Rauws EA, et al. Long-term follow-up and risk factors for strictures after hepaticojejunostomy for bile duct injury: an analysis of surgical and percutaneous treatment in a tertiary center. Surgery. 2018;163(5):1121-7.
25. Cuendis-Velázquez A, Trejo-Ávila M, Bada-Yllán O, Cárdenas-Lailson E, Morales-Chávez C, Fernández-Álvarez L, et al. A new era of bile duct repair: robotic-assisted versus laparoscopic hepaticojejunostomy. J Gastrointest Surg. 2019;23(3):451-9.
26. Ai C, Wu Y, Xie X, Wang Q, Xiang B. Roux-en-Y hepaticojejunostomy or hepaticoduodenostomy for biliary reconstruction after resection of congenital biliary dilatation: a systematic review and meta-analysis. Surg Today. 2023;53(1):1-11.
27. Furtado R, Yoshino O, Muralidharan V, Perini MV, Wigmore SJ. Hepatectomy after bile duct injury: a systematic review. HPB. 2022;24(2):161-8.
28. Vilatobá M, Chávez-Villa M, Figueroa-Méndez R, Domínguez-Rosado I, Cruz-Martínez R, Leal-Villalpando RP, et al. Liver transplantation as definitive treatment of post-cholecystectomy bile duct injury: experience in a high-volume repair center. Ann Surg. 2022;275(5):e729-32.
29. Inamdar S, Slattery E, Sejpal DV, Miller LS, Pleskow DK, Berzin TM, et al. Systematic review and meta-analysis of single-balloon enteroscopy-assisted ERCP in patients with surgically altered GI anatomy. Gastrointest Endosc. 2015;82(1):9-19.

30. Lindström O, Udd M, Rainio M, Nuutinen H, Jokelainen K, Kylänpää L. Benign biliary strictures treated with biodegradable stents in patients with surgically altered anatomy using double balloon enteroscopy. Scand J Gastroenterol. 2020;55(10):1225-33.
31. Kumar S, Vignesh S, Boruah DK, Gupta A, Yadav RR, Kapoor VK, et al. The utility of biliary manometry in assessing early catheter removal after percutaneous balloon dilatation of hepaticojejunostomy strictures. Cureus. 2022;14(3):e22761.
32. Pasha SF, Harrison ME, Das A, Nguyen CC, Vargas HE, Balan V, et al. Endoscopic treatment of anastomotic biliary strictures after deceased donor liver transplantation: outcomes after maximal stent therapy. Gastrointest Endosc. 2007;66(1):44-51.
33. Sung MJ, Jo JH, Lee HS, Park JY, Bang S, Park SW, et al. Optimal drainage of anastomosis stricture after living donor liver transplantation. Surg Endosc. 2021;35(11):6307-17.
34. Jang SI, Lee KH, Yoon HJ, Lee DK. Treatment of completely obstructed benign biliary strictures with magnetic compression anastomosis: follow-up results after recanalization. Gastrointest Endosc. 2017;85(5):1057-66.
35. Barbaro F, Tringali A, Larghi A, Baldan A, Onder G, Familiari P, et al. Endoscopic management of non-anastomotic biliary strictures following liver transplantation: long-term results from a single-center experience. Dig Endosc. 2021;33(5):849-57.
36. Siiki A, Helminen M, Sand J, Laukkarinen J. Covered self-expanding metal stents may be preferable to plastic stents in the treatment of chronic pancreatitis-related biliary strictures: a systematic review comparing 2 methods of stent therapy in benign biliary strictures. J Clin Gastroenterol. 2014;48(7):635-43.
37. Ramchandani M, Lakhtakia S, Costamagna G, Tringali A, Püspöek A, Tribl B, et al. Fully covered self-expanding metal stent vs multiple plastic stents to treat benign biliary strictures secondary to chronic pancreatitis: a multicenter randomized trial. Gastroenterology. 2021;161(1):185-95.
38. Regimbeau JM, Fuks D, Bartoli E, Fumery M, Hanes A, Yzet T, et al. A comparative study of surgery and endoscopy for the treatment of bile duct stricture in patients with chronic pancreatitis. Surg Endosc. 2012;26(10):2902-8.
39. European Society of Gastrointestinal Endoscopy, European Association for the Study of the Liver, European Association for the Study of the Liver. Role of endoscopy in primary sclerosing cholangitis: European Society of Gastrointestinal Endoscopy (ESGE) and European Association for the Study of the Liver (EASL) clinical guideline. J Hepatol. 2017;66(6):1265-81.
40. Natt N, Michael F, Michael H, Dubois S, Al Mazrou'i A. ERCP-related adverse events in primary sclerosing cholangitis: a systematic review and meta-analysis. Can J Gastroenterol Hepatol. 2022;2022:2372257.
41. Lanzillotta M, Della-Torre E, Wallace ZS, Stone JH, Karadag O, Fernández-Codina A, et al. Efficacy and safety of rituximab for IgG4-related pancreato-biliary disease: a systematic review and meta-analysis. Pancreatology. 2021;21(7):1395-401.
42. Miyazawa M, Takatori H, Kawaguchi K, Kitamura K, Arai K, Matsuda K, et al. Management of biliary stricture in patients with IgG4-related sclerosing cholangitis. PLoS One. 2020;15(4):e0232089.

43. Hirano K, Tada M, Isayama H, Sasahira N, Umefune G, Akiyama D, et al. Outcome of long-term maintenance steroid therapy cessation in patients with autoimmune pancreatitis: a prospective study. J Clin Gastroenterol. 2016;50(4):331-7.

SUGGESTED READING

1. Kapoor VK. Safe Cholecystectomy A-to-Z (Forewords by John G Hunter and L Michael Brunt). New Delhi: SELSI; 2021. pp. 1-310.
2. Kapoor VK (Ed). Post-cholecystectomy Bile Duct Injury (Foreword by Henri Bismuth, John L Cameron, Steven M Strasberg). Singapore: Springer; 2020. pp. 1-244.
3. Kapoor VK (Ed). Surgery of Bile Ducts. New Delhi: Elsevier; 2013. pp. 1-172.

CHAPTER 8

Obscure Gastrointestinal Bleed

RA Sastry

■ INTRODUCTION

Considerable developments have taken place in the last 25 years in the investigation and management of patients presenting with obscure intestinal bleeding. Widespread use of video-capsule endoscopy, enteroscopy, computed tomography/magnetic resonance (CT/MR) enterography, CT angiography, etc., has changed our approach dramatically, reducing the number of diagnostic laparotomies to a great extent. However, diagnostic precision has not been proportionately matched by therapeutic improvements, although new therapies, particularly in the fields of interventional endoscopy and imageology, are helpful in many cases. Some of these investigative and therapeutic procedures, however, lack general applicability and are still reserved for specialized centers. Many guidelines have been published in Europe and Japan and by the American College of Gastroenterology.[1,2] The discussion that follows is consistent with those guidelines.

■ DEFINITION

In the past, the term "obscure" was used if no source of bleeding was found after an endoscopic evaluation. However, more recently, it has been proposed that the term obscure be used if patients have not had a source of bleeding identified after a panendoscopy and a thorough examination of the entire gastrointestinal (GI) tract, including the small bowel.[1] In this chapter, however, the term is used only in the traditional sense when a source of bleeding cannot be identified with routine upper GI endoscopy and colonoscopy. It covers both occult and overt GI bleeding: Overt (visible) when there is visible bright red blood or altered blood (such as coffee grounds, melena, or clots) in vomiting or stool and occult when there is no visible blood. In approximately half cases, GI bleeding originates in the upper GI tract (esophagus, stomach, and/or duodenum—proximal to the ligament of Treitz), 40% originate from the lower GI tract (colon and rectum) and 10% from the small bowel.[2,3]

■ WHY SOME GASTROINTESTINAL BLEEDS ARE OBSCURE?

Some GI bleeds are obscure because the lesions may have stopped bleeding and are overlooked. Significant anemia and volume contraction or very slow bleeding or intermittent bleeding may make them look less obvious. Routine examinations may not always detect lesions in small bowel because of difficult access. Obscure GI bleed accounts for 10–20% of all GI bleeds;[4] 5% of them are recurrent and remain obscure. Some of the general characteristics that stand out include that they are always recurrent; the majority are due to lesions in the small bowel (40–75%),[5,6] and the remaining are missed lesions on upper GI endoscopy and colonoscopy.

■ ETIOLOGY

Etiologically, the bleeding lesions could be classified as vascular, tumoral, and miscellaneous. They could also be classified into lesions occurring in those above 40 years of age and those below 40 years of age **(Table 1)**. Thus, inflammatory bowel disease (IBD), Meckel's diverticulum, and tumors of the small intestine such as stromal tumor **(Figs. 1A and B)**, carcinoid tumor, adenocarcinoma, and lymphoma represent the main causes before the age of 40 years, while vascular lesions such as angiodysplasia **(Figs. 2A and B)** and ulcerations secondary to nonsteroidal anti-inflammatory drugs (NSAIDs) predominate after 40 years. Of these, some tend to be more difficult to identify than others, for example, hemosuccus pancreaticus, hemobilia, Dieulafoy's

TABLE 1: Common causes of obscure GI bleed.

Vascular	Tumors of small bowel	Miscellaneous	Above 40 years	Below 40 years
Angiodysplasias	GIST	Medication-related	Angiodysplasias	Small bowel tumors
Vascular ectasia	Carcinoid	Infections—TB, typhoid	GAVE	Crohn's disease
Gastric antral vascular ectasia (GAVE)	Carcinoma	Meckel's diverticulum	Small bowel tumors	Infections—TB, typhoid
Dieulafoy's lesion		Vasculitis	Drug-induced small bowel injury	Meckel's diverticulum
		Radiation enteritis	Dieulafoy's lesion	Polyposis syndromes
		Jejunal diverticula		Vascular malformations
		Chronic mesenteric ischemia		

(GI: gastrointestinal; GIST: gastrointestinal stromal tumor; TB: tuberculosis)

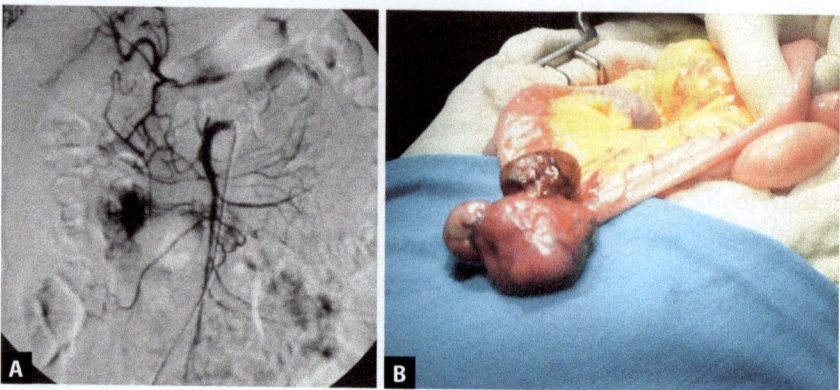

Figs. 1A and B: Obscure overt lower GI bleed from a GIST in a young adult, localized only on a selective angiogram. (GI: gastrointestinal; GIST: gastrointestinal stromal tumor)

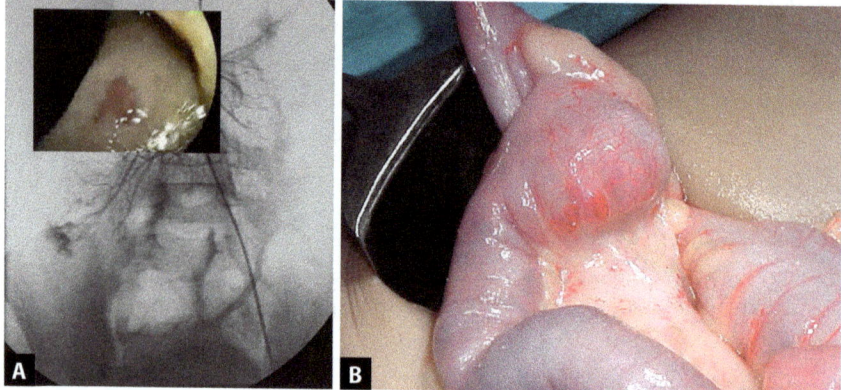

Figs. 2A and B: Angiomatous malformations in the small intestine of a 25-year-old woman demonstrated on a selective angiogram. The inset shows the initial capsule endoscopic image.

ulcer (stomach and other sites), Meckel's diverticulum, jejunal diverticula **(Figs. 3A and B)**, and extraesophageal varices. One study that reviewed the literature identified the main causes of obscure GI bleed as angiodysplasia, tumors, IBD, and mucosal ulcerations secondary to the use of NSAIDs.[7] The other rare causes of obscure GI bleed include hemorrhagic telangiectasia, hereditary polyposis syndromes (familial adenomatous polyposis, Peutz–Jeghers syndrome), small bowel varices, and aortoenteric fistula.[1,3]

Angioectasia: It is the formation of aberrant blood vessels that may be seen in any segment of GI tract in advanced age or in patients having comorbidities such as rheumatologic disorders, chronic renal disease, cirrhosis, and severe cardiovascular disease. The lesions are usually multiple. It may cause overt or occult GI bleeding, particularly in elderly individuals who are on antiplatelet

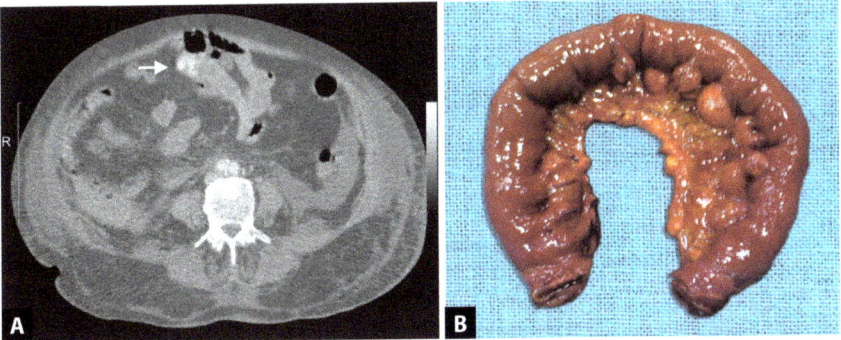

Figs. 3A and B: (A) Obscure bleeding from jejunal diverticulum in a 30-year-old man demonstrated on a CT angiogram; (B) Resected specimen of jejunum showing multiple diverticula.

agents and/or anticoagulants. On endoscopy, it appears as erythematous lesions of size 2–10 mm with arborizing ectatic blood vessels that emanate from a central vein.[3]

Meckel's diverticulum: It is a congenital anomaly that appears as an intestinal pouch located in the distal ileum. It characteristically follows "the rule of 2s"; that is, it is present in 2% of population, seen within 2 feet from ileocecal valve, 2 inches long in size, the complications develop in 2% cases, mostly contains 2 types of ectopic tissue (gastric or pancreatic), clinically present usually at 2 years of age, and male-to-female ratio is also reported >2:1. The most common complications of Meckel's diverticulum are bleeding, bowel obstruction, and diverticulitis.[3,8]

Nonsteroidal anti-inflammatory drug-induced small intestinal erosions and ulcers: These are reported as high as 25–55% in patients taking nonselective NSAIDs in high doses. However, the incidence is lower in patients taking selective cyclooxygenase (COX)-2 inhibitors.[9]

Small bowel neoplasms: The common lesions are adenoma, GI stromal tumor, carcinoids, lymphoma, hamartoma, juvenile polyp, and adenocarcinoma.[3]

Dieulafoy lesion: It is most commonly present in the stomach; however, it may be seen in any part of the GI tract. In younger age, it is usually present in small intestine, and in older individuals, it is common in the stomach.[3,9]

■ CLINICAL EVALUATION

The diagnostic strategy aiming to locate the origin of the occult GI bleeding is a real challenge. A good history and physical examination, as in all the other clinical situations, is an essential prerequisite. Of particular importance in history are age, nature, and duration of bleeding, as well as stool color and frequency. Associated symptoms of significance are abdominal pain, change in bowel habits, fever, urgency, tenesmus, and weight loss. The relevant past history typically includes previous bleeding episodes, surgical operations, acid peptic disease, tuberculosis, inflammatory bowel disease, and pelvic or abdominal radiation. Other comorbid conditions that should be looked for are cardiac or liver disease, iron deficiency anemia, clotting disorders, and history of medications such as NSAIDs and anticoagulants.

It is important to ascertain whether the bleeding is occult or overt. If overt, is it hematemesis, hematochezia, or melena? Hematemesis or dysphagia suggests an upper GI source, whereas hemodynamically stable hematochezia suggests a lower GI source. A history of cirrhosis or risk factors for liver disease suggests varices, which may occur anywhere in the GI tract, as well as portal hypertensive gastropathy, enteropathy, and colopathy. In addition to history of bleeding disorders, factors contributing to acquired coagulopathy or thrombocytopenia should be investigated. For example, patients with increased circulatory turbulence from mechanical valves, left ventricular-assist devices, hypertrophic cardiomyopathy, and severe mitral regurgitation are more likely to develop angiodysplasias, as are patients with aortic stenosis with Heyde syndrome and acquired von Willebrand syndrome. Family history of polyposis syndromes (including Gardner syndrome, Cowden disease, Cronkhite–Canada syndrome, Peutz–Jeghers syndrome, and familial adenomatosis polyposis) and malignancies is important in the investigation of obscure or occult GI bleeding.

Based on the pattern of bleeding, three clinical profiles may be identified:
1. Elderly patient, a nonoperative candidate with significant comorbid diseases
2. Young patient with no underlying medical problems
3. Patient without GI symptoms but iron-deficient anemia

The priority of investigations should proceed according to the clinical profile.

■ INITIAL MANAGEMENT

Initial management of overt-obscure GI bleeding is similar to any GI bleeding and is focused on resuscitation and achievement of hemodynamic stability. In a rare instance after an initial bidirectional endoscopy, it is confirmed that the bleeding is obscure but massive; there is a place for direct operative exploration, particularly when more advanced investigations are not readily accessible. Thus, emergency surgical intervention is indicated when hemodynamic instability persists despite aggressive resuscitation and when there is blood transfusion requirement of more than three units to maintain hemodynamic stability. In such desperate circumstances, operative enteroscopy aids significantly in the localization of the bleeding. A gentle saline wash of the colon and small intestine through a cecostomy on the operating table, followed by a bidirectional enteroscopy of serial occluded segments of small and large bowel, helps in many of such patients and avoids blind resections. Peroral operator-guided enteroscopy is a useful alternative. In addition to direct intraluminal vision, transillumination through the serosal surface is an added advantage of operative enteroscopy. This could be a definitive way of management in desperate situations in resource-deficient facilities. Laparoscopic operative enteroscopy is another described option attractive for its minimal invasiveness. However, one should be wary of the traumatic artifacts created by the invasive procedures and possible overdiagnoses of angiomatous malformations.

Relook Endoscopy

If initial upper GI endoscopy and colonoscopy are negative, patients can be considered as having a possible small bowel bleed. However, before resorting to extensive small bowel evaluation, a repeat second-look endoscopy is proved to have a definite value, particularly if the initial examinations were inadequate or if overt bleeding that had stopped has recurred.[10] The most common lesions missed on initial endoscopy include Cameron's erosions, arteriovenous malformations (AVMs) of the stomach and proximal duodenum, and peptic ulcer disease, especially with recent NSAID use.[11] For patients with risk factors for hemobilia or hemosuccus pancreaticus, the upper endoscopy should include evaluation with a side-viewing duodenoscope. An upper GI endoscopy and colonoscopy should be performed in asymptomatic men and postmenopausal women presenting with iron deficiency anemia with no obvious cause. Upper GI malignancy in 2% and colonic malignancy in 9% of patients were detected in such patients in one study.[12]

Nongastrointestinal Sources

Evaluation for non-GI sources of blood loss should be pursued for patients with symptoms or signs such as nosebleeds, oral lesions, or lymphadenopathy. One of the author's patients with recurrent lower GI bleeding after a sigmoid polypectomy, and when the bleeding recurred even after anterior resection, was ultimately found to have hemophilia B with factor IX deficiency. History of previous surgery needs special mention. With the advent of more and more radical dissections and vascular divestments and resections, an increasing number of vascular pseudoaneurysms with obscure luminal bleeds are seen. **Figures 4A to F** illustrate one such patient, who presented 1 year after a Whipple's operation with recurrent obscure GI bleed from a pseudoaneurysm of the right hepatic artery that could be localized only with a selective angiogram. When the bleeding recurred 1 month after a successful embolization, he required open surgery.

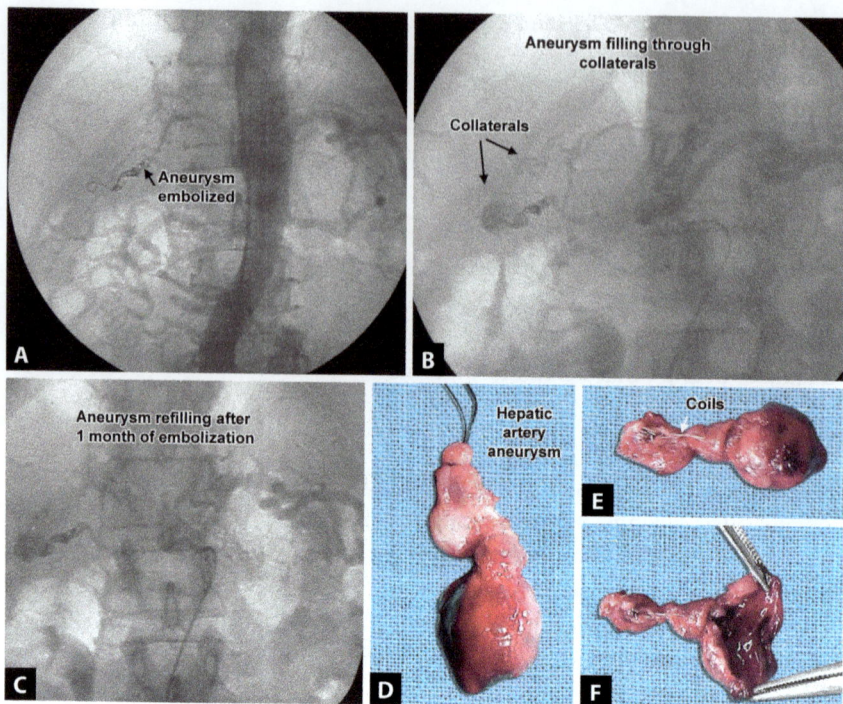

Figs. 4A to F: Obscure recurrent bleed after Whipple operation from an eroding pseudoaneurysm of the right hepatic artery requiring surgery after a partial success of angioembolization.

Evaluation of Small Intestine

When the relook endoscopy has failed to localize the cause of bleed, further strategies to evaluate the small intestinal source should be proceeded with. They include wireless video capsule endoscopy (VCE), deep enteroscopy, CT/MR enterography including angiography, tagged red blood cell (RBC) scan, Meckel scan, and provoked endoscopy. Majority of the GI bleeding occurs between the ampulla of Vater and the ileocecal valve, with angiodysplasia accounting for 30–40% of bleeding lesions.[1] The American College of Gastroenterology (ACG) and the European Society of Gastrointestinal Endoscopy recommend VCE as the next diagnostic procedure if small bowel bleeding is suspected, following exclusion of the source of bleeding from upper and lower GI tracts. It also recommends push enteroscopy for the lesion suspected in duodenum and jejunum as capsule endoscopy has a lower detection rate for the lesion in these areas.[3]

Capsule Endoscopy

Video capsule endoscopy is generally the first test after a negative bidirectional endoscopy. It is noninvasive and allows examination of the entire intestinal tract, providing a useful road map for a deep enteroscopy if needed later. Capsule endoscopy (CE) has a diagnostic accuracy of 40–80% in obscure gastrointestinal bleeding (OGIB) as compared with double-balloon endoscopy, which is the gold standard for detection of lesion in small bowel.[4,6] The device is basically a capsule fitted with a disposable mini video camera. The video data is transmitted and stored in a recorder worn on a belt. The video capsule is swallowed with water. Following capsule ingestion, recorded images are downloaded and processed on workstations. The capsules are disposable and are excreted with bowel movements. The advantages are that it is painless; no sedation is required, it provides three-dimensional (3D) color images of the small intestine without surgery, and it allows clinicians to make early, accurate diagnosis of problems so that they can recommend the most appropriate treatment. CE images are recorded through a transparent dome; magnified images are captured when the capsule is in contact with the bowel wall. Thus, it easily detects vascular and ulcerative lesions; however, submucosal lesions (like tumors) with an intact mucosal surface are difficult to diagnose. These submucosal lesions are detected with high accuracy on balloon endoscopy and cross-sectional imaging.[4] Angiomatous malformations, small bowel gastrointestinal stromal tumors (GISTs), and inflammatory and infective lesions such as tuberculosis, Crohn's disease, and polyps can be easily recognized. The disadvantages are that it cannot be used when there is partial or intermittent intestinal obstruction, gastroparesis, in the presence of any swallowing disorders, in patients who are inoperable because of severe comorbid conditions, and in pregnant women. The other disadvantage is that the test does not permit a biopsy or any therapeutic intervention. The diagnostic yield, as in other diagnostic modalities, depends on whether it is an overt bleeding, the intensity of bleeding, and the timing of the test after an active bleed. When the initial study is suboptimal, a repeat capsule endoscopy is advised in resource-rich facilities, and it may unravel any hidden lesions. VCE should be performed as soon as possible after overt bleeding, preferably within 14 days, for high diagnostic yield.[1,10] An area of active development and research is the use of artificial intelligence (AI) to improve detection of GI lesions by capsule endoscopy. Once these algorithms are fully validated, they should substantially reduce reading times and are likely to enhance the accuracy of capsule reads.

Enteroscopy

When capsule endoscope is not able to localize the bleed or the source of bleed, further invasive endoscopic interventions such as push enteroscopy or device-assisted enteroscopy (single-balloon, double-balloon, and spiral endoscopy) are the next choice. Push enteroscopy can be performed with a dedicated enteroscope or pediatric colonoscope. It can assess small bowel approximately 100 cm distal to ligament of Treitz.[3] Initial device-assisted enteroscopy may be appropriate if there is a massive bleed or when capsule endoscopy is contraindicated. Device-assisted enteroscopy, also called deep enteroscopy, can be performed using different types of enteroscopes. The first device-assisted deep enteroscopy used the double-balloon technique [double-balloon enteroscopy (DBE)], which uses two balloons. The distal tip of the enteroscope has one balloon and the other at the distal end of a flexible overtube. Both balloons allow anchoring to the small bowel wall and advancing the enteroscope through the small bowel. By serial inflation of the balloon(s) and pleating, the enteroscope is advanced, the looping of the small intestine is minimized, and one can reach up to the terminal ileum. Single-balloon enteroscopy is similar to DBE; however, it has lower diagnostic yield. The new technique is spiral enteroscopy, in which the motor rotates an overtube equipped with spiral fins supporting continuous pleating or folding of the small bowel. Thus, maneuverability becomes easy, and it also decreases the procedure time.[3] Although deep enteroscopy is typically done antegrade, a combination of antegrade and retrograde enteroscopy may allow complete enteroscopy, helped by a clip or tattoo mark marked at the deepest extent of visualization antegrade. The types of bleeding lesions seen on capsule endoscopy and enteroscopy are listed in **Table 2**. Availability of therapeutic options is an advantage with deep enteroscopy over capsule endoscopy. However, both CE and enteroscopy are essential and play complementary roles in the diagnosis and treatment of obscure bleed. Pennazio et al. evaluated CE in overt and occult bleeding and reported diagnostic yield of 92 and 44%, respectively.[13] Shinozaki et al. reported diagnostic yield of DBE as 77 and 67% in overt and occult bleeding, respectively.[14] Thus, it may be concluded that overt bleeding CE may be a suitable investigation; however, in occult bleed, DBE may be preferred.

Comparison of enteroscopies: A meta-analysis of 39 studies of the capsule endoscopy and deep enteroscopy demonstrated a combined diagnostic yield of 44–100% when done during ongoing bleeding.[15] According to a systematic

TABLE 2: Types of bleeding lesions seen on enteroscopy/capsule endoscopy.

Type	Bleeding lesions
Type 1a	Punctate erythema (<1 mm) with or without oozing
Type 1b	Punctate erythema (a few millimeters) with or without oozing
Type 2a	Punctate lesions (<1 mm) with pulsatile bleeder
Type 2b	Pulsatile red protrusions without surrounding venous dilatation
Type 3	Pulsatile red protrusions with surrounding venous dilatation
Type 4	Other lesions not classified into any of the above categories

review and meta-analysis of studies comparing these two procedures, capsule enteroscopy was shown to have a higher diagnostic yield than device-assisted deep enteroscopy for identifying the source of obscure GI bleeding. However, device-assisted deep enteroscopy may be more effective in certain cases, such as when there is a high suspicion of small bowel tumors or strictures.[16] A cost-effective analysis comparing the two found that initial deep enteroscopy was cost-effective, but the capsule-directed deep enteroscopy may be associated with even better long-term outcomes.[17] It is important to note that both procedures have their own advantages and disadvantages, and the choice of procedure depends on several factors such as the patient's medical history, symptoms, and other clinical factors.

■ IMAGING MODALITIES

Imaging modalities that are available in the evaluation of occult GI bleeding include CT and MR enterography, CT angiography, conventional angiography, and radionuclide scintiscans. Barium follow-throughs have no place in the current evaluation of GI bleeds.

Computed Tomography and Magnetic Resonance Enterography

It involves administration of a high volume of oral contrast along with intravenous contrast and acquisition of CT or MR images in all the vascular phases. These are particularly useful to detect small space-occupying lesions in the small bowel or when other evaluations such as capsule endoscopy or deep enteroscopy are contraindicated. The disadvantages include lack of therapeutic options, exposure to high radiation, contrast allergies and toxicities, pregnancy, and noncompatible metal implants for MR examination. When compared with capsule endoscopy in the evaluation of obscure GI bleeding, a meta-analysis of seven studies found a positive yield of 34% for CT enterography compared with 53% for capsule endoscopy.[18]

Computed Tomography Angiography

Computed tomography angiography is most useful during brisk bleeding episodes and acts as a guide before selective angiography, particularly in hemodynamically unstable patients where the risks are high for a blind conventional angiogram. The sensitivity is 85% for bleeding rates of even 0.3–0.5 mL/min and a specificity of 92% for acute bleeding.[19] Active contrast extravasation is considered a positive finding, which may manifest as a blush within the bowel lumen, a jet of contrast, or contrast extravasation on delayed imaging that may be seen moving owing to peristalsis. The disadvantages of

CT angiography are radiation exposure and the need for a large amount of iodinated contrast with its attending risks.

Angiography

Angiography is an invasive technique mostly used after the bleeding site is localized on CT angiogram or enteroscopy when endoscopic intervention has failed to contain the bleeding, or when the lesion identified cannot be intervened by endoscopy. It is also used when all other investigations have failed to localize the bleeding site, particularly during brisk bleeding episodes. The sensitivity is lower than CT angiogram. It does not have any significant role in occult bleeding and requires expertise and is accessible only at major hospitals. The ability to intervene even in an unprepared gut is the main advantage. Angiography may detect lesions that are bleeding or nonbleeding lesions (as AVM, it has characteristic angiographic features including a dilated artery, a nidus, and early venous return). In the presence of active bleeding, mesenteric angiography will show extravasation of contrast into the bowel lumen (if bleed is ≥0.5 mL/min).[20] Transarterial embolization (TAE) is an effective procedure in such cases; however, bowel infarction is a well-known complication (4.3%).[21]

Provoked Angiography and Endoscopy

Provoked techniques of enterography and endoscopy involve administration of provocation agents such as anticoagulants, fibrinolytics, and vasodilators. Heparin is commonly used as the effects can be easily reversed. A recent study of 27 patients with provoked endoscopies showed a diagnostic yield of 27–71%.[22] The results are, however, not uniform, and the risks of provoked bleeding are not completely addressed.

Radionuclide Scan

Computed tomography angiography has largely supplanted scintigraphy in the evaluation of obscure GI bleeding, and the current role is limited. RBCs from the patient are tagged with technetium-99m and are reinfused. A general area of blush may be observed, potentially guiding other studies. Theoretically, scintigraphy is sensitive to detect bleeding at 0.1 mL/min if performed earlier (80%) than later (40%). Scintigraphy can detect bleeding at bleeding rates as low as 0.04 mL/min.[3] It has low specificity to localize the bleeding site, 22% false-positive rate due to bowel motility, no therapeutic facility, no widespread availability, and has no predictive value for angiography success. The follow-up serial scans may also be obtained as radiolabeled RBCs remain in circulation for 24 hours.[3] The other scintigraphic technique that is used involves scanning with Tc-99m pertechnetate to detect ectopic gastric mucosa within Meckel's diverticulum. In pediatric patients,

TABLE 3: Comparison of different investigative modalities for obscure GI bleed.

Study	Advantages	Disadvantages	Diagnostic success rate
Video capsule endoscopy	• Noninvasive • Entire GI tract visualized • Mucosal lesions well visualized	• Contraindicated when obstruction is suspected • No therapeutic option	>90% when done close to the time of bleed
Deep enteroscopy	Permits therapeutic option	• Invasive • Chance of incomplete visualization of the entire intestine due to technical difficulties	78–84%
CT enterography	• Good for diagnosis of tumors and inflammatory lesions • Preferred investigation when obstruction is suspected	• Radiation exposure • Contrast allergies and toxicity • Poor results for mucosal lesions	34%
Scintigraphy	Useful for young patients with suspicion of Meckel's diverticulum	• Not very effective for localizing the occult bleed • Low sensitivity and specificity	21–54%
Operative enteroscopy	• Maximum sensitivity. • Highest potential for therapeutic efficacy	• Highly invasive • High morbidity	>90%

(CT: computed tomography; GI: gastrointestinal)

sensitivity and specificity of scan for detection of ectopic gastric mucosa in Meckel's diverticulum were 75-94% and 97-98%, respectively.[23,24] However, in adults, the scan was less sensitive and specific because the prevalence of heterotopic gastric mucosa declines with age in symptomatic patients. Thus, it is the less invasive test to rule out Meckel's diverticulum, especially in pediatrics age.[25] However, the scan provides only circumstantial evidence of the source of bleeding and needs to be followed up by capsule enteroscopy, enteroscopy, or surgery when the suspicion is strong. A comparison of the various diagnostic modalities is charted in **Table 3**.

Intraoperative enteroscopy: With the advent and routine use of advanced endoscopic techniques, including VCE and device-assisted deep enteroscopy, the diagnosis and management of overt OGIB have become more accurate. Today, intraoperative enteroscopy is largely reserved for patients with negative extensive evaluation and with ongoing overt-obscure GI bleeding and a continuing need for blood transfusions.[3]

■ IF THE BLEEDING REMAINS OBSCURE

Patients without an obvious source of bleeding, even after capsule endoscopy and enteroscopy, account for 5-10% in various studies. The decision to pursue diagnostic evaluation depends on the intensity of comorbidities and whether there are signs of continuous bleeding. It may be reasonable to stop evaluation in elderly patients with significant comorbid illnesses with a slow rate of blood loss and treat them with expectant management, replacing blood or iron as needed. Aggressive management with operative enteroscopy may be warranted in young patients who are in good health and have ongoing bleeding. If the bleeding appears to have stopped and recurred, a repeat evaluation in the same order as above is appropriate.

■ CONCLUSION

Evaluation and management of obscure GI bleeding can be a challenge despite the continuous advances in endoscopic techniques. In the management of

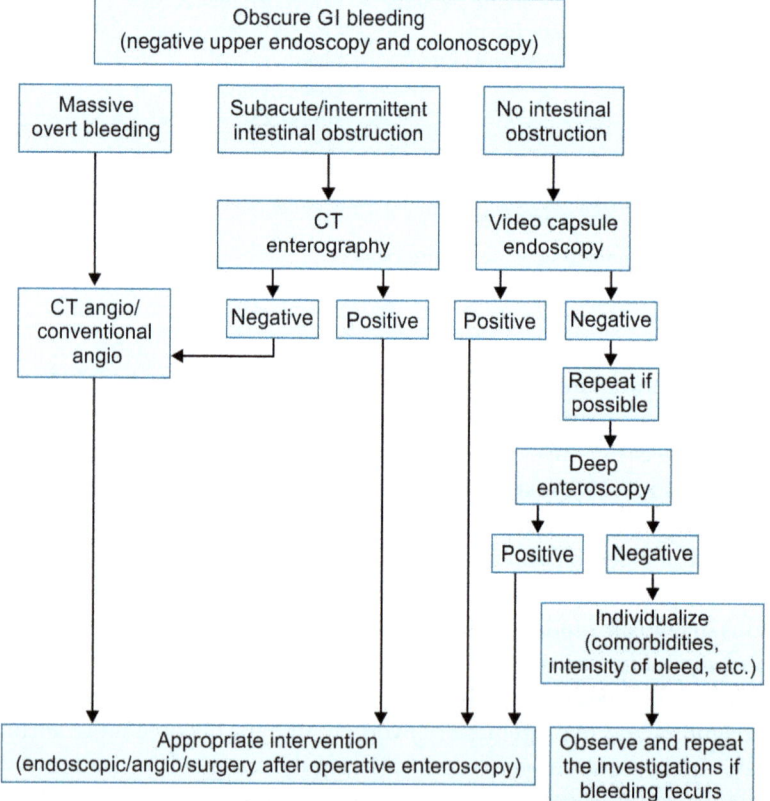

Flowchart 1: A suggested management algorithm for obscure GI bleeding.

(CT: computed tomography; GI: gastrointestinal)

obscure GI bleeding, it is good to follow a set algorithm involving history, physical examination, and preliminary resuscitation as required, assessing the intensity of bleed by serial hemoglobin and hematocrits, assessing the coagulation profile, and ruling out upper GI sources and colonic sources by appropriate re-endoscopy and treat them if found. If no source is found, plan advanced imaging techniques such as capsule enteroscopy, deep enteroscopy, and contrast-enhanced cross-sectional imaging as detailed above and employ appropriate therapeutic maneuver such as endoscopic, angiographic, or surgical technique. It is, however, important to remember that the selection of a specific maneuver often depends more on local availability and expertise than a rigid algorithmic approach to the problem.

■ REFERENCES

1. Gerson LB, Fidler JL, Cave DR, Leighton JA. ACG clinical guideline: diagnosis and management of small bowel bleeding. Am J Gastroenterol. 2015;110(9):1265-87.
2. Pennazio M, Rondonotti E, Despott EJ, Dray X, Keuchel M, Moreels T, et al. Small-bowel capsule endoscopy and device-assisted enteroscopy for diagnosis and treatment of small-bowel disorders: European Society of Gastrointestinal Endoscopy (ESGE) Guideline - update 2022. Endoscopy. 2023;55:58.
3. Awadie H, Zoabi A, Gralnek IM. Obscure-overt gastrointestinal bleeding: a review. Pol Arch Intern Med. 2022;132(5):16253.
4. Tanabe S. Diagnosis of obscure gastrointestinal bleeding. Clin Endosc. 2016;49:539-41.
5. Zuckerman GR, Prakash C, Askin MP, Lewis BS. AGA technical review on the evaluation and management of occult and obscure gastrointestinal bleeding. Gastroenterology. 2000;118:201-21.
6. Raju GS, Gerson L, Das A, Lewis B. American Gastroenterological Association (AGA) Institute technical review on obscure gastrointestinal bleeding. Gastroenterology. 2007;133:1697-717.
7. Rockey DC. Occult and obscure gastrointestinal bleeding: causes and clinical management. Nat Rev Gastroenterol Hepatol. 2010;7:265-79.
8. Triantafyllou K, Gkolfakis P, Gralnek IM, Oakland K, Manes G, Radaelli F, et al. Diagnosis and management of acute lower gastrointestinal bleeding: European Society of Gastrointestinal Endoscopy (ESGE) guideline. Endoscopy. 2021;53(8):850-68.
9. Yano T, Yamamoto H, Sunada K, Miyata T, Iwamoto M, Hayashi Y, et al. Endoscopic classification of vascular lesions of the small intestine (with videos). Gastrointest Endosc. 2008;67(1):169-72.
10. Pennazio M, Spada C, Eliakim R, Keuchel M, May A, Mulder CJ, et al. Small-bowel capsule endoscopy and device-assisted enteroscopy for diagnosis and treatment of small-bowel disorders: European Society of Gastrointestinal Endoscopy (ESGE) Clinical Guideline. Endoscopy. 2015;47(04):352-86.
11. Leighton JA, Goldstein J, Hirota W, Jacobson BC, Johanson JF, Mallery JS, et al. Obscure gastrointestinal bleeding. Gastrointest Endosc. 2003;58(5):650-5.
12. Rockey DC, Altayar O, Falck-Ytter Y, Kalmaz D. AGA technical review on gastrointestinal evaluation of iron deficiency anemia. Gastroenterology. 2020;159(3):1097-119.

13. Pennazio M, Santucci R, Rondonotti E, Abbiati C, Beccari G, Rossini FP, et al. Outcome of patients with obscure gastrointestinal bleeding after capsule endoscopy: report of 100 consecutive cases. Gastroenterology. 2004;126:643-53.
14. Shinozaki S, Yamamoto H, Yano T, Sunada K, Miyata T, Hayashi Y, et al. Long-term outcome of patients with obscure gastrointestinal bleeding investigated by double-balloon endoscopy. Clin Gastroenterol Hepatol. 2010;8:151-8.
15. Estevinho MM, Pinho R, Fernandes C, Rodrigues A, Ponte A, Gomes AC, et al. Diagnostic and therapeutic yields of early capsule endoscopy and device-assisted enteroscopy in the setting of overt GI bleeding: a systematic review with meta-analysis. Gastrointest Endosc. 2022;95(4):610-25.e9.
16. Uchida G, Nakamura M, Yamamura T, Furukawa K, Kawashima H, Honda T, et al. Systematic review and meta-analysis of the diagnostic and therapeutic yield of small bowel endoscopy in patients with overt small bowel bleeding. Dig Endosc. 2021;33(1):66-82.
17. Gerson L, Kamal A. Cost-effectiveness analysis of management strategies for obscure GI bleeding. Gastrointest Endosc. 2008;68:920.
18. Wang Z, Chen JQ, Liu JL, Qin XG, Huang Y. CT enterography in obscure gastrointestinal bleeding: a systematic review and meta-analysis. J Med Imaging Radiat Oncol. 2013;57(3):263-73.
19. Kim G, Soto JA, Morrison T. Radiologic assessment of gastrointestinal bleeding. Gastroenterol Clin N Am. 2018;47(3):501-14.
20. Baum S, Athanasoulis CA, Waltman AC, Ring EJ. Gastrointestinal hemorrhage. II. Angiographic diagnosis and control. Adv Surg. 1973;7:149-98.
21. Hongsakul K, Pakdeejit S, Tanutit P. Outcome and predictive factors of successful transarterial embolization for the treatment of acute gastrointestinal hemorrhage. Acta Radiol. 2014;55:186-94.
22. Raines DL, Jex KT, Nicaud MJ, Adler DG. Pharmacologic provocation combined with endoscopy in refractory cases of GI bleeding. Gastrointest Endosc. 2017;85(1):112-20.
23. Sinha CK, Pallewatte A, Easty M, De Coppi P, Pierro A, Misra D, et al. Meckel's scan in children: a review of 183 cases referred to two paediatric surgery specialist centres over 18 years. Pediatr Surg Int. 2013;29:511-7.
24. Hosseinnezhad T, Shariati F, Treglia G, Kakhki VRD, Sadri K, Kianifar HR, et al. 99mTc-Pertechnetate imaging for detection of ectopic gastric mucosa: a systematic review and meta-analysis of the pertinent literature. Acta Gastroenterol Belg. 2014;77:318-27.
25. Levy AD, Hobbs CM. From the archives of the AFIP. Meckel diverticulum: radiologic features with pathologic correlation. Radiographics. 2004;24:565-87.

CHAPTER 9

Management of Adrenal Incidentaloma

Rinelle Mascarenhas, Gaurav Agarwal

■ INTRODUCTION

Incidentally detected tumors or lesions in various organs or glands are increasingly being detected on imaging for unrelated reasons. The adrenal glands are small, paired, triangular-shaped organs located on top of each kidney. They play a crucial role in producing hormones such as cortisol, aldosterone, and adrenaline, which regulate various body functions and metabolism. An adrenal incidentaloma, by definition, is an unexpected finding of a mass or tumor ≥1 cm in one or both adrenal glands while conducting cross-sectional imaging for unrelated reasons. Adrenal tumor or pathology discovered on imaging performed for evaluating symptoms of hormone hypersecretion, or other symptoms attributable to the adrenal mass itself, or while staging a cancer patient are not considered "incidentalomas".[1]

These lesions are common, estimated to be present in 4% of patients on imaging series and up to 10% of the elderly population.[2,3] The prevalence of incidentally discovered adrenal masses has grown substantially with the increasing use of cross-sectional imaging. Adrenal incidentalomas are usually discovered during imaging studies such as computed tomography (CT) scans, magnetic resonance imaging (MRI) scans, or ultrasound examinations performed for unrelated medical issues. These imaging procedures may have been done during evaluation of a patient involved in road traffic accident or other forms of trauma, fever of unknown origin, for evaluation of a nonspecific abdominal symptom that is not attributable to an adrenal pathology, and for various other clinical conditions unrelated to a known adrenal pathology. Management of adrenal incidentalomas requires close coordination between various specialists to chalk out an evidence-based comprehensive management plan for each patient. An overview of management protocols commonly used and advocated is shown in **Flowchart 1**.

Discovery of an adrenal lesion raises two important questions that determines the plan of management:[1]
1. Is it malignant?
2. Is it functional?

Flowchart 1: Approach to management of incidentally detected adrenal masses.

```
Adrenal Incidentaloma
           │
           ▼
Assessment of symptoms/signs of:
• Adrenal hormone hypersecretion
• Manifestation of metastatic disease
           │
           ▼
Biochemical and hormonal assessment and evaluation of
imaging characteristics
```

- Biochemical/hormonal evaluation
  - Confirmation of hormone hypersecretion with overt clinical manifestations

- Non-functional or subclinical hypercortisolism
  - Suspicious >/= 10 HU, contrast enhancement, complex/heterogeneous enhancement
    - Unilateral → Unilateral suspicious mass → Surgery
    - Unilateral → Consider characterization on alternative radiology such as CECT, MRI, FDG-PET
      - Uncertainty? → Ambiguous results or in decision regarding surgery
    - Bilateral, history of malignancy or immune suppression
      - Concern for metastases or infection → Image-guided percutaneous biopsy

- Imaging characteristics
  - Benign Features <10 HU, <4 cm, lacking contrast enhancement, homogeneous

Repeat Evaluation in 3–6 months:
- Growth >1 cm/year
- Suspicious imaging features
- New or worsening hormonal hypersecretion

A. No strong indication for surgery
B. Consideration for active surveillance:
If initially 'non-functional':
• No need for repeated biochemical testing
• Consider repeating biochemical testing if worsening comorbidities (Diabetes Mellitus 2, Hypertension) as may be indicator for worsening hypersecretion
If subclinical or overt hypersecretion:
• Individualized consideration for surgery based on comorbidities and other factors, low threshold for surgery
• Patient's preference (surgery/surveillance)
• No strong indication for further imaging

(CT: computed tomography; FDG-PET: fluorodeoxyglucose positron emission tomography; HU: Hounsfield units; MRI: magnetic resonance imaging)

DIFFERENTIAL DIAGNOSIS OF ADRENAL INCIDENTALOMA

Majority of adrenal incidentalomas are benign nonfunctioning adrenal adenomas, which account for 75% of all adrenal incidentalomas. Benign functional tumors and malignant tumors are less common. Other rare causes of incidentally detected adrenal lesions are hemorrhage, infections,

TABLE 1: Differential diagnosis of an adrenal incidentaloma, and relative incidence of the causative pathology.

Type	Range (%)
Benign	
Non-functional:	
• Non-functional adenomas	71–84 (Majority)
• Ganglioneuroma	0–8
• Myelolipoma	7–15
• Cysts	4–22
Functional (Hormone hypersecretion):	
• Cushing's adenoma	1–30
• Conn's adenoma	2–7
• Pheochromocytoma	1.5–14
Malignant	
Adrenocortical carcinoma	1.2–12
Metastases	0–21
Malignant Pheochromocytoma	1.5–14

and granulomatous diseases (tuberculosis, fungal infections, sarcoidosis) in varying proportions **(Table 1)**. Functional tumors can present with features of hypersecretion of cortisol, aldosterone, or catecholamines and rarely with hypersecretion of more than one of these adrenal cortical or medullary hormones. Adrenal incidentalomas can also represent primary adrenal malignancy such as adrenocortical carcinoma (ACC) or metastases from malignant tumors arising from other organs (lung, breast, melanoma, renal).[2-4] Rarely, nonadrenal pathology of retroperitoneum, such as soft-tissue tumors and sarcomas, ganglioneuromas, neuroblastoma, and other miscellaneous tumors may mimic an adrenal pathology, which can be diagnosed and treated appropriately with careful evaluation by clinical, biochemical, and imaging means.

EVALUATION OF A PATIENT WITH ADRENAL INCIDENTALOMA

The beginning point of evaluation of such a patient is a detailed clinical history and physical examination to determine the nature of an incidentally detected adrenal mass. A careful focused history for any symptoms or manifestations of hypersecretion and adrenal/extra-adrenal malignancy needs to be taken, and a thorough head-to-toe clinical examination must be carried out **(Table 2)**.[5]

Biochemical and Hormonal Evaluation

Adrenal lesions can be hormonally active and may secrete cortisol, aldosterone, catecholamines, sex hormones, or steroid precursors in

TABLE 2: Clinical manifestations of common adrenal pathologies.

Tailored and focused history and physical examination for evaluation of the potential etiology of an adrenal mass

From adrenal medulla: Pheochromocytoma (catecholamine hypersecretion)	Headaches, anxiety attacks, sweating, palpitations, anger outbursts Or Family history of young-onset stroke, hypertension, abdominal surgeries Or Known familial syndromic association of: • Von Hippel–Lindau disease • Multiple endocrine neoplasia type 2 • Familial paraganglioma syndrome • Neurofibromatosis type 1	Severe hypertension, tachycardia, arrhythmias, congestive heart failure, excessive sweating, anxiety, and pallor
From adrenal cortex: Cushing's syndrome (cortisol hypersecretion)	Weight gain, central obesity, easy bruising, hypertension, diabetes, fatigue, proximal muscle weakness, depression, sleep disturbances, menstrual irregularities and virilization (in females), or fractures after trivial trauma	Hypertension, central obesity, buffalo hump, moon facies, facial plethora, thinned-out skin, purple and wide (>1 cm) abdomen striae, acne, ecchymoses, hirsutism, skin infections, and proximal muscle weakness or muscle wasting
Conn's syndrome (aldosterone hypersecretion)	Hypertension, hypokalemia, muscle cramping and weakness, headaches, intermittent or periodic paralysis	Severe hypertension, fluid retention
Adrenocortical carcinoma (nonfunctioning or functional)	Flank pain, vague abdominal discomfort, hypercortisolism, virilization, feminization, or aldosteronism	Weight loss, hirsutism, gynecomastia, signs of hypercortisolism
Metastases	Personal and family history of malignancy, constitutional symptoms such as loss of weight and appetite, unexplained fevers	Lymphadenopathy, lung mass, breast mass, renal mass or skin lesion suspicious for melanoma, as well as other cancer-specific findings

excessive amounts,[5,6] and rarely a combination of more than one of these. The optimal tests to be performed to assess hypersecretion of each of these adrenal pathologies and their interpretation are outlined in **Table 3**.

TABLE 3: Biochemical testing of patients with adrenal incidentaloma.

Hormone excess	Patients to test	Tests	Abnormal values	Ancillary tests
Autonomous cortisol secretion	All adrenal incidentalomas	Dexamethasone suppression test: 1 mg of Tab. Dexa is taken at 11 PM and serum cortisol measured at 8 AM the following morning	*Nonfunctional:* ≤50 nmol/L; *possibly functional:* 51–138 nmol/L; *autonomous hypercortisolism:* >138 nmol/L	- LDDST - ACTH-independent mass should be confirmed in all patients who are considered for intervention by measuring plasma ACTH - 24-hr urinary-free cortisol, 11 PM salivary cortisol
Pheochromocytoma	Lipid-poor, contrast-avid, heterogeneous adrenal masses	Plasma or urinary fractionated metanephrines	>2X to 4X higher than the upper normal limit of the reference range	N/A
Primary aldosteronism	Hypertension and/or hypokalemia	Serum aldosterone to plasma renin activity estimation	- Serum aldosterone to plasma renin activity ratio (ARR) >20–30 - Suppressed renin	- Saline suppression, and salt loading with 24-hr aldosterone estimation in urine - Adrenal vein sampling for lateralization
Androgen excess	Suspected ACC or hirsutism/virilization	DHEAS	Total testosterone higher than the upper limit of the reference range	17β-estradiol, 17-OH progesterone, androstenedione, 17-OH pregnenolone, 11-deoxycorticosterone, progesterone, and estradiol

(ACC: adrenocortical carcinoma; ACTH: adrenocorticotropic hormone; DHEAS: dehydroepiandrosterone sulfate; LDDST: low-dose dexamethasone suppression test; N/A: not applicable)

The first step in diagnosis of cortisol hypersecretion is to confirm the diagnosis and then determine the source/cause of hypercortisolism. The most widely accepted screening test to identify cortisol excess is the overnight dexamethasone suppression test (ONDST). The patient is administered 1 mg of dexamethasone at 11 PM, and serum cortisol levels are measured the following morning at 8 AM. A result of ≤50 nmol/L (≤1.8 µg/dL) excludes autonomous cortisol excess (sensitivity >95%). Cortisol levels >138 nmol/L (>5.0 µg/dL) denote autonomous cortisol secretion, and levels between 51 and 138 nmol/L (1.9–5.0 µg/dL) are considered equivocal.[7-9] There are a few important factors to consider when interpreting the results of a 1-mg ONDST. Dexamethasone is metabolized by CYP3A4 enzyme, and several interacting medications can impact the results. Women on oral contraceptive pills (OCPs) can have a 50% false-positive ONDST. Patients with critical illness, depression, or shift workers may have a blunted circadian rhythm of cortisol secretion. Thus, alternatively, a 24-hour urinary-free cortisol or midnight salivary cortisol may be considered **(Table 3)**. If hypercortisolism is confirmed on ONDST, additional biochemical tests are warranted. This generally includes confirmatory testing such as low-dose dexamethasone suppression test (LDDST) and confirmation of adrenocorticotropic hormone (ACTH)-independent cortisol secretion.

While evaluating for aldosteronism, serum aldosterone and plasma renin activity (PRA) need to be assayed to determine the aldosterone to PRA ratio (ARR). An ARR >20 ng/dL per ng/mL/h has high sensitivity and specificity of >90% for the diagnosis of hyperaldosteronism.[10] False-positive results may be seen in patients being treated with β-adrenergic blockers and central agonists, angiotensin-converting enzyme inhibitors (ACEI), angiotensin II receptor blockers (ARB) which increase plasma aldosterone and decrease plasma renin levels; thus it is imperative that these drugs be stopped at least two weeks prior to testing. Stopping anti-hypertensive medication like calcium channel blockers like verapamil, hydralazine, alpha blockers like prazosin and doxazosin is not required and can be used as substitutes for interfering medications.[11] In a patient with biochemical confirmation of primary hyperaldosteronism, lateralization of aldosterone hypersecretion to the side of the functional adrenal lesion with adrenal vein sampling (AVS) is the most reliable method. Though not universally essential, it is employed frequently in patients with unequivocal imaging findings and those with bilateral adrenal lesions.

Adrenocortical carcinoma is responsible for the majority of androgen hypersecretion and can be confirmed by testing serum levels of dehydroepiandrosterone sulfate (DHEAS), testosterone, 17β-estradiol, 17-OH progesterone, androstenedione, 17-OH pregnenolone, 11-deoxycorticosterone, progesterone, and estradiol.[5] A pleuri-hormonal picture, where there is a simultaneous hypersecretion of cortisol, aldosterone, and testosterone or estradiol, is highly indicative of a malignant adrenal tumor.

Depending on the availability of center-specific testing, screening for pheochromocytoma is primarily done by measuring plasma-free metanephrines (PfMN) or 24-hour urinary fractionated metanephrines (UfMN). A 24-hour UfMN level two times greater than the upper limit of normal is highly sensitive and specific for diagnosis of hypercatecholaminism or pheochromocytoma. Likewise, plasma normetanephrine levels >2.2 nmol/L or metanephrine levels >1.2 nmol/L are also highly specific for catecholamine hypersecretion.[12-14] Traditionally, it has been a practice to test all patients with adrenal incidentalomas for hypercatecholaminism to rule out pheochromocytomas. However, recent evidence from observational studies suggests that biochemical testing for pheochromocytoma is not essential in normotensive patients that have no clinical suspicion of pheochromocytoma and in those patients having adrenal incidentalomas with unenhanced attenuation of up to 10 Hounsfield units (HU) upon review retrospectively.[15,16]

Adrenal Imaging

The primary imaging modalities performed to characterize incidental adrenal masses are contrast-enhanced CT (CE-CT) and MRI scans **(Figs. 1A to D)**. The initial step in characterization of an adrenal mass is to determine if it is benign or malignant **(Table 4)**. **Box 1** lists features on noncontrast and CE-CT scan that are suggestive of malignancy.[17,18] These masses can be further evaluated with CE-CT (adrenal protocol) or MRI. The most validated initial imaging for adrenal masses is noncontrast CT. A homogeneous mass that is well circumscribed and measures <10 HU can be considered benign. Presence of large areas of macroscopic fat (measuring between −10 to −15 HU) is diagnostic of a benign myelolipoma.[18] Adrenal masses with >10 HU are considered indeterminate and do not fit the radiological criteria to rule out malignancy.

A benign adrenal adenoma will characteristically show rapid uptake of contrast and have a rapid loss of contrast or "washout" whereas malignant lesions typically display a slower contrast washout. These parameters are exploited in contrast-enhanced and washout CTs, which quantify the amount of "contrast washout" by measuring lesion attenuation at specific time points during the CT.

Contrast-enhanced CT adrenal protocol involves dynamic imaging, with documentation of the CT attenuation values at the following time points:
- Precontrast—before injection of contrast medium (HU NC)
- Postcontrast (arterial phase) at 70 seconds following injection of contrast medium (HU A), and then
- Delayed phase, i.e., 15 minutes after contrast injection (HU D).

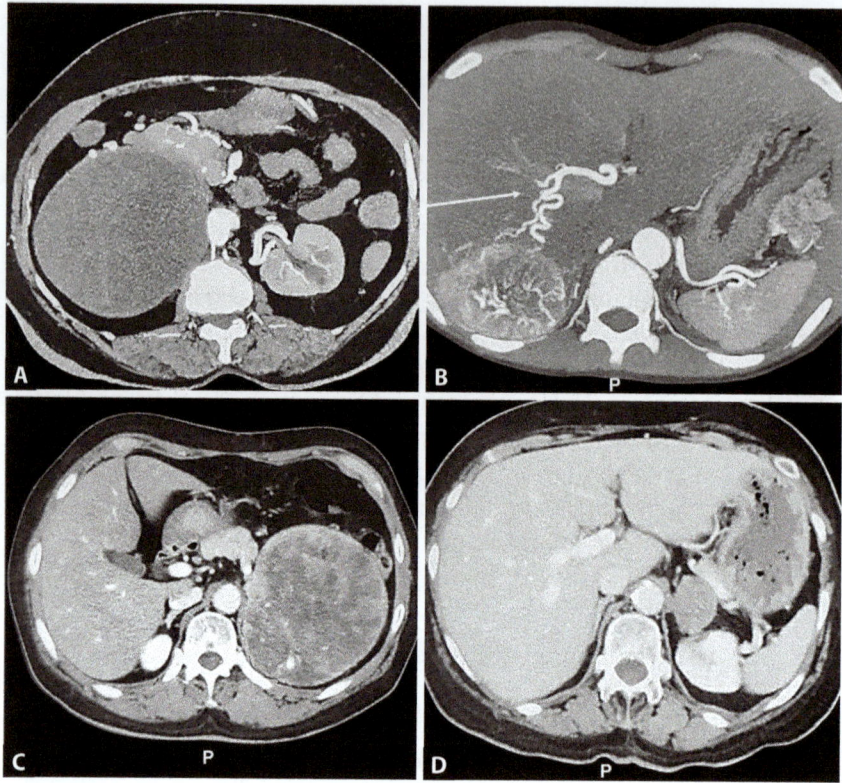

Figs. 1A to D: Contrast-enhanced computed tomography of (A) adrenal myelolipoma; (B) Pheochromocytoma, (C) Adrenocortical carcinoma; (D) Adrenal adenoma.

TABLE 4: Radiographic characteristics suggestive of benign versus malignant adrenal masses.

Features	Likely to be benign	Malignant potential
Irregularity	✗	✓
Heterogeneity/Complexity	✗	✓
Necrosis and/or calcifications	✗	✓
Size in cm	<4	>6
Rate of increase in size	<1 cm/year	>/= 1 cm/year
Noncontrast CT	<10 HU	>/= 10 HU
Washout on CT adrenal protocol at 15 minutes in %	Absolute >60 Relative >40	Absolute ≤60 Relative ≤40
Lipid-rich content on MRI	✓	✗
FDG-PET avidity	✗	✓

CT = computed tomography; HU = Hounsfield units; FDG = fluorodeoxyglucose; PET= positron emission tomography

BOX 1: Features of malignancy of CT scan in an adrenal incidentaloma.

Noncontrast:
- >6 cm
- Unilateral nonhomogenous mass
- Irregular margins
- Necrosis and occasionally calcifications
- >/= 10 HU

Contrast enhancement:
- </= 40% relative washout
- Relation to surrounding vasculature
- Lymphadenopathy

(HU: Hounsfield units)

The absolute washout and relative washout are then calculated using the following formulae:
- Absolute washout = (HU A − HU D)/(HU A −HU NC)
- Relative washout = (HU A − HU D)/HU A.

Benign adrenal masses typically show a relative and absolute washout of >40% and >60%, respectively.[19] Around one-third of pheochromocytomas may exhibit contrast washout in the characteristic range of an adenoma.[19,20] Although pheochromocytomas are usually heterogeneous and show higher CT attenuation in the arterial phase compared to adenoma, there is significant overlap between groups, preventing a confident imaging diagnosis.[21] When using washout CT scans for characterization of indeterminate adrenal masses, one should be aware of these limitations.

A second-line option for imaging an indeterminate on CT scan adrenal mass is MRI. Chemical-shift MRI exploits the different frequency of protons in water and fat and is used to detect microscopic fat.[22] On T2-weighted MRI, adenomas have characteristically low signal intensity compared with liver. Metastases and carcinoma have moderate signal intensity, whereas pheochromocytomas are extremely bright (light bulb sign). MRI is highly sensitive for microscopic fat and can detect microscopic fat in adrenal adenomas that measure 10–30 HU on a noncontrast CT.[23] When microscopic fat is identified as a homogeneous signal intensity drop on chemical-shift MRI, these features are diagnostic of lipid-rich adrenal adenoma. Heterogeneous signal intensity drop is a more controversial imaging finding since minute amounts of microscopic fat have been identified in pheochromocytoma, ACC, and some fat-containing metastases.[22,24] Size criteria for malignancy are not definitive, though a cutoff of 6 cm is frequently used as high (>25%) probability for malignancy in adrenal cortical tumors. The actual size of tumors is underestimated by at least 1 cm by CT and MRI scans.

■ IS THERE A ROLE FOR BIOPSY IN ADRENAL MASSES?

Biopsy of an adrenal mass is rarely indicated in the workup of an incidental adrenal lesion. In patients with imaging characteristics of a benign lesion or operable malignancy in an adrenal mass, there is no role for adrenal biopsy.[6] Biopsy may be considered when the diagnosis of metastatic disease from an extra-adrenal malignancy is highly probable. An image-guided core needle biopsy is the preferred method as fine needle aspiration cytology alone cannot distinguish adenomas from carcinomas. A core biopsy is useful only in setting of a patients with history of extra-adrenal carcinoma or nonoperable infiltrative adrenal mass performed under CT guidance after pheochromocytoma has been ruled out with appropriate biochemical testing. A 2016 systematic review found that adrenal mass biopsy was associated with a low risk of complication (2.5%) and good diagnostic performance (sensitivity of 87%, specificity 100%).[25] Biopsy of suspected ACC should not be routinely performed due to potential risk of tumor seeding the needle tract.[26]

■ MANAGEMENT OF ADRENAL INCIDENTALOMA

Surgery versus Observation

Management of adrenal incidentalomas often involves a multidisciplinary approach with input from endocrine surgeons, endocrinologists, radiologists, pathologists, and oncologists. Various types of adrenal tumors and pathologies present with distinct to overlapping gross **(Figs. 2A to D)** and microscopic pathology features, and an expert pathologist with experience in reporting endocrine pathology is a vital member of the multidisciplinary team for management of adrenal tumors. Collaboration among specialists helps tailor the management plan to the individual patient's needs. The vital decision this team has to take is whether to offer surgical treatment or conservative observational follow-up to an individual patient. This is based on the clinical, biochemical, and imaging characteristics in an individual patient, and in certain cases with an equivocal picture, the patient's own desire to choose one form of management plan after having been counseled regarding the pros and cons of the two approaches.

Indications of surgery in incidentaloma:
- All lesions >4 cm
- Functional tumor
- Primary operable malignancy
- Metastasis

In the era of laparoscopic surgery, surgery can be also offered to:
- Patients with laboratory testing confirmed subclinically functional tumor
- Patients desirous of operative management rather than observation and close follow-up.

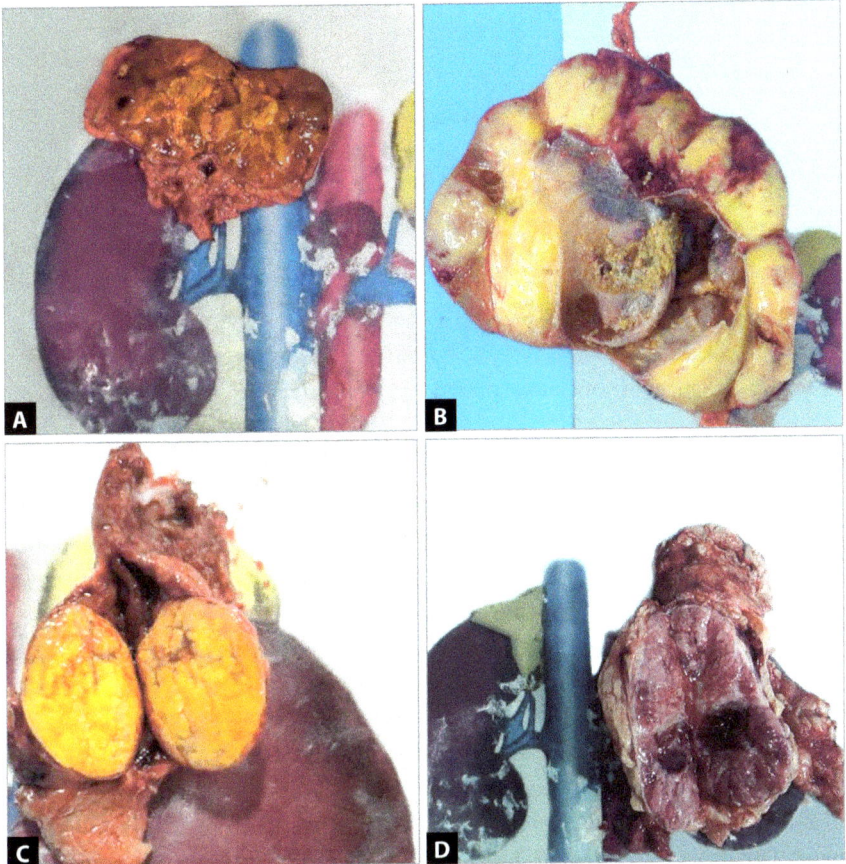

Figs. 2A to D: Gross appearance of (A) Cushing's adenoma; (B) Myelolipoma; (C) Conn's adenoma showing "Canary yellow" appearance on cut section; (D) Pheochromocytoma showing fleshy appearance with hemorrhage and necrosis on cut section.

Benign Functional Lesions

Cortisol-secreting Lesions

Patients with unilateral cortisol-secreting adenomas and clinical features of Cushing's syndrome such as hypertension, moon facies, buffalo hump, plethora, central obesity, and acne should undergo surgical resection of the hypersecreting adrenal gland. Laparoscopic adrenalectomy, first performed by Gagner in 1991, or other forms of minimally invasive adrenalectomy is the current gold standard procedure for small benign adrenal masses.[27] The most commonly practiced procedure is a lateral transabdominal laparoscopic adrenalectomy **(Fig. 3)**, which provides a good access to the adrenal vasculature, and the largest evidence base for safety and efficacy of surgical management for almost all small organ contained adrenal pathology.

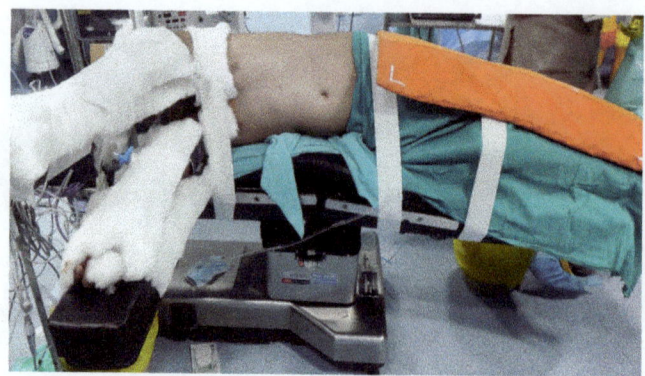

Fig. 3: Patient in right lateral position for laparoscopic left adrenalectomy.

Patients with Cushing's syndrome need aggressive and careful preoperative preparation and optimization of their cardiorespiratory risk. Early institution of respiratory capacity-building exercises and spirometry, achieving good blood pressure and blood sugar control, and of any other metabolic and infective morbidities is highly desirable before surgery.

Subclinical Cushing's syndrome is a distinct clinical entity, characterized by cortisol-secreting adrenal lesions without symptoms and signs of Cushing's syndrome. This entity is now labeled as "mild autonomous cortisol secretion" (MACS). These patients have an unsuppressed ONDST results. In a recent systematic review, comprising low-quality observational studies, none of the patients with subclinical Cushing's syndrome progressed to develop overt Cushing's syndrome. Although subclinical Cushing's syndrome is regarded as having a low risk of progression to overt Cushing's syndrome, it can contribute to medical comorbidities such as diabetes mellitus type 2, hypertension, and cardiovascular events. A systematic review and meta-analysis showed that without operative management, none of the patients with subclinical Cushing's syndrome had improvement with respect to diabetes, hypertension, or dyslipidemia. However, patients undergoing adrenalectomy benefited with lower rates of diabetes and lesser severity of hypertension and dyslipidemia. Thus, adrenalectomy is a beneficial management option for patients with subclinical Cushing's syndrome, particularly those who are young or those who have progressive metabolic comorbidities attributable to cortisol excess.[27]

Pheochromocytoma

It is well accepted that patients with pheochromocytomas should undergo surgical resection. Careful and comprehensive preoperative management using alpha-adrenoceptor blockers, prazosin or phenoxybenzamine, is considered highly desirable for control of blood pressure, prevention of any cardiac dysrhythmia, and achieving blood volume expansion with extra-oral fluids and salt supplementation, and when necessary intravenous fluids. Additionally, beta blockers, if needed for management of tachycardia and/or dysrhythmia, and other antihypertensive medications including calcium channel blockers for good blood pressure control are a must.

Laparoscopic or minimally invasive excision is preferred for small noninvasive pheochromocytoma over an open approach. In a 20-year retrospective study on 137 pheochromocytoma patients managed in a single tertiary care endocrine unit, the outcomes of open and laparoscopic procedures for 101 unilateral organ-contained pheochromocytoma patients were compared. There were no significant differences in perioperative hemodynamic events; however, mean blood loss, blood transfusion and analgesic requirements, and postoperative ICU and hospital stay were significantly lesser in the laparoscopic group than the open pheochromocytoma surgery group. Laparoscopic procedures have resulted in lesser morbidity and shorter convalescence and provided equal chance for cure of pheochromocytoma and hypertension as conventional open surgical procedures.[28] The most preferred form of minimally invasive adrenalectomy procedure is the transabdominal laparoscopic approach described by Gagner.[27] The posterior retroperitoneoscopic adrenalectomy approach was first performed by Walz.[29] It is now the preferred approach in some institutes due to complete isolation from the peritoneal cavity.[30] Recently, robotic adrenalectomy has been adopted in many high-volume tertiary centers with the advantage of better ergonomics and 3D visualization of the operative field. However, whether robotic adrenalectomy offers any benefits over conventional laparoscopic adrenalectomy is still a matter of debate. With the current high costs of robotic surgery, these procedures cannot be considered cost-effective.

A proposed term "subclinical pheochromocytoma" refers to a totally asymptomatic incidentaloma that is histologically proven to be a pheochromocytoma. A large retrospective study of adrenal incidentalomas in a developing country reported that majority of incidentalomas, i.e., 37.7% had hypercatecholaminism, while only 1.9% had hypercortisolism. The incidence of pheochromocytoma was high among large adrenal incidentalomas.[31] Following adrenalectomy, majority of patients are cured of hypercatecholaminism. All patients should be followed up to detect persistent or recurrent pheochromocytoma using a standard protocol **(Flowchart 2)**.

Pheochromocytoma in pregnancy: Pheochromocytoma during pregnancy is very rare and can be misdiagnosed as gestational hypertension. It can have detrimental effects and be potentially fatal for the mother and fetus. Such patients should be treated at centers of excellence with demonstrated

Flowchart 2: Algorithm for long-term follow-up of patients with pheochromocytoma.

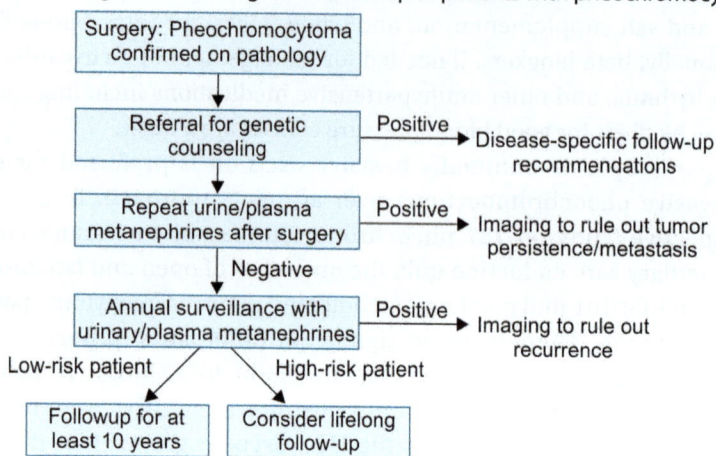

expertise and experience in managing pheochromocytoma and high-risk pregnancies. Multidisciplinary team management, including the endocrine surgeon, gynecologist and obstetrician, neonatologist, endocrinologist, and anesthesiologist, should be carried out. If the diagnosis is made within the first 24 weeks of pregnancy, adrenalectomy is recommended in the second trimester, while surgery should be postponed until after delivery if the diagnosis is made in the third trimester.[32,33] The pregnancy should be closely monitored, and institutional delivery, preferably via an elective cesarean section, should be ensured.

Aldosterone-secreting lesions: Patients should be managed preoperatively to achieve good blood pressure control and correction of hypokalemia, if present. Spironolactone is the drug of choice, though associated with certain postoperative events. The perioperative considerations for removal of a functional adrenal lesion are beyond the scope of this chapter. Unilateral aldosterone-producing adenomas or aldosteronomas and bilateral adrenal hyperplasia can be the cause for primary hyperaldosteronism. The term subclinical primary aldosteronism refers to a patient with an incidentaloma who may be normotensive or hypertensive with normokalemia. Around 30–40% of patients with primary hyperaldosteronism have normal serum potassium levels. In patients with a high index of suspicion such as patients who are hypertensive on multiple antihypertensive medications, screening for subclinical primary aldosteronism should be done by estimating the plasma aldosterone concentration (PAC) and plasma renin activity (PRA). An upright PAC to PRA ratio (ARR) is calculated. The commonly used ARR cut-off to diagnose primary hyperaldosteronism is 30 (when PAC is expressed in ng/mL/h, and PRA in ng/dL). However, some advocate using a lower threshold of 20 to increase sensitivity of diagnosis, at the cost of specificity.[10,34,35]

Laparoscopic adrenalectomy is the procedure of choice for the management of aldosteronomas. The overall cure rates are 75-95%. Cure is defined as clinical and biochemical end points. Reduction in blood pressure readings, in the number of antihypertensive medications required, and in plasma and urine aldosterone levels and resolution of hypokalemia (if previously present) are observed as soon as 24 hours after successful surgery. The primary aldosteronism surgical outcome (PASO) study established an international consensus for outcomes after adrenalectomy.[36] Clinical success is defined as complete (normalization of blood pressure without antihypertensive medication), partial (decrease in antihypertensive medication or reduction in blood pressure with the same medication), or absent. Biochemical success is defined as complete (correction of hypokalemia and normalization of aldosterone to renin ratio), partial (correction of hypokalemia and ≥50% decrease in plasma aldosterone but persistently elevated aldosterone to renin ratio), or absent. More than 80% of patients can expect either normalization of blood pressure or a significant reduction in antihypertensive medication requirements (i.e., from three to four medications, down to one). For those patients who continue to be hypertensive in the short term, medications may be added back temporarily, as needed, until the blood pressure gradually reaches a new equilibrium over time. Hyperkalemia due to transient suppression of the contralateral adrenal gland may occur in 5-10% of patients following adrenalectomy for hyperaldosteronism.[36] Renal insufficiency and suppression of aldosterone secretion from the contralateral adrenal gland at AVS are predictors of hyperkalemia. Hyperkalemia occurs within 1-3 weeks after surgery. Thus, patients should be monitored with weekly serum potassium levels for 1 month postresection. Persistent hyperkalemia can be treated with fludrocortisone, i.e., mineralocorticoid replacement therapy.

Some patients continue to require antihypertensive medications even after operation. The risk factors for these subsets of patients include men older than 45 years, family history of hypertension, long-standing hypertension, requirement of more than two antihypertensive medications preoperatively, and those nonresponsive to spironolactone. These patients could also have some component of essential hypertension. Based on these features, patients should be appropriately counseled as to what they should expect to gain from surgery. Following resection of Conn's adenomas, postoperative imaging is not required, and postoperative hormonal workup is only done in the short term to confirm the resolution of hypersecretion. Lack of biochemical cure should raise concern for bilateral disease, or removal of the nonhypersecreting adrenal gland if lateralization using AVS was not done prior to surgery.[37]

Nonfunctional Benign Adrenal Tumors

This group of lesions includes a nonfunctional adrenocortical adenoma, myelolipoma, and other miscellaneous benign adrenal pathologies. It is generally accepted that tumors > 4 cm in size, irrespective of their functional status, be surgically resected. Tumors with sizes ranging from 1 to 4 cm, or those lesions with a high suspicion for malignancy on clinical or imaging characteristics, or in patients who are desirous of surgical resection rather than being on periodic evaluation and close follow-up, should be offered surgery. Almost all such patients with benign adrenal masses are best treated with laparoscopic or other forms of minimally invasive adrenalectomy. An exception to this is anecdotal patients with massive myelolipoma, which may warrant a conventional open surgical approach, rather than a minimally invasive one.

■ MANAGEMENT OF ADRENOCORTICAL CARCINOMA

Adrenocortical carcinoma is an orphan malignancy, with an annual incidence of 0.7–2 cases/million/year. There are two distinct age distribution peaks, namely early adulthood and 40–50 years age. There exists a slightly female predominance of ~55–60%. However, in the German ACC registry, there is no absolute peak in childhood, and the median age is 46 years (range 0.3–86 years). Interestingly, this female predominance seems to be true only for functional tumors.[38] Cushing's syndrome is the most frequent presentation in functional ACC. Management requires a multidisciplinary approach. In patients with suspected ACC, resection is recommended, as complete surgical resection is the only potentially curative treatment for resectable stages I to III ACCs. The aim of surgery is to achieve a complete margin-negative (R0) resection as patients with an R0 resection have a 5-year survival rate of 40–50% compared to the <1 year survival of those with incomplete resection.[39] ACCs are large at presentation and measure >6 cm in >90% cases, with the median size being 10–11 cm. A CT attenuation value of >10 HU has a high sensitivity, but relatively low specificity to define an adrenal mass as malignant.[40,41] In early series, the majority of patients were diagnosed with advanced disease. In a meta-analysis by Wooten and King, including more than 600 patients, published between 1952 and 1992, around 49% of patients were described as stage IV. In contrast, in more recent studies, the percentage of patients in stage I or II is much higher, reflecting earlier diagnosis due to widely available advanced imaging technology.[38] The overall survival (OS) rates of stages I, II, III, and IV were 82%, 61%, 50%, and 13%, respectively.[25]

The European Society of Endocrine Surgeons (ESES) and the European Network for the Study of Adrenal Tumors (ENSAT) recommend thoracoabdominal CT imaging with contrast or fluorodeoxyglucose (FDG) positron emission tomography (PET) CT scan to be done within 6 weeks of planned adrenalectomy for suspicious ACC.[25] Molecular imaging is now available using cytochrome P450 enzymes CYP11B1 and CYP11B2. ^{11}C metomidate is an adrenocortical specific tracer under evaluation. Metomidate labeled with ^{123}I (iodometomidate [^{123}I] IMTO) has the advantage of identifying adrenocortical lesions with high specificity, identifying patients suitable for specific targeted radioactive treatment, besides being useful for detection of distant metastasis before surgery and in follow-up. However, it is unable to differentiate benign versus malignant adrenal masses.[42]

When a preoperative diagnosis or high level of suspicion of ACC exists, open surgical oncological resection is recommended. Minimally invasive approaches in the scenario of a suspected or confirmed ACC are highly contentious, and the majority view is to rely on conventional open surgery to ensure R0 resection without any breach in the tumor capsule and tumor seedings in the operative field. The evidence suggesting that locoregional lymph removal might improve diagnostic accuracy and therapeutic outcome is limited. Any contiguously infiltrated organs and structures, if resectable, should also be resected en bloc. Kidney, liver, pancreas, the psoas muscle and other abdominal wall muscle resection, removal of renal vessels and inferior vena cava (IVC) thrombus are sometimes resorted to, as the most proven curative and palliative option available is en bloc and radical surgical resection.[43]

Oncological standards to be maintained are:[44]
- Complete en bloc resection of the ACC with the peritumoral/periadrenal retroperitoneal fat.
- Enucleation and partial adrenal resection are contraindicated.
- Avoid intraoperative tumor capsule rupture or spillage.

Laparoscopic surgery has been explored but is highly debated. Concerns have been regarding the quality of surgical resection and related oncological risks. In ACC, several laparoscopic series have been reported and have reported conflicting results. According to contemporary guidelines, open surgery should be regarded as the standard treatment localized (stage I-II)/locally advanced (stage III) ACC, whereas laparoscopic adrenalectomy can be pursued in selected patients with small ACCs (<8 cm) with no preoperative evidence for invasion beyond adrenal boundaries. A conservative open approach is recommended for all adrenocortical lesions that cannot be classified as benign before surgery.[44,45]

Lymph node involvement in ACC has been reported in 4 to 73% patients, implying that regional lymphadenectomy is neither formally performed by all surgeons nor accurately assessed or reported by all pathologists.[39,45] Routine locoregional lymphadenectomy can be performed with adrenalectomy for highly suspected or proven ACC, and it should include, as a minimum, the periadrenal and renal hilum nodes. Excision of the tumor with intact tumor capsule is essential, whereas involvement of the IVC or renal vein with tumor thrombus is not a contraindication for surgery. However, even following an apparently complete surgical resection, 50–80% of patients develop locoregional or metastatic recurrence. Although such patients may be candidates for aggressive surgical resection, routine debulking is not recommended except for control of hormonal hypersecretion.[39,40] Ablative therapies, particularly targeting hepatic disease, are used to decrease tumor load and the hypersecretory syndromes. Individualized treatment decisions are made in cases of tumors with extension into large vessels based on a multidisciplinary surgical team. Such tumors should not be regarded "unresectable" until reviewed in an expert center. Adrenalectomy can be considered in select cases of metastatic ACC when complete resection of the primary tumor and all metastases is feasible at the time of primary diagnosis.[25]

In patients with inoperable, locally invasive or metastatic ACC, medical treatment as an adjuvant or salvage strategy has been used, though there continues to be considerable debate on their utility. The most common and most effective therapy is use of the adrenolytic agent "mitotane", which needs to be used with close monitoring for toxicity. Combination cytotoxic chemotherapy has been used with limited success. Adjuvant radiotherapy does not seem to offer any survival benefits but can be used for symptom control in a selective manner.[25]

CONSERVATIVE MANAGEMENT OR ACTIVE SURVEILLANCE OF BENIGN NONFUNCTIONAL LESIONS

Active surveillance is recommended in those patients with adrenal incidentalomas with
- No clinical or laboratory evidence of hypersecretion
- No suspicion of ACC
- No other associated symptoms in relation to the adrenal mass.

Small, nonfunctional adrenal incidentalomas that are unlikely to be malignant or those who do not have any suspicion of malignancy may be monitored periodically with imaging studies to assess growth and biochemically to assess future hyperfunction. For benign-appearing incidentalomas on imaging, a repeat imaging after 6–12 months should be performed to reconfirm the initial diagnosis of a benign adrenal lesion.[45] Factors that should be considered in surgical decision-making in benign nonfunctioning tumors <4 cm include suspicious imaging characteristics, the patient's age and surgical risk, growth on interval imaging, and the patient's preference. Characteristics suggestive of a benign lesion on CT scan include homogeneous appearance, <10 HU, well-defined borders, high lipid content, and rapid washout of contrast (relative washout >40 and absolute washout >60).

Studies have found that CT and MRI underestimate adrenal tumor size by approximately 20%, an effect that is exaggerated in smaller tumors. Therefore, it is advisable to remove all tumors measuring 4 cm or larger. Most experts would consider resecting any tumor that enlarges by >1 cm in diameter during the follow-up period. However, most adrenal masses that grow are not malignant. Nonetheless, surgical removal should be considered for masses ≥4 cm to avoid missing adrenal carcinomas, particularly in younger patients and in patients developing features of hormonal excess.

■ SUMMARY

Incidental adrenal masses are common, and most of these lesions are benign. Identification and timely management of functional and malignant lesions are crucial. This chapter provides a contemporary approach to the appropriate clinical, radiographical, and endocrine assessments required for the evaluation, management, and follow-up of patients with such lesions.

■ REFERENCES

1. Grumbach MM, Biller BM, Braunstein GD, et al. Management of the clinically inapparent adrenal mass ("incidentaloma"). Ann Intern Med. 2003;138(5):424-9. doi:10.7326/0003-4819-138-5-200303040-00013.
2. Song JH, Chaudhry FS, Mayo-Smith WW. The incidental adrenal mass on CT: prevalence of adrenal disease in 1049 consecutive adrenal masses in patients with no known malignancy. Am J Roentgenol. 2008;190:1163-8. https://doi.org/10.2214/AJR.07.2799.
3. Young Jr WF. Management approaches to adrenal incidentalomas: a view from Rochester, Minnesota. Endocrinol Metab Clin North Am. 2000;29:159-85. https://doi.org/10.1016/S0889-8529(05)70122-5.
4. Kapoor A, Morris T, Rebello R. Guidelines for the management of the incidentally discovered adrenal mass. Can Urol Assoc J. 2011;5:241-7. https://doi.org/10.5489/cuaj.657.
5. Rowe NE, Kumar RM, Schieda N, et al. Canadian Urological Association guideline: diagnosis, management, and followup of the incidentally discovered adrenal mass. Can Urol Assoc J. 2023;17(2):12-24. http://dx.doi.org/10.5489/cuaj.8248.
6. Vaidya A, Hamrahian A, Bancos I, Fleseriu M, Ghayee HK. The evaluation of incidentally discovered adrenal masses. Endocrine Practice. 2019;25(2):178-92. doi:10.4158/dscr-2018-0565.
7. Di Dalmazi G, Vicennati V, Rinaldi E, et al. Progressively increased patterns of subclinical cortisol hypersecretion in adrenal incidentalomas differently predict major metabolic and cardiovascular outcomes: a large, cross-sectional study. Eur J Endocrin. 2012;166:669-77. https://doi.org/10.1530/EJE-11-1039.
8. Debono M, Bradburn M, Bull M, et al. Cortisol as a marker for increased mortality in patients with incidental adrenocortical adenomas. J Clin Endocrinol Metab. 2014;99:4462-70. https://doi.org/10.1210/jc.2014-3007.
9. Di Dalmazi G, Vicennati V, Garelli S, et al. Cardiovascular events and mortality in patients with adrenal incidentalomas that are either non-secreting or associated

with intermediate phenotype or subclinical Cushing's syndrome: a 15-year retrospective study. Lancet Diabetes Endocrinol. 2014;2:396-405. https://doi.org/10.1016/ S2213-8587(13)70211-0.

10. Funder JW, Carey RM, Fardella C, et al (Endocrine Society). Case detection, diagnosis, and treatment of patients with primary aldosteronism: an Endocrine Society Clinical Practice Guideline. J Clin Endocrinol Metab. 2008;93:3266-81. https://doi.org/10.1210/ jc.2008-0104.

11. Seifarth C, Trenkel S, Schobel H, et al. Influence of antihypertensive medication on aldosterone and renin concentration in the differential diagnosis of essential hypertension and primary aldosteronism. Clin Endocrinol. 2002;57:457-65. https://doi.org/10.1046/j.1365-2265.2002.01613.x.

12. Van Berkel A, Lenders JW, Timmers HJ. Diagnosis of endocrine disease: biochemical diagnosis of phaeochromocytoma and paraganglioma. Eur J Endocrinol. 2014;170:R109-19. https://doi. org/10.1530/EJE-13-0882.

13. Perry CG, Sawka AM, Singh R, et al. The diagnostic efficacy of urinary fractionated metanephrines measured by tandem mass spectrometry in detection of pheochromocytoma. Clin Endocrinol. 2007;66:703-8. https://doi.org/10.1111/j.1365- 2265.2007.02805.x.

14. Canu L, Van Hemert JA, Kerstens MN, et al. CT characteristics of pheochromocytoma: relevance for the evaluation of adrenal incidentaloma. J Clin Endocrinol Metab. 2019;104:312-8. https:// doi.org/10.1210/jc.2018-01532.

15. Buitenwerf E, Korteweg T, Visser A, et al. Unenhanced CT imaging is highly sensitive to exclude pheochromocytoma: a multicenter study. Eur J Endocrinol. 2018;178:431-7. https://doi.org/10.1530/EJE-18-0006.

16. Gruber LM, Strajina V, Bancos I, et al. Not all adrenal incidentalomas require biochemical testing to exclude pheochromocytoma: Mayo clinic experience and a meta-analysis. Gland Surg. 2020;9:362. https://doi.org/10.21037/gs.2020.03.04.

17. Allolio B, Fassnacht M. Clinical review: adrenocortical carcinoma; clinical update. J Clin Endocrinol Metab. 2006;91:2027-37. https://doi.org/10.1210/jc.2005-2639.

18. Young WF Jr. The incidentally discovered adrenal mass. N Engl J Med. 2007;356:601-10. https://doi.org/10.1056/NEJMcp065470.

19. Pena CS, Boland GW, Hahn PF, et al. Characterization of indeterminate (lipid-poor) adrenal masses: use of washout characteristics at contrast-enhanced CT. Radiology. 2000;217:798-802. https://doi.org/10.1148/radiology.217.3.r00dc29798.

20. Szolar DH, Kammerhuber FH. Adrenal adenomas and non-adenomas: assessment of washout at delayed contrast-enhanced CT. Radiology. 1998;207:369-75. https://doi.org/10.1148/radiology.207.2.9577483.

21. Akbulut S, Erten O, Kahramangil B, et al. A critical analysis of computed tomography washout in lipid-poor adrenal incidentalomas. Ann Surg Oncol. 2021;28:2756-62. https://doi.org/10.1245/s10434-020-09329-1.

22. Schieda N, Siegelman ES. Update on CT and MRI of adrenal nodules. Am J Roentgenol. 2017;208:1206-17. https://doi.org/10.2214/AJR.16.17758.

23. Schieda N, Al Dandan O, Kielar AZ, et al. Pitfalls of adrenal imaging with chemical shift MRI. Clin Radiol. 2014;69:1186-97. https://doi. org/10.1016/j.crad.2014.06.020.

24. Haider MA, Ghai S, Jhaveri K, et al. Chemical-shift MR imaging of hyperattenuating (>10 HU) adrenal masses: does it still have a role? Radiology. 2004;231:711-6. https://doi.org/10.1148/radiol.2313030676.
25. Fassnacht M, et al. European Society of Endocrinology Clinical Practice Guidelines on the Management of Adrenocortical Carcinoma in Adults, in collaboration with the European Network for the Study of Adrenal Tumours. Eur J Endocrinol. 2018;179:1–46
26. Mody MK, Kazerooni EA, Korobkin M. Percutaneous CT-guided biopsy of adrenal masses: immediate and delayed complications. J Comp Assist Tomograph. 1995;19:434-9. https://doi. org/10.1097/00004728-199505000-00017.
27. Gagner M, Lacroix A, Bolté E. Laparoscopic adrenalectomy in Cushing's syndrome and pheochromocytoma. N Engl J Med. 1992;327(14):1033
28. Agarwal G, Dhalapathy S, Aggarwal V, Chand G, Mishra A, Agarwal A, Verma AK, Mishra SK. Surgical management of organ contained unilateral pheochromocytoma: comparative outcomes of laparoscopic and conventional open surgical procedures in a large single institution series. "Langenbeck's Arch Surg" 2012.
29. Walz M. Posterior retroperitoneoscopic adrenalectomy. In: Linos D, van Heerden J (Eds). Adrenal Glands. Berlin: Springer-Verlag; 2005.
30. Kiriakopoulos A, Economopoulos KP, Poulios E, et al. Impact of posterior retroperitoneoscopic adrenalectomy in a tertiary care center: a paradigm shift. Surg Endosc. 2011;25(11):3584-9.
31. Bhargav PRK, Mishra A, Agarwal G, Agarwal A, Verma AK, Mishra SK. Adrenal incidentalomas: experience in a developing country. 2008;32(8):1802-08. doi:10.1007/s00268-008-9550-8.
32. Townsend CM. In: Sabiston Textbook of Surgery: The Biological Basis of Modern Surgical Practice. St Louis, MO: Elsevier; 2022. p. 976–8.
33. Mohanta B, Anbarasu KR, Dabadghao P, Agarwal G, Pradhan M. Abstract 52: Pheochromocytoma in pregnancy. Indian Journal of Endocrinology and Metabolism. 2022;26(8):22. doi: 10.4103/2230-8210.363740.
34. Linos DA. Management approaches to adrenal incidentalomas (adrenalomas). A view from Athens, Greece. Endocrinol Metab Clin North Am. 2000;29(1): 141-57.
35. Funder JW, Carey RM, Mantero F, et al. The management of primary aldosteronism: case detection, diagnosis, and treatment: an Endocrine Society clinical practice guideline. J Clin Endocrinol Metab. 2016;101:1889-916.
36. Williams TA, Lenders JWM, Mulatero P, et al. Outcomes after adrenalectomy for unilateral primary aldosteronism: an international consensus on outcome measures and analysis of remission rates in an international cohort. Lancet Diabetes Endocrinol. 2017;5:689-99.
37. Pasternak JD, Epelboym I, Seiser N, et al. Diagnostic utility of data from adrenal venous sampling for primary aldosteronism despite failed cannulation of the right adrenal vein. Surgery. 2016;159:267-73.
38. Wooten MD, King DK: Adrenal cortical carcinoma: epidemiology and treatment with mitotane and a review of the literature. Cancer. 1993;72(11):3145-55.
39. Kassi E, Kaltsas G, Zografos G, Chrousos G. Current issues in the diagnosis and management of adrenocortical carcinomas. Expert Review of Endocrinology and Metabolism. 2010;5(3):451-66. Doi:10.1586/eem.10.6.

40. Zini L, Porpiglia F, Fassnacht M. Contemporary management of adrenocortical carcinoma. Eur Urol. 2011;60:1055-65.
41. Zhang HM, Perrier ND, Grubbs EG, Sircar K, Ye ZX, Lee JE et al. CT features and quantification of the characteristics of adrenocortical carcinomas on unenhanced and contrast-enhanced studies. Clin Radiol. 2012;67:38-46.
42. Hahner S, Stuermer A, Kreissl M, Reiners C, Fassnacht M, Haenscheid H et al. [123I]iodometomidate for molecular imaging of adrenocortical cytochrome P450 family 11B enzymes. J Clin Endocrinol Metab. 2008;93:2358-65.
43. Ip JC, Pang TC, Glover AR, Soon P, Clarke S, Richardson A, et al. Improving outcomes in adrenocortical cancer: an Australian perspective. Ann Surg Oncol. 2015;22:2309-16. Adrenal Surgery Practice Guidance for the UK, 2016.
44. Autorino R, Bove P, De Sio M, Miano R, Micali S, Cindolo L, et al. Open versus laparoscopic adrenalectomy for adrenocortical carcinoma: a meta-analysis of surgical and oncological outcomes. Ann Surg Oncol. 2016;23(4):1195-202. doi: 10.1245/s10434-015-4900-x. Epub 2015 Oct 19. PMID: 26480850.
45. Terzolo M, Stigliano A, Chiodini I, Loli P, Furlani L, Arnaldi G, et al. Italian Association of Clinical Endocrinologists. Eur J Endocrinol. 2011;164(6):851. Epub 2011 Apr 6.

CHAPTER 10

Enhanced Recovery After Surgery for Gastrointestinal Surgery

Vikram Kate, Likhita Subhash Singh, Gurushankari Balakrishnan, N Ananthakrishnan

■ INTRODUCTION

The revolutionary concept of promoting Early Recovery After Surgery (ERAS), postulated by Henrik Kehlet, was first documented in colonic surgery in the 1990s. It soon became popular as these measures translated into faster patient recovery after different types of surgery across various specialties. Surgery performed to ameliorate a disease condition induces a stress response in patients, which, in turn, can lead to complications.[1] Generations of surgeons have devised protocols to avoid these complications. Some of these include the need for preoperative prolonged fasting, mechanical bowel preparation (MBP) to prevent intraoperative contamination, prolonged gastric decompression with nasogastric (NG) tube, and postoperative prolonged fasting after surgery to allow anastomotic site healing. Intra-abdominal drain placement following gastrointestinal (GI) surgery in order to prevent intra-abdominal collection and for early detection of complications such as gastrointestinal and biliary leak and hemorrhage. Prolonged immobilization and indwelling urinary catheter were recommended to facilitate abdominal wall healing. These abovementioned principles were often based on individual or group experiences and were not supported by appropriate evidence. Several multi-institutional studies have deemed these practices unnecessary and detrimental.[2]

Recent advancements in the field of surgery and anesthesia along with multimodal treatment approaches have led to path-breaking interventions and ERAS protocols that are evidence-based.[3] In the era of evidence-based medicine, the current protocols streamline perioperative care, minimizing surgical pain and enhancing recovery, diminishing complications, facilitating early hospital discharge, improving overall outcomes, and further working toward advances and betterment of patient care. ERAS protocols need advanced planning and forethought with several healthcare professionals and patients working in synergy with each other. This poses a challenge to ERAS in certain elective surgeries due to different surgical demands and in emergency settings where the preoperative period is limited.[4] Hence, adaptation to the standard ERAS Society guidelines is imperative for implementing them to diverse surgical specialties and different populations. The adapted ERAS protocols have been practiced and have documented better outcomes in a wide range of elective and emergency surgeries.[5]

SURGICAL STRESS RESPONSE AND ROLE OF EARLY RECOVERY AFTER SURGERY

Surgical interventions trigger a reflex response pathway that is mediated by the autonomic nervous system (sympathetic) and by the endocrine system (hypothalamic–pituitary–adrenal axis), increasing the production of catecholamines, glucagon, and glucocorticoids.[1] This integrated and coordinated metabolic response to stress is characterized by changes in cardiovascular tone, respiratory pattern, GI dysfunction, immune depression, inflammatory reaction, protein catabolism, and alterations in intermediary metabolism, which leads to a state of postoperative insulin resistance and hyperglycemia resulting in delayed recovery.[6] Effectively modifying these responses to attenuate the impact of surgery can help to reduce postoperative complications and promote early recovery. The factors involved in surgical stress response are depicted in **Flowchart 1**.

Post surgical stress, there is an increase in the levels of various counter-regulatory hormones such as adrenaline, adrenocorticotropic hormone (ACTH), cortisol, and glucagon as a result of the neurohormonal response, which leads to a catabolic state.[1] Interleukin-6 (IL-6) and tumor necrosis factor (TNF), which are hepatic acute phase response mediators, diminish the responsiveness of insulin-regulated peripheral transport proteins and when coupled with low insulin production can lead to temporary insulin resistance in peripheral tissues. This leads to organ dysfunction and thus postoperative morbidity.[6] Several factors such as pain, starvation, tissue edema, hypothermia, and immobilization compound the response to

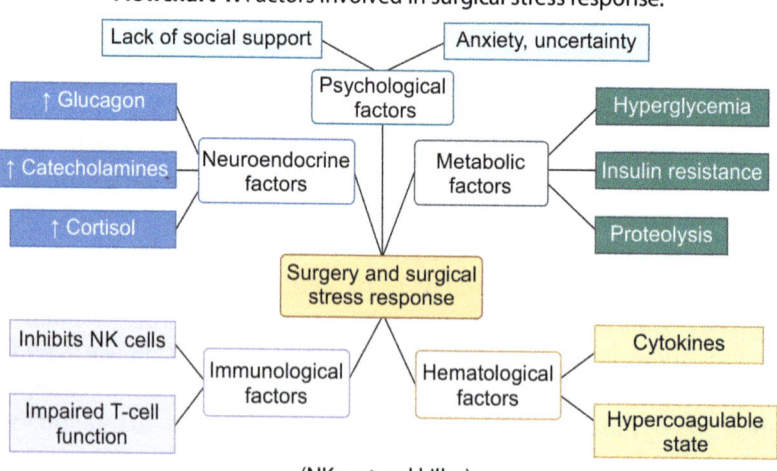

Flowchart 1: Factors involved in surgical stress response.

(NK: natural killer)

injury. ERAS program aims at modifying these factors by suppressing the neurohormonal responses.

The ERAS protocol utilizes specific regional anesthesia techniques that suppress these neuroendocrine responses, thus reducing protein breakdown and glucose intolerance. This neurogenic blockade, however, has no effect on the inflammatory and immunological response.[3] Minimizing preoperative starvation by administration of clear carbohydrate-rich liquids 2 hours prior to surgery, early resumption of enteral feeds, and early mobilization postoperatively help in reducing insulin resistance.[6] Muscle wasting is reduced by early mobilization, which also decreases the risk of thromboembolic events. This protocol has proven benefits in cardiopulmonary functions and in pain management in the postoperative period. The use of minimally invasive techniques reduces the inflammatory response and may not have an effect on the endocrine response. Preoperative optimization, which is a key component of the ERAS protocol, aids in coping with stress better and alleviates anxiety, thus resulting in enhanced recovery.[7]

COMPONENTS OF EARLY RECOVERY AFTER SURGERY

The core principles of ERAS are based on the prevention of catabolism in the perioperative period and the reduction of any intervention that may be deemed avoidable or may impede patient mobilization in any way.

The recommendations for care at every step of surgery are provided by the ERAS protocol, which was developed by the ERAS Society and is constantly evolving.[8] Traditionally, ERAS pathways are divided into the following components:
- Preoperative
- Intraoperative
- Postoperative

Preoperative

Preoperative Counseling

A well-informed patient is a less anxious patient. Counseling provided to the patient prior to the surgery, either orally or in written form, has been shown to improve recovery. Providing the patient with easily understandable information about the procedure, expected postoperative recovery time, and day-specific targets with respect to oral feeding, mobilization, and other aspects of perioperative care, empowers the patient to be a stakeholder in their recovery and has been shown to reduce the rate of complications.[9]

Risk Stratification

It has been shown that the majority of postoperative mortality occurs in high-risk groups, which are susceptible to complications following major surgery.

Therefore, it becomes important to identify these patients beforehand. The American Society of Anesthesiologists' (ASA) physical status score, early warning scores, and certain case-specific scores such as P-POSSUM (Portsmouth Physiological and Operative Severity Score for the enUmeration of Mortality) score and Mannheim peritonitis index (MPI) help us predict the risk of mortality and morbidity in a patient. The cardiovascular risk in patients undergoing noncardiac surgery can be assessed with the help of Lee index, cardiovascular risk calculator, etc.[10] It is also important to assess the functional capacity of the individual in terms of metabolic equivalents (METs) or by using dynamic tests such as walk tests, handgrip dynamometry, or cardiopulmonary exercise testing (CPET).

Optimization of Comorbidities and Addictions

Smoking and alcohol consumption have shown to have a higher risk of intraoperative bleeding and delayed wound healing.[7,11] A minimum period of abstinence from alcohol and smoking for 4 weeks preoperatively is recommended to minimize these effects on the body. Anemia has also been linked to adverse postoperative outcomes and its correction preoperatively has been advised. Preoperative correction of anemia based on the etiology is advised.[12] Other comorbidities such as uncontrolled hypertension, diabetes mellitus, and asthma should also be brought under control prior to surgery. Malnutrition in patients planned for surgery is an important concern, particularly in the Indian context, and requires proper assessment and optimization.[13]

Avoidance of Fasting and Carbohydrate Loading

One of the key elements in the ERAS protocol is the elimination of overnight fasting prior to surgery, which has been shown to increase intraoperative hypoglycemia and insulin resistance, leading to adverse outcomes postoperatively.[6] The current recommendation is that patients can take clear fluids up to 2 hours prior to induction. Preoperative loading with a drink made of simple or complex carbohydrates (maltodextrin) has been shown to be beneficial in this regard, to counteract the effects of perioperative insulin resistance.[14] However, caution should be exercised while administering the same in patients with disorders causing delayed gastric emptying (DGE).

Preanesthetic Medications

Prophylactic intravenous antibiotics should be administered 60 minutes prior to skin incision. Using a chlorhexidine-based solution, decontamination of the skin should be performed prior to incision.[8] It is recommended that long-acting sedatives and opioids be avoided as they prolong the time taken for mobilizing the patient postoperatively. Analgesics such as gabapentinoids (gabapentin/pregabalin) and acetaminophen are recommended in colorectal surgeries and in certain emergency surgeries.[8]

Bowel Preparation

Historically, the role of preoperative bowel preparation has been controversial. Present guidelines state that there is no benefit to using MBP alone; on the other hand, it may result in dehydration. Although there is a doubtful advantage of using MBP along with oral antibiotics, ERAS guidelines do not recommend MBP.[15]

Prevention of Postoperative Nausea/Vomiting

Scoring systems such as Apfel score have been developed to identify patients at a high risk of developing postoperative nausea/vomiting (PONV).[16] It is recommended that patients with ≥2 risk factors receive two to three prophylactic antiemetics.[8] If there is PONV despite prophylaxis, then rescue therapy with a different class of antiemetics is recommended.

Intraoperative

Standard Anesthetic Protocol

Short-acting agents are preferred as they tend to have less residual effects at the end of the procedure.[8] Rapid sequence of induction and intubation has shown better outcomes with a lower risk of aspiration after induction and better control of airway in compromised high-risk patients in emergency laparotomy (EL). Monitoring of depth of anesthesia and cerebral function using bispectral index/alternatives such as electroencephalogram (EEG) and maintaining it within the target range may aid in better anesthetic delivery. Neuromuscular blockade must be monitored using ulnar nerve stimulation with quantitative train of four (TOF) assessment in abductor pollicis longus and should be completely reversed at the end of the procedure, to avoid postoperative respiratory complications.[17]

Goal-directed Fluid Therapy

The ERAS protocol aims to avoid fluid overload, which usually occurs due to intraoperative crystalloid administration. Goal-directed fluid therapy (GDFT) is based on the principle of using cardiac output monitoring to assess the volume status and guide administration of fluid and vasopressors with a target to maintain mean arterial pressure (MAP) of 60–65 mm Hg and cardiac index of 2.2 L/min/m^2.[17] Recent advances in technology and ultrasonography techniques make cardiac output monitoring, measurements of stroke volume, stroke volume variation (SVV), pulse pressure variation (PVV), and cardiac index feasible through modalities such as minimally invasive cardiac output devices, transthoracic echocardiography (TTE), and bedside ultrasound by trained personnel. Studies have shown that applying GDFT in patients is associated with a reduced hospital stay, morbidity, and faster recovery of bowel functions. Perioperative weight gain should be restricted below 2.5 kg in elective surgery.[8] Patients with reduced cardiac contractility may be considered for receiving inotropes therapy.[18]

Intraoperative Normothermia

Perioperative hypothermia is strongly associated with increased mortality and morbidity. Monitoring of core body temperature and deploying measures to maintain normothermia using warm intravenous fluids, warming blankets, and humidification of anesthetic gases are important.

Surgical Approaches

Minimally invasive approaches have been consistently shown to be associated with better postoperative recovery and earlier discharge when compared to the traditional or open approach. Minimally invasive techniques also aid in better delivery of ERAS protocol elements, such as avoiding opioid analgesia and giving GDFT.[8]

Usage of Abdominal Drains

It has been shown in multiple large trials that the routine usage of abdominal drains does not confer any benefit with respect to anastomotic leakage, wound infection, or mortality.[3]

Postoperative

Removal of Drain and Tubes

Routine usage of NG drainage by means of an NG tube increases the chance of respiratory infections and pharyngolaryngitis postoperatively, leading to a delay in starting oral feeds. Avoidance of routine NG tube usage is also associated with faster bowel recovery.[19] Hence, routine usage of NG tube is not recommended, and if placed, they must be removed before reversing the anesthesia.[8] Earlier removal of urinary catheters is associated with lower rates of urinary tract infection (UTI). Ideally, catheters should be removed on the day following surgery, unless otherwise indicated by patient-specific or surgery-specific concerns.[8] It is also advisable to remove the abdominal drains if placed at the earliest.

Postoperative Pain Relief

Usage of analgesic drugs from different classes and avoidance of opioids form the cornerstone of pain management under ERAS. Paracetamol and nonsteroidal anti-inflammatory drugs (NSAIDs) should be given initially. Infiltration of the surgical site with local anesthetic agents may also be of use.[20] While usage of thoracic epidural analgesia has shown clear benefit in case of laparotomy, its advantage over other modes of analgesia in case of laparoscopic procedures is unclear.[8] Spinal anesthesia with long-acting opioids, when used as an adjunct with general anesthesia, allows reduction of postoperative opioid use. Perioperative continuous infusion of lidocaine also helps reduce PONV and postoperative opioid consumption.[21]

Recently, local anesthetic blockade of the abdominal wall has been studied extensively. Of these, transversus abdominis plane (TAP) blocks have shown benefits in a wide range of surgical procedures and are also associated with earlier recovery of bowel functions.[22] Patient-controlled analgesia (PCA) is also one of the modalities to relieve postoperative pain.

Thromboprophylaxis

Current guidelines state that patients undergoing major abdominal surgery must receive both pharmacological and mechanical thromboprophylaxis, in the form of low-molecular-weight heparin (single daily dose) and compression stockings and/or intermittent pneumatic compression, until the patient is fully mobilized.[8]

Prevention of Postoperative Ileus

Several components of the ERAS protocol such as limiting opioids, minimally invasive approaches, GDFT, and avoiding routine use of NG tube act synergistically to reduce the development of postoperative ileus.[8] In addition to these, interventions such as chewing gum and peripheral opioid antagonists such as alvimopan, bisacodyl, and coffee have also been tried, but with doubtful benefit.[23]

Achievement of Early Milestones of Functional Recovery

A Cochrane review has concluded that there is no obvious benefit in keeping the patients "nil per oral" following GI surgery.[24] The current guidelines recommend that the patient be started on orals on the day of surgery. In fact, it has been shown that it is safe to start orals as early as 4 hours following colorectal surgery.[25] Rather than starting patients on a clear liquid diet after surgery, a low residue diet has shown an advantage in terms of less PONV and ileus.[26] Even for patients undergoing gastrectomy, it is advised that they be allowed food and drink according to their tolerance, from the day following surgery.

Prolonged immobilization following surgery is associated with several life-threatening complications such as respiratory infections, bedsores, and pulmonary thromboembolism. Therefore, it is crucial that patients start mobilizing as soon as possible in the postoperative period. Critically ill patients who are unable to walk may be subjected to simple activities such as sitting or standing. It is also important to address other factors that may be confining the patient to the bed, such as inadequate analgesia, tubes, drains, and catheters, continuous intravenous fluids, lack of awareness, and lack of encouragement.[8] Early mobilization of the patient has been significantly associated with a successful outcome in patients in an ERAS pathway.

A comparison of conventional practices in perioperative care and ERAS protocols is depicted in **Table 1**. Adherence to these elements is important and it involves a multidisciplinary team approach, a collaboration in diversity for a successful outcome **(Figs. 1 and 2)**.

EARLY RECOVERY AFTER SURGERY IN ELECTIVE ABDOMINAL SURGERIES

Early Recovery After Surgery in Elective Colorectal Surgeries

Colorectal surgeries were one of the first areas where a fast-track pathway was studied, and it still remains the most studied with respect to ERAS. The ERAS Society has released a set of standard guidelines to be followed in colorectal surgeries, first in 2013 and a revised version in 2018.[8] There is strong evidence to suggest that implementation of ERAS in elective colorectal surgeries reduces the length of hospital stay significantly without increasing the readmission rates, supported by multiple meta-analyses.[27,28] Other observational studies showed a decrease in UTIs with the implementation of ERAS.[29] It is also seen that the effectiveness of ERAS protocol strongly correlates with the number of items implemented and adhered to, to the extent that adherence to five or less items in the protocol led to threefold prolongation of the length of hospitalization (LOH).[30]

Madan et al., carried out a study on the application of ERAS protocols on patients undergoing elective stoma reversal and it was found that the LOH was significantly shorter by 1.73 days in the ERAS arm.[31] The ERAS group had early functional recovery when compared to standard care in terms of early enteral feeds, time to first defecation, and early mobilization along with no increase in postoperative complications. Currently, the focus is on measures to increase the adherence to the ERAS protocol in colorectal surgeries by extensive data collection and audit and also to develop institute-specific protocols that are locally appropriate, using the standard guidelines as a blueprint.

Early Recovery After Surgery in Elective Upper Gastrointestinal Surgeries

Though surgeries performed in the upper GI tract may be considered a "late adopter" of ERAS protocols, recent years have seen growing evidence in

TABLE 1: Elements of enhanced recovery protocols versus conventional care.

Enhanced recovery after surgery	Standard care

Preadmission/preoperative:
• Preadmission information, education, and counseling
• *Preoperative optimization:*
  – Risk assessment
  – Smoking cessation and abstinence from alcohol for at least 4 weeks prior to surgery
• Prehabilitation
• Preoperative nutritional care
• Management of anemia based on etiology over routine preoperative blood transfusions
• Postoperative nausea and vomiting prophylaxis based on Apfel score
• Antimicrobial prophylaxis
• Bowel preparation—no MBP
• Avoid salt and water overload
• No prolonged fasting. Allow carbohydrate-rich clear liquids till 2 hours prior to surgery
• Preanesthetic medication—short-acting anxiolytics
	• Information about surgical procedure is usually given just 1 day prior to surgery while taking consent
	• Preanesthetic checkup and risk stratification as per ASA classification
	• *Optimization:* Focused only on major comorbidities (HTN, DM, asthma). Smoking cessation and abstinence from alcohol is not given much consideration
	• Prolonged preoperative fasting—as solids are restricted 8–12 hours prior to surgery
	• Maintenance of IV fluids
	• MBP based on surgeon's decision
	• Antibiotic prophylaxis
	• Anxiolytics—long-acting benzodiazepines

Intraoperative: • *Anesthesia:* Use short-acting anesthetic agents and opioid-free analgesics. Prefer NMB with agents that have SRBA for reversal, e.g., rocuronium which can be reversed by sugammadex • GDFT • Normothermia • Minimally invasive surgery • No abdominal drains	• Standard anesthetic protocols do not have restrictions on the use of opioids for analgesia and benzodiazepines for sedation • IV fluid therapy is guided by endpoints such as urine output, BP, HR, and clinical judgment • NG tube insertion • Routine use of abdominal drains
Postoperative: • No NG drain • Multimodal analgesia—epidural/TAP block • Thromboprophylaxis • *Postoperative fluid and electrolyte therapy:* Balanced crystalloids to achieve net "near-zero" fluid balance • Early removal of urinary catheter • Prevention of postoperative ileus—chewing gums, peripheral opioid receptor blockers, prokinetics • Early enteral nutrition • Early mobilization • Audit of compliance and outcomes	• Removal of NG tube on surgeon's discretion • Abdominal drains are usually once the patient tolerates unrestricted liquid diet for at least 24 hours and drain output shows a reducing trend • Urinary catheters are removed after patient maintains urine output of 1 mL/kg/h for 24 hours • Use of opioid analgesics in the immediate postoperation is a common practice, which can later be difficult to wean

(ASA: American Society of Anesthesiologists; BP: blood pressure; DM: diabetes mellitus; GDFT: goal-directed fluid therapy; HR: heart rate; HTN: hypertension; IV: intravenous; MBP: mechanical bowel preparation; NG: nasogastric; NMB: neuromuscular blockade; SRBA: selective relaxant binding agent; TAP: transversus abdominis plane)

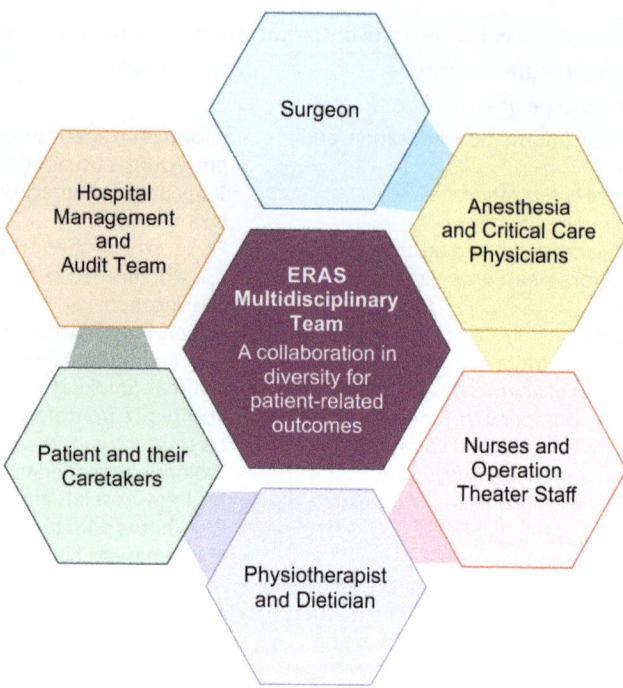

Fig. 1: Enhanced recovery after surgery (ERAS) is a multidisciplinary team approach.

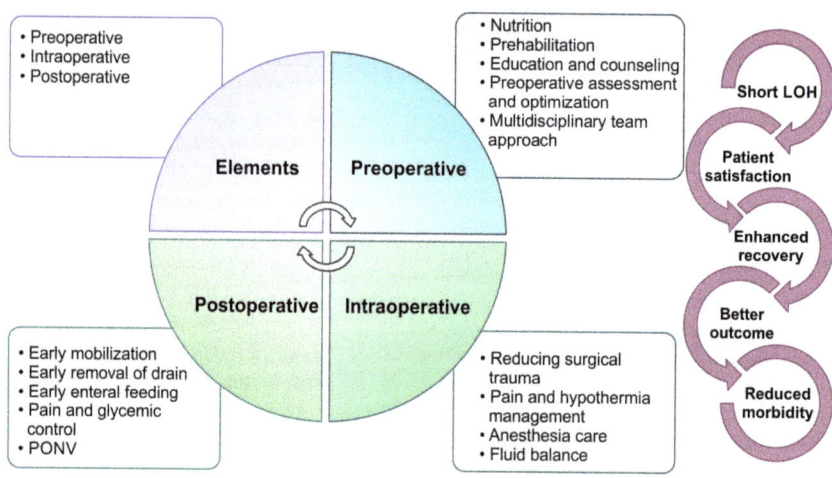

Fig. 2: Elements of Enhanced Recovery After Surgery. (LOH: length of hospitalization; PONV: postoperative nausea/vomiting)

this area. One of the early procedures for the ERAS protocol was gastrectomy. A recent meta-analysis of 18 randomized controlled trials (RCTs) has shown that patients in the ERAS arm had a reduction in the length of hospital stay and that the difference was more pronounced in open surgeries than in laparoscopic procedures.[32] Hospital costs too were found to be significantly lesser in case of ERAS patients in all these trials. Functional bowel recovery was faster, with a shorter time to first flatus, first stool, first walk, and oral intake. Apart from a reduction in pulmonary complications, rates of other complications remained the same between ERAS and standard care groups. However, the rate of readmissions was found to be higher in case of ERAS patients in one meta-analysis.[33] This could possibly be attributed to poor or incomplete compliance to the ERAS protocol. There is also inadequate evidence regarding the outcomes for individual components of the ERAS protocol for gastric resections. Swaminathan et al., highlighted the implementation of respiratory prehabilitation with the ERAS protocol in elective gastrectomy.[34] A total of 58 patients were randomized into two groups, conventional perioperative care and ERAS care. The ERAS group had a significantly shorter LOH (11 vs. 13 days) and a better pulmonary function test profile indicated by smaller fall in postoperative peak expiratory flow rate (PEFR) from baseline postoperatively.

Early Recovery After Surgery in esophagectomy is a relatively new concept as it is associated with relatively higher mortality and morbidity. In 2019, the ERAS Society guidelines for perioperative care in esophagectomy were released.[35] Among others, it recommended starting early enteral nutrition and routine use of NG tube for decompression but advising an early removal [on postoperative day 2 (POD2)] when possible. A meta-analysis showed that ERAS in esophagectomy lowered the cost, days of hospital stay, and pulmonary complications but not other morbidities.[36] More studies are needed for ERAS in esophagectomy before concrete, procedure-specific conclusions can be drawn.

Early Recovery After Surgery in Hepatopancreaticobiliary Surgeries

The ERAS protocol has been considered in liver resections and pancreaticoduodenectomies (PD). With respect to PD, there have been a few trials and meta-analyses with conflicting results.[37] A recent meta-analysis, with a total of 22 trials, with 3 RCTs showed that minor morbidity (Clavien–Dindo grades I and II) was significantly lower in the ERAS group.[37] Major complications and the rate of postoperative pancreatic fistula were comparable between the ERAS group and the control group. Few studies showed that the length of hospital stay and readmission rates were comparable between the two groups.[38,39] Implementing ERAS also reduced the rates of surgical site infection (SSI) and DGE postoperatively.

The ERAS Society guidelines for hepatectomy (in noncirrhotic patients) were published in 2016 with 23 items. Among other recommendations, they advocated for using an omental flap to prevent the development of DGE and a minimally invasive approach wherever applicable.[40] Though we are still in the nascent stage with respect to liver resection, a meta-analysis of trials published so far showed a decrease in hospital stay, intensive care unit (ICU) stay, and complications with the implementation of ERAS.[41]

ROLE OF EARLY RECOVERY AFTER SURGERY IN EMERGENCY GASTROINTESTINAL SURGERIES

The possible role of ERAS in emergency setting was realized as early as 2009 when the ERAS guideline stated that "every attempt should be made to implement as many components as possible in the context of emergency setting," though the extent of its implementation is not certain. In an emergency, implementing most of the components of the ERAS protocol has several challenges. One major challenge is the execution of the preoperative components, which may not always be feasible owing to the nature of the disease in emergency settings. However, many of the intra- and postoperative elements are applicable to most emergency patients.[42] It has been reported that the mortality rates of emergency surgeries are higher compared to elective surgeries even in developed countries. Therefore, it is necessary that we improve the standard of care of emergency surgeries. Mohsina et al., reported a lower hospital mortality in patients undergoing emergency simple closure of a perforated duodenal ulcer.[43] Procedures similar to various components of fast-track protocols were used by the above three studies, thus proving that with a good understanding of current practices and identifying the barriers and enablers, the benefits of ERAS protocols can be extended to emergency patients. In 2020, a meta-analysis on ERAS in emergency abdominal surgeries reported reduction of LOH, lower rate of complications, earlier resumption of bowel functions and oral intake, with similar mortality and 30-day readmission rate.[44] Preoperative elements such as full optimization of comorbidities and preoperative carbohydrate loading cannot be implemented in the emergency setting, while a brief counseling of the patient, opioid-free analgesics, and premedication is feasible. Hence, a modified protocol may be applied in emergencies.

Data on ERAS in emergency is limited, which needs to be the focus of future research. Gonec et al., in 2013 published the first RCT which studied the feasibility of ERAS pathways on patients who underwent repair of perforated peptic ulcer disease laparoscopically. This study showed a significant reduction in the LOH from 6.9 days (control) to 3.8 days in the ERAS arm. Small sample size and exclusion of high-risk patients, however, limited the value of the study.[45] Following this, a larger study by Mohsina et al., on ERAS in perforated duodenal ulcer patients was done. The study showed a significant reduction of LOH by 4.41 days in the ERAS arm, with the patients in that arm having a significantly earlier resolution of ileus, resumption of orals, with lesser rates of PONV, superficial SSI, UTI, and pulmonary complications. ERAS also reduced the need for extra analgesia postoperatively.[43] The first study on the application of ERAS protocol in emergency colorectal surgery reported significant reduction in the hospital stay. They also found that the patients in the ERAS arm were able to receive adjuvant chemotherapy earlier, when compared to the controls. Shida et al., published a similar study, which also studied a subjective parameter—the patient's assessment of quality of recovery—which was found to be similar to those undergoing elective colorectal surgery.[46]

A propensity-matched case–control study from China, across four centers, over a period of 8 years, on 839 patients with colorectal malignancy undergoing emergent resection showed a significant reduction in postoperative complications, a 3-day reduction in LOH, reduced time to GI recovery, and diminished interval between surgery and adjuvant chemotherapy.[47] Wisely and Barclay performed a retrospective records-based analysis on 370 patients who underwent major lower GI surgeries as an emergency, before and after the implementation of the ERAS protocol in their center. They found a reduction in the rates of urinary and pulmonary complications but did not find any reduction in the LOH or GI recovery.[48]

A recent review noted that there were no RCTs pertaining to ERAS in colorectal surgeries.[49] Apart from comparing ERAS versus standard care in emergency colorectal resections, the review also looked at the ERAS protocol as applied to elective colorectal surgery and emergency colorectal surgery. Both the studies in this regard showed a shorter hospital stay in the ERAS group and overall lesser compliance with ERAS protocols in emergency.

Saurabh et al., used an adapted ERAS protocol in patients operated primarily for acute intestinal obstruction, perforation, or gut gangrene, undergoing resection and anastomosis, simple closure of perforation, or ileostomy.[50] A reduced LOH by 2.83 days, with a significant decrease in time to resumption of bowel function, orals, and mobilization, was documented. The rate of complications was comparable across the groups. Pranavi et al., used adapted ERAS protocols in patients undergoing emergency surgeries for perforation peritonitis.[51] A total of 120 patients were randomized into 2 arms, 61 in ERAS group and 59 in control group, and it was noted that LOH reduced by 3 days in the ERAS group when compared to the standard protocol group. Certain factors such as high output stoma, preexisting malignancies, and respiratory complications were associated with delayed discharge.[51] In a recent study by Likhita, adapted ERAS protocols were used in the entire spectrum of patients with acute abdomen requiring emergency surgery.[52] A reduction in LOH without any significant increase in postoperative complications or morbidity was seen. Furthermore, despite the study being conducted during the COVID-19 pandemic, it was observed that a lower incidence of postoperative pulmonary complications in patients who were treated with the adapted ERAS protocol was noted. These findings suggest that ERAS protocols could represent a valuable tool in the management of patients with acute abdomen requiring emergency surgery while also minimizing postoperative complications. Further, it has been suggested that the ERAS protocol in emergency colorectal surgeries be tailored on the basis of whether intra-abdominal sepsis is present or not.

Early Recovery After Surgery in Emergency Laparotomy—Guidelines

Recently in 2021, the ERAS Society held a meeting to formulate guidelines to establish the role of ERAS in EL.[53] These guidelines have been divided into three parts, with the first part dedicated to preoperative care. Emphasis was given on early warning scores, early diagnosis, and resuscitation in these guidelines. Furthermore, these guidelines highlighted novel aspects such as geriatric care, screening for perioperative neurocognitive disorders, and frailty.[53]

Due to the delay caused by the COVID-19 pandemic, the guideline development group could only be reconvened in 2022 and parts two and three of the ERAS guidelines were published in 2023.[17,54] Part two of these guidelines deals with elements of ERAS in intraoperative and postoperative care. It has a total of 23 components, and the importance of rapid-sequence induction and intubation, depth of anesthesia monitoring, assessment of neuromuscular blockade, and reversal were the focus of the guidelines. Other factors such as restrictive blood transfusion, integrated assessment at the end of surgery for patient evaluation, endotracheal extubation, and utilization of risk scores to protocolize admission to ICU were highlighted.[17]

Part three of the guidelines focuses on the organizational aspects of ERAS implementation in EL and end-of-life care in the "NoLap" population.[54] These guidelines pave way for future scope of development for EL bundle, which consists of high-impact components of ERAS rather than all components, as few studies have shown higher compliance and better outcomes when selected high-impact components of ERAS were implemented.[55] A compilation of all three parts of ERAS-EL guidelines amounts to a total of 40 plus elements. However, some of the important elements are succinctly highlighted in **Box 1**.

A summary of our experience with ERAS pathways in the elective and emergency settings is briefly outlined in **Table 2**. In implementing ERAS, we can encounter impediments that can lead to suboptimal inclusion of ERAS elements, which can result into an unsuccessful outcome. These have been

BOX 1: Adapted enhanced recovery protocols in emergency laparotomy.

Preoperative:
- Identifying physiological derangement rapidly and risk stratification with the aid of early warning scores. Escalation of care to senior personnel on call when high-risk patients are identified
- Screen for sepsis and implement surviving sepsis guidelines without any delay
- Source control by surgery/bedside interventions/interventional radiology-aided procedures—in patients with septic shock <3 hours and in patients with sepsis without shock <6 hours
- Cognitive assessment and evaluation of frailty
- Utilization of point-of-care tests for assessing glycemic status and coagulation profile
- Reversal of anticoagulant medication if any
- Time to surgery after the decision to operate is made should be <6 hours
- *Shared decision-making and improvement of end-of-life care:* Treatment escalation and advance care plans should be discussed and documented after educating the patient and family members about the emergent condition. Consider the patient's goals of care when surgery is palliative or high risk
- Nasogastric intubation is recommended considering the risk of aspiration and gastric distension due to GI dysfunction

Intraoperative:
- Antibiotic prophylaxis, unless already receiving appropriate therapy based on surviving sepsis guidelines
- *Anesthesia:* Rapid-sequence induction, monitoring of depth of anesthesia in patient above 60 years of age considering risk of anesthesia-induced hypotension and postoperative delirium and lung ventilation strategy with low tidal volume and PEEPs (TV = 6–8 mL/kg predicted body weight and PEEP ≥5 cm H_2O)
- Chlorhexidine and alcohol are considered for optimal skin asepsis
- *Measure to reduce SSI:* Use of wound protector, peritoneal lavage in contaminated cases, and change of gloves for abdominal closure
- GDFT
- Restrictive blood transfusion
- *Multimodal analgesia:* Consider abdominal wall blocks, wound catheters or epidural analgesia in cases where sepsis and coagulation abnormalities are ruled out
- Mechanical thromboprophylaxis in patients when pharmacological thromboprophylaxis is not feasible
- End of surgery evaluation and extubation considering high risk of postoperative complication and reintubation
- To prevent postoperative pulmonary complications, consider CPAP/NIV if end-operative ABG shows evidence of hypoxemia
- Establishment of preoperative risk score to determine ICU admission

Postoperative:
- Postoperative delirium screening and prevention (in patients with age >65 years)
- Nasogastric tube removal based on risk of aspiration and gastric stasis on a case-to-case basis
- VTE risk assessment and treatment
- Early removal of urinary catheter
- Enteral feeds initiated within 24 hours post surgery. When enteral feeds are contraindicated/nutrition needs are not met (<50% of calorie requirement) for 7 days, parenteral nutrition is considered
- Early ambulation

(ABG: arterial blood gas; CPAP: continuous positive airway pressure; GDFT: goal-directed fluid therapy; GI: gastrointestinal; ICU: intensive care unit; NIV: noninvasive ventilation; PEEP: positive end-expiratory pressure; SSI: surgical site infection; TV: tidal volume; VTE: venous thromboembolism)

TABLE 2: Enhanced recovery protocol-based studies—our experience.

Trial	Study design	Study population	Sample size			Primary outcome LOH		
			Total	Standard care	ERAS	ERAS vs. standard care (days)	Mean/median difference (in days)	p-value
Emergency:								
Mohsina et al.[43] (2018)	RCT	Perforated duodenal ulcer—emergency open repair	99	49	50	9.78 vs. 5.36	4.42	<0.001
Saurabh et al.[50] (2020)	RCT	Small bowel pathology	70	35	35	10.83 vs. 8	2.83	<0.001
Pranavi et al.[51] (2021)	RCT	Perforation peritonitis (across GI tract)	120	59	61	11 vs. 8	3	<0.001
Likhita[52] (2023)	RCT	Emergency abdominal surgeries	96	47	49	16 vs. 10	6	<0.001
Elective:								
Swaminathan et al.[34] (2020)	RCT	Respiratory prehabilitation in gastrectomy	58	29	29	13 vs. 11	2	0.003
Madan et al.[31] (2023)	RCT	Stoma reversal	80	40	40	7 vs. 5.27	1.73	0.0008

(ERAS: Enhanced recovery after surgery; GI: gastrointestinal; LOH: length of hospitalization; RCT: randomized controlled trial)

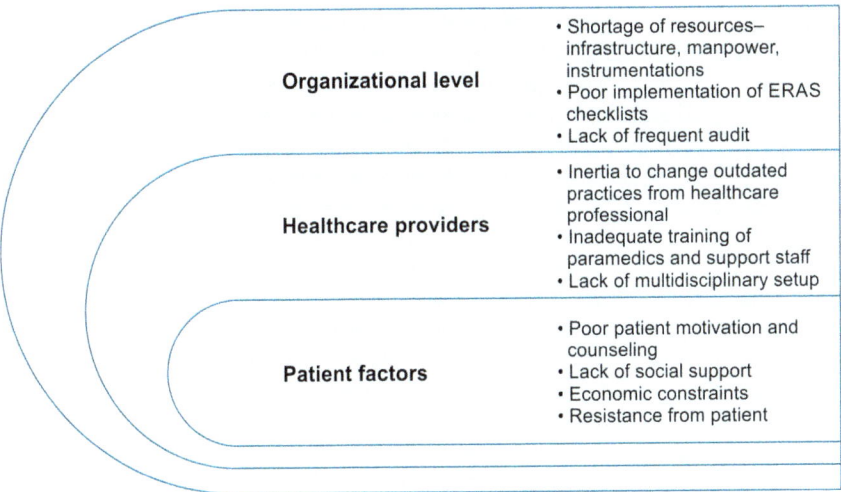

Fig. 3: Impediments that can lead to suboptimal inclusion of enhanced recovery after surgery (ERAS) elements.

summarized in **Figure 3**. Proper actions at the organizational, healthcare provider, and patient levels are important to overcome these for a successful outcome.

CONCLUSION

In the era of evidence-based medicine, the ERAS protocols streamline perioperative care while maintaining normal homeostasis, reducing postsurgical inflammatory response, minimizing surgical pain, and enhancing recovery. These lead to diminishing complications, facilitating early hospital discharge, improved overall outcomes, and betterment of patient care. It also reduces the financial burden and helps in optimizing healthcare resources. ERAS pathways, initiated with elective colorectal surgeries few decades back, now have been extended into emergency procedures and subspecialties. ERAS protocols are now available for upper GI and hepatopancreatobiliary surgeries. The ERAS protocol needs advanced planning and forethought with healthcare professionals and patients working in synergy with each other. Although there are barriers and limitations in implementing ERAS, these can be overcome. A change in practice comes with a change in the thought process and it is time to change practice.

REFERENCES

1. Desborough JP. The stress response to trauma and surgery. Br J Anaesth. 2000;85(1):109-17.

2. Brady M, Kinn S, Stuart P. Preoperative fasting for adults to prevent perioperative complications. Cochrane Database Syst Rev. 2003;(4):CD004423.
3. Carli F, Kehlet H, Baldini G, Steel A, McRae K, Slinger P, et al. Evidence basis for regional anesthesia in multidisciplinary fast-track surgical care pathways. Reg Anesth Pain Med. 2011;36(1):63-72.
4. Quiney N, Aggarwal G, Scott M, Dickinson M. Survival after emergency general surgery: what can we learn from enhanced recovery programmes? World J Surg. 2016;40(6):1283-7.
5. Lyon A, Payne CJ, Mackay GJ. Enhanced recovery programme in colorectal surgery: does one size fit all? World J Gastroenterol. 2012;18(40):5661-3.
6. Ljungqvist O, Jonathan E. Rhoads lecture 2011: insulin resistance and Enhanced Recovery After Surgery. JPEN J Parenter Enteral Nutr. 2012;36(4):389-98.
7. Lindström D, Sadr Azodi O, Wladis A, Tønnesen H, Linder S, Nåsell H, et al. Effects of a perioperative smoking cessation intervention on postoperative complications: a randomized trial. Ann Surg. 2008;248(5):739-45.
8. Gustafsson UO, Scott MJ, Hubner M, Nygren J, Demartines N, Francis N, et al. Guidelines for perioperative care in elective colorectal surgery: Enhanced Recovery After Surgery (ERAS®) Society recommendations: 2018. World J Surg. 2019;43(3):659-95.
9. Clarke HD, Timm VL, Goldberg BR, Hattrup SJ. Preoperative patient education reduces in-hospital falls after total knee arthroplasty. Clin Orthop. 2012;470(1):244-9.
10. Lee TH, Marcantonio ER, Mangione CM, Thomas EJ, Polanczyk CA, Cook EF, et al. Derivation and prospective validation of a simple index for prediction of cardiac risk of major noncardiac surgery. Circulation. 1999;100(10):1043-9.
11. Tonnesen H, Kehlet H. Preoperative alcoholism and postoperative morbidity. Br J Surg. 1999;86(7):869-74.
12. Hare GMT, Baker JE, Pavenski K. Assessment and treatment of preoperative anemia: continuing professional development. Can J Anaesth J Can Anesth. 2011;58(6):569-81.
13. Lawson CM, Daley BJ, Sams VG, Martindale R, Kudsk KA, Miller KR. Factors that impact patient outcome: nutrition assessment. JPEN J Parenter Enteral Nutr. 2013;37(5 Suppl):30S-8S.
14. Karimian N, Kaneva P, Donatelli F, Stein B, Liberman AS, Charlebois P, et al. Simple versus complex preoperative carbohydrate drink to preserve perioperative insulin sensitivity in laparoscopic colectomy: a randomized controlled trial. Ann Surg. 2020;271(5):819-26.
15. Bucher P, Gervaz P, Soravia C, Mermillod B, Erne M, Morel P. Randomized clinical trial of mechanical bowel preparation versus no preparation before elective left-sided colorectal surgery. Br J Surg. 2005;92(4):409-14.
16. Apfel CC, Läärä E, Koivuranta M, Greim CA, Roewer N. A simplified risk score for predicting postoperative nausea and vomiting: conclusions from cross-validations between two centers. Anesthesiology. 1999;91(3):693-700.
17. Scott MJ, Aggarwal G, Aitken RJ, Anderson ID, Balfour A, Foss NB, et al. Consensus guidelines for perioperative care for emergency laparotomy Enhanced Recovery After Surgery (ERAS®) Society recommendations part 2—emergency laparotomy: intra- and postoperative care. World J Surg. 2023;47(8):1850-80.
18. Feldheiser A, Conroy P, Bonomo T, Cox B, Garces TR, Spies C, et al. Development and feasibility study of an algorithm for intraoperative

goaldirected haemodynamic management in noncardiac surgery. J Int Med Res. 2012;40(4):1227-41.
19. Nelson R, Edwards S, Tse B. Prophylactic nasogastric decompression after abdominal surgery. Cochrane Database Syst Rev. 2007;2007(3):CD004929.
20. Hamilton TW, Athanassoglou V, Mellon S, Strickland LH, Trivella M, Murray D, et al. Liposomal bupivacaine infiltration at the surgical site for the management of postoperative pain. Cochrane Database Syst Rev. 2017;2(2):CD011419.
21. Kranke P, Jokinen J, Pace NL, Schnabel A, Hollmann MW, Hahnenkamp K, et al. Continuous intravenous perioperative lidocaine infusion for postoperative pain and recovery. Cochrane Database Syst Rev. 2015;(7):CD009642.
22. Walter CJ, Maxwell-Armstrong C, Pinkney TD, Conaghan PJ, Bedforth N, Gornall CB, et al. A randomised controlled trial of the efficacy of ultrasound-guided transversus abdominis plane (TAP) block in laparoscopic colorectal surgery. Surg Endosc. 2013;27(7):2366-72.
23. Müller SA, Rahbari NN, Schneider F, Warschkow R, Simon T, von Frankenberg M, et al. Randomized clinical trial on the effect of coffee on postoperative ileus following elective colectomy. Br J Surg. 2012;99(11):1530-8.
24. Andersen HK, Lewis SJ, Thomas S. Early enteral nutrition within 24h of colorectal surgery versus later commencement of feeding for postoperative complications. Cochrane Database Syst Rev. 2006;(4):CD004080.
25. Gustafsson UO, Hausel J, Thorell A, Ljungqvist O, Soop M, Nygren J, et al. Adherence to the Enhanced Recovery After Surgery protocol and outcomes after colorectal cancer surgery. Arch Surg. 2011;146(5):571-7.
26. Lau C, Phillips E, Bresee C, Fleshner P. Early use of low residue diet is superior to clear liquid diet after elective colorectal surgery: a randomized controlled trial. Ann Surg. 2014;260(4):641-7; discussion 647-9.
27. Lv L, Shao YF, Zhou YB. The Enhanced Recovery After Surgery (ERAS) pathway for patients undergoing colorectal surgery: an update of meta-analysis of randomized controlled trials. Int J Colorectal Dis. 2012;27(12):1549-54.
28. Tan SJ, Zhou F, Yui WK, Chen QY, Lin ZL, Hu RY, et al. Fast track programmes vs. traditional care in laparoscopic colorectal surgery: a meta-analysis of randomized controlled trials. Hepatogastroenterology. 2014;61(129):79-84.
29. Miller TE, Scott MJ. Enhanced recovery and the changing landscape of major abdominal surgery. Anesthesiol Clin. 2015;33(1):xv-vi.
30. Ban KA, Berian JR, Ko CY. Does implementation of Enhanced Recovery After Surgery (ERAS) protocols in colorectal surgery improve patient outcomes? Clin Colon Rectal Surg. 2019;32(2):109-13.
31. Madan S, Sureshkumar S, Anandhi A, Gurushankari B, Keerthi AR, Palanivel C, et al. Comparison of Enhanced Recovery After Surgery (ERAS) pathway versus standard care in patients undergoing elective stoma reversal surgery—a randomized controlled trial. J Gastrointest Surg. 2023.
32. Lee Y, Yu J, Doumouras AG, Li J, Hong D. Enhanced Recovery After Surgery (ERAS) versus standard recovery for elective gastric cancer surgery: a meta-analysis of randomized controlled trials. Surg Oncol. 2020;32:75-87.
33. Wee IJY, Syn NLX, Shabbir A, Kim G, So JBY. Enhanced recovery versus conventional care in gastric cancer surgery: a meta-analysis of randomized and non-randomized controlled trials. Gastric Cancer. 2019;22(3):423-34.

34. Swaminathan N, Kundra P, Ravi R, Kate V. ERAS protocol with respiratory prehabilitation versus conventional perioperative protocol in elective gastrectomy—a randomized controlled trial. Int J Surg. 2020;81:149-57.
35. Low DE, Allum W, De Manzoni G, Ferri L, Immanuel A, Kuppusamy M, et al. Guidelines for perioperative care in esophagectomy: Enhanced Recovery After Surgery (ERAS®) Society recommendations. World J Surg. 2019;43(2):299-330.
36. Pisarska M, Małczak P, Major P, Wysocki M, Budzyński A, Pędziwiatr M. Enhanced Recovery After Surgery protocol in oesophageal cancer surgery: systematic review and meta-analysis. PLoS One. 2017;12(3):e0174382.
37. Wang XY, Cai JP, Huang CS, Huang XT, Yin XY. Impact of Enhanced Recovery After Surgery protocol on pancreaticoduodenectomy: a meta-analysis of non-randomized and randomized controlled trials. HPB (Oxford). 2020;22(10):1373-83.
38. Takagi K, Yoshida R, Yagi T, Umeda Y, Nobuoka D, Kuise T, et al. Effect of an Enhanced Recovery After Surgery protocol in patients undergoing pancreaticoduodenectomy: a randomized controlled trial. Clin Nutr Edinb Scotl. 2019;38(1):174-81.
39. Hwang DW, Kim HJ, Lee JH, Song KB, Kim MH, Lee SK, et al. Effect of Enhanced Recovery After Surgery program on pancreaticoduodenectomy: a randomized controlled trial. J Hepatobiliary Pancreat Sci. 2019;26(8):360-9.
40. Melloul E, Hübner M, Scott M, Snowden C, Prentis J, Dejong CHC, et al. Guidelines for perioperative care for liver surgery: Enhanced Recovery After Surgery (ERAS) Society recommendations. World J Surg. 2016;40(10):2425-40.
41. Lei Q, Wang X, Tan S, Xia X, Zheng H, Wu C. Fast-track programs versus traditional care in hepatectomy: a meta-analysis of randomized controlled trials. Dig Surg. 2014;31(4-5):392-9.
42. Paduraru M, Ponchietti L, Casas IM, Svenningsen P, Zago M. Enhanced recovery after emergency surgery: a systematic review. Bull Emerg Trauma. 2017;5(2):70-8.
43. Mohsina S, Shanmugam D, Sureshkumar S, Kundra P, Mahalakshmy T, Kate V. Adapted ERAS pathway vs. standard care in patients with perforated duodenal ulcer—a randomized controlled trial. J Gastrointest Surg. 2018;22(1):107-16.
44. Hajibandeh S, Hajibandeh S, Bill V, Satyadas T. Meta-analysis of Enhanced Recovery After Surgery (ERAS) protocols in emergency abdominal surgery. World J Surg. 2020;44(5):1336-48.
45. Gonenc M, Dural AC, Celik F, Akarsu C, Kocatas A, Kalayci MU, et al. Enhanced postoperative recovery pathways in emergency surgery: a randomised controlled clinical trial. Am J Surg. 2014;207(6):807-14.
46. Shida D, Tagawa K, Inada K, Nasu K, Seyama Y, Maeshiro T, et al. Modified Enhanced Recovery After Surgery (ERAS) protocols for patients with obstructive colorectal cancer. BMC Surg. 2017;17(1):18.
47. Shang Y, Guo C, Zhang D. Modified Enhanced Recovery After Surgery protocols are beneficial for postoperative recovery for patients undergoing emergency surgery for obstructive colorectal cancer: a propensity score matching analysis. Medicine (Baltimore). 2018;97(39):e12348.
48. Wisely JC, Barclay KL. Effects of an Enhanced Recovery After Surgery programme on emergency surgical patients. ANZ J Surg. 2016;86(11):883-8.

49. Lohsiriwat V, Jitmungngan R. Enhanced Recovery After Surgery in emergency colorectal surgery: review of literature and current practices. World J Gastrointest Surg. 2019;11(2):41-52.
50. Saurabh K, Sureshkumar S, Mohsina S, Mahalakshmy T, Kundra P, Kate V. Adapted ERAS pathway versus standard care in patients undergoing emergency small bowel surgery: a randomized controlled trial. J Gastrointest Surg. 2020;24(9):2077-87.
51. Pranavi AR, Sureshkumar S, Mahalakshmy T, Kundra P, Kate V. Adapted ERAS pathway versus standard care in patients undergoing emergency surgery for perforation peritonitis—a randomized controlled trial. J Gastrointest Surg. 2022;26(1):39-49.
52. Likhita SS. Adapted Enhanced Recovery After Surgery (ERAS) Pathway Versus Standard Care in Patients Undergoing Emergency Abdominal Surgery—A Randomized Controlled Trial [Dissertation]. Puducherry: Jawaharlal Institute of Postgraduate Medical Education and Research; 2023.
53. Peden CJ, Aggarwal G, Aitken RJ, Anderson ID, Bang Foss N, Cooper Z, et al. Guidelines for perioperative care for emergency laparotomy Enhanced Recovery After Surgery (ERAS) Society recommendations: part 1—preoperative: diagnosis, rapid assessment and optimization. World J Surg. 2021;45(5):1272-90.
54. Peden CJ, Aggarwal G, Aitken RJ, Anderson ID, Balfour A, Foss NB, et al. Enhanced Recovery After Surgery (ERAS®) Society consensus guidelines for emergency laparotomy part 3: organizational aspects and general considerations for management of the emergency laparotomy patient. World J Surg. 2023;47(8):1881-98.
55. Aggarwal G, Peden CJ, Mohammed MA, Pullyblank A, Williams B, Stephens T, et al. Evaluation of the collaborative use of an evidence-based care bundle in emergency laparotomy. JAMA Surg. 2019;154(5):e190145.

CHAPTER 11: Recent Trends in Thoracic Surgery

Belal Bin Asaf, Mohan V Pulle, Arvind Kumar

■ INTRODUCTION

Thoracic surgery has evolved immensely from just being a side hustle of cardiothoracic surgery. Gone are the days when thoracic surgery was considered tuberculosis surgery. The advances in the surgical treatment of noncardiac chest organs, including lungs, pleura, mediastinum, tracheobronchial tree, esophagus, chest wall and diaphragm, and strides, made in the field of lung transplantation have brought thoracic surgery to the forefront and have established it as a separate specialty in many institutions both in India and abroad. There has been a paradigm shift in the thoracic surgical world from *"More is better to Lesser the better".* The crux has shifted to organ preservation and minimally invasive techniques, including video-assisted thoracic surgery (VATS) and robotic-assisted thoracic surgery (RATS). A further trend is developing in minimally invasive thoracic surgery, moving toward fewer ports as in uniportal VATS and RATS. A better understanding of the disease process in oncology and screen-detected early lung cancers have allowed thoracic surgeons to push the envelope toward anatomical sublobar lung resections, including segmentectomy and even subsegmentectomy.[1,2] Technological developments in instrumentation and imaging such as virtual-assisted lung mapping, the use of augmented reality using indocyanine green (ICG), and surgeon-friendly three-dimensional (3D) computed tomography (CT) image analysis systems are helping surgeons in mapping the lung lesion and segmental borders more accurately, thereby improving the accuracy of surgery.

In this chapter, we will discuss these future trends in the field of thoracic surgery. Knowing about the latest developments helps us to stay at the forefront by developing new skills and adapting these skills to evolving techniques and technologies for improved patient outcomes.

■ MINIMALLY INVASIVE THORACIC SURGERY

Advances in:
- Video-assisted thoracic surgery
- Robotic-assisted thoracic surgery

Video-assisted Thoracic Surgery

Video-assisted thoracic surgery has revolutionized thoracic surgery. It is used for various diagnostic and therapeutic interventions for infective, inflammatory, and oncological conditions involving the noncardiac thoracic organs. From the evaluation of undiagnosed pleural effusions, management of recurrent pneumothorax, empyema thoracis, and emphysematous lung disease to complex oncological operations, including mediastinal tumors, esophageal and lung cancer, VATS has emerged as an essential tool in the thoracic surgical armamentarium.

The basic principle of any minimally invasive surgery lies in its ability to perform complete and adequate surgery without the trauma of access caused by conventional open approaches such as thoracotomy and sternotomy. VATS reduces the incidence of postoperative morbidity by causing less pain, fewer pulmonary complications due to preserved chest wall mechanics, less blood loss, and shorter intensive care unit (ICU) and hospital stays. The reduction in morbidity becomes particularly relevant in patients with borderline cardiopulmonary function, where VATS has been demonstrated to reduce postoperative morbidity.[3] The oncological adequacy of VATS for lung cancer has been debated. A recent systematic review comparing VATS and thoracotomy in lung cancer shows that VATS is a highly efficient alternative to thoracotomy in both early and locally advanced lung cancer.[4]

Indications of Video-assisted Thoracic Surgery

Virtually, any thoracic surgery performed by open technique can be performed by VATS in appropriately selected patients. The indications of VATS can be summarized as follows.

Diagnostic
- Evaluation of undiagnosed pleural effusion
- Pleural biopsies
- Staging thoracoscopy for lung cancer
- Lymph node biopsy
- Lung biopsy/lung nodule biopsy

Therapeutic
- Pleural diseases—recurrent pleural effusion, empyema thoracis, pleurodesis, thoracic duct ligation for chylothorax
- Lung—wedge resection, lobectomy, segmentectomy, pneumonectomy, lung bullectomy, lung volume reduction surgery
- Mediastinum—thymectomy for myasthenia gravis/thymoma, excision of mediastinal tumors including thymoma, mediastinal germ cell tumors and posterior mediastinal tumors, sympathectomy for hyperhidrosis, excision of cysts—esophageal duplication/bronchogenic cyst

- Chest wall—excision of rib tumors
- Esophagus—esophagectomy for esophageal cancer, enucleation of esophageal leiomyoma, tracheo-broncho-esophageal fistula
- Diaphragm—diaphragmatic plication for eventration, diaphragmatic hernia repair
- Trauma—clot evacuation

Types of Video-assisted Thoracic Surgery

- *Multiport VATS:* It involves placement of three to four ports (small incisions) for performing a procedure. One port is used for inserting the thoracoscope, and two additional ports ranging from 1 to 5 cm are used to insert specialized long instruments.
- *Biportal VATS:* It involves placement of only two incisions.
- *Needlescopic VATS:* This technique utilizes only 3–5-mm instruments to perform the surgery and has been mainly used for dorsal sympathectomy.
- *Uniportal VATS:* Only a single 3–5-cm incision is used in this type of VATS. The thoracoscope and the surgeon's instrument go through a single incision to perform the surgery **(Fig. 1A)**. At the end of the procedure, a single chest tube is placed through the same incision as shown in **Figure 1B**.
- *Nonintubated VATS (NIVATS)*

As is evident from the above-mentioned types, VATS has evolved from multiport to single-port surgery. Dr Gaetano Rocco brought in the early version of uniportal VATS for simple intrathoracic procedures such as pneumothorax and wedge resections.[5,6] The technique of uniportal VATS

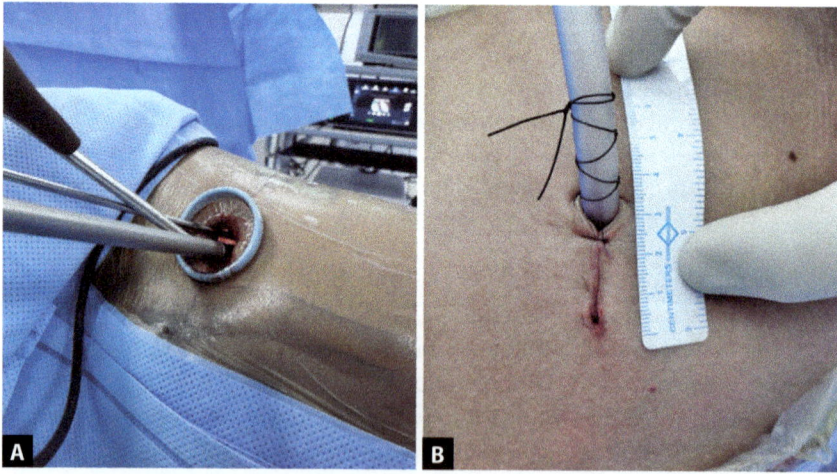

Figs. 1A and B: Uniportal video-assisted thoracic surgery (VATS). (A) Single incision for camera and instruments; (B) Chest tube through the same incision.

for lobectomy was developed and popularized by Dr Diego Gonzalves-Rivas from Spain.[7] Today, the most complex oncological resection of lung tumors involving tracheobronchial and vascular reconstruction, i.e., bronchovascular sleeve resection including carinal resections, can be performed using the uniportal approach.[8-10]

The advantages of uniportal surgery as popularized by expert groups include the following:
- The technique involves the anterior surgical approach, which provides direct visualization of target tissue.
- A 30° thoracoscope is used and is held in the upper part of the incision giving a vision that simulates the normal vision, allowing for better hand–eye coordination.
- A single 3–4-cm incision with no muscle disruption and no rib spreading reduces the number of intercostal space utilization, thereby reducing the injury to intercostal nerves. All this transforms into faster recovery of patients, shorter postoperative hospital stays, and better cosmetic results.

The reduction in morbidity is proven beyond doubt when thoracotomy has been compared to multiport VATS.[11,12] Extrapolating this finding, it is only natural to expect a further decrease in morbidity when the trauma of surgical access is reduced by decreasing the number of incisions as in uniportal VATS. It should, in theory, lead to a decrease in pain, paresthesia, and morbidity and lead to faster recovery.[5] In a systematic review and meta-analysis by Harris et al. comparing multiportal VATS with uniportal VATS, there was a statistically significant shorter hospital stay, decreased postoperative drainage duration, and reduced overall morbidity.[13] On the other hand, Perna et al.[14] published a prospective randomized study comparing uniportal VATS with different styles of VATS. They concluded that uniportal VATS offers no measurable benefits compared with other VATS approaches when performing lung lobectomy. There is no clear-cut answer to the question of the superiority of uniportal VATS compared to conventional multiport technique. More studies with larger sample sizes and multicentric collaboration are needed to answer this conclusively. Nonetheless, uniportal VATS is a well-established technique and is being widely adopted for carrying out most complex of the oncological resections and may become the dominant technique in VATS.

Nonintubated VATS
Thoracic surgeons across the globe are pushing the boundaries by performing major lung resections with VATS (multiport/uniportal technique) to reduce morbidity. However, all these procedures require general anesthesia with lung isolation using a double-lumen endotracheal tube with their own adverse effects. These include intubation-related trauma, increased risk

of pulmonary complications such as pneumonia, ventilator-associated lung injury (VALI), impaired cardiac performance, adverse effects of the neuromuscular blocking agents, and postoperative nausea and vomiting.[15] Evidence suggests that GA and one-lung ventilation can negatively impact immunity by affecting the response of lymphocytes and natural killer cells, pivotal in fighting against tumors and infections.[16] Advances in minimally invasive thoracic surgery have opened a whole new possibility of avoiding the adverse effects of GA and one-lung ventilation by performing minimally invasive thoracic surgery in nonintubated spontaneously breathing patients. This technique is called NIVATS. NIVATS involves conducting thoracoscopic procedures under regional anesthesia (local anesthesia, intercostal nerve blocks, paravertebral blocks, or thoracic epidural anesthesia) in spontaneously breathing patients.[17,18]

The safety and feasibility of NIVATS were reported by Pompeo et al. in 2004 by performing thoracoscopic resection of pulmonary nodules.[19] Gonzalez-Rivas et al. published the first report of a single-port thoracoscopic major pulmonary resection in a patient with spontaneous ventilation (nonintubated surgery) in 2014.[20] Since then, NIVATS has been successfully used to perform a plethora of surgical procedures, ranging from recurrent pneumothorax[21-24] malignant pleural effusion,[25] empyema thoracis,[26] lung volume reduction[27] to major pulmonary resections,[7,28-31] with the potential benefits of faster postoperative recovery times, fewer complications, and shorter hospital stays.

For successful outcomes, NIVATS (particularly major lung resections) should only be done by experienced surgical teams who can perform the surgery efficiently and quickly and have the technical prowess to control catastrophic bleeding from major pulmonary vessels. Case selection is also equally important, and NIVATS should not be used in patients with a difficult airway as intraoperative conversion to GA might be challenging and troublesome. Some of the common contraindications for NIVATS are as follows:

- Allergy to local anesthetics
- Coagulation disorders
- Active neurologic disorders
- An American Society of Anesthesiologists (ASA) score higher than 3
- Sleep apnea
- Unfavorable spinal anatomy
- Uncooperative patients or
- Obesity [body mass index (BMI) >30 kg/m^2]

The published data on NIVATS is relatively small. Available reports suggest it to be safe and feasible in selected patients. Prospective studies with large numbers are needed to prove its efficacy and superiority over conventional VATS.

Robotic-assisted Thoracic Surgery

Minimally invasive thoracic surgery has advanced by leaps and bounds, with proven advantages over conventional open surgery in short- and long-term outcomes. Despite all the apparent advantages, the thoracic surgical fraternity has been relatively slow in adopting the technique. If one looks at the European Society of Thoracic Surgeon Database, the proportion of all lung resections done by VATS was only 42.2%. Although this is better than the previous years, it still shows that even after nearly three decades of its existence, less than half of thoracic surgeons perform VATS for lung resection. This data forces one to think about why the results claimed by expert surgical groups are not replicated by all.

The answer comes from understanding the limitations of conventional VATS. Most surgical teams use a two-dimensional imaging system that limits depth perception. This has been addressed by introducing 3D imaging systems, which are still not commonly used. All the movements in VATS are counterintuitive because of the use of long rigid instruments that work on a fulcrum, forcing surgeons to move in a direction opposite to the intended movement of the instrument tip. This leads to difficult hand–eye coordination, translating to more extended learning curves. The surgeon in VATS is in an ergonomically taxing position that puts strain on the shoulders in long surgeries. Complex maneuvers in difficult-to-reach areas such as the anterior mediastinum and extremes of the thoracic cavity become tricky.

To overcome these limitations, a robotic surgical system was designed to allow the instrument tips to move like a human hand. This has been made feasible by incorporating an EndoWrist **(Fig. 2)** function into the instruments. These instruments allow 7 degrees of freedom of movement and 540 degrees of rotation, even more than the human hand. The robotic systems have a built-in tremor filtration feature, which filters any tremors at the surgeon's

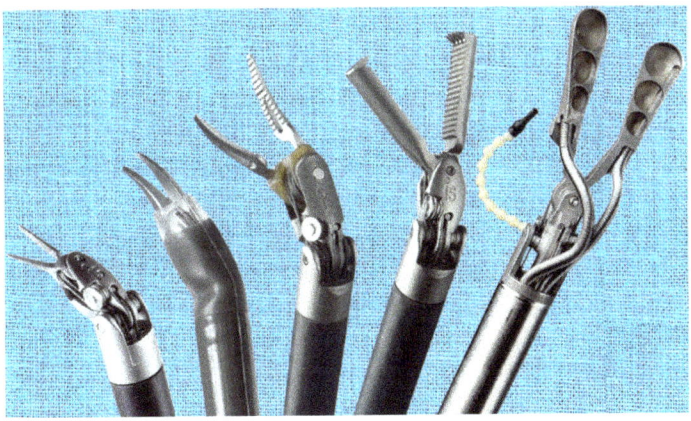

Fig. 2: EndoWrist instruments used in robotic surgery.

level. The lead surgeon is seated comfortably at a console during the surgery, offering exceptional ergonomics. All these translate into more precise movements, the ability to perform complex suturing maneuvers, and a relatively shorter learning curve.

Like VATS, virtually any procedure possible with VATS can be performed using the surgical robot. However, the most common use of the robot has been in thoracic surgical oncology. Robotic-assisted lung surgery for lung cancer, robotic esophagectomy for esophageal cancer, robotic mediastinal surgery for thymoma, middle mediastinal tumors/cysts, posterior mediastinal tumors, and diaphragmatic plication are some of the common surgeries performed using robotic assistance.[32-35]

There is a good amount of literature available on RATS. The initial reports concentrated on safety, feasibility, and technique and primarily focused on lung resections and thymectomy.[36,37] Various studies demonstrated good short-term outcomes in terms of lesser morbidity, equivalent rates of complete resection, and slightly better lymph node dissection with RATS.[38] At the same time, other studies also have demonstrated fair long-term oncological outcomes.[39] The comparison of VATS with RATS is a point of constant debate. More precise dissection, especially in narrow spaces like the anterior mediastinum and better mediastinal lymphadenectomy, is cited as an example in favor of RATS. On the other hand, proponents of VATS claim that the benefits offered are not significant enough to affect short- or long-term outcomes and hence cannot justify the added cost.

Studies comparing RATS and VATS have shown conflicting results. In a study based on a large database, Kent et al. compared the results of robotic lobectomies or segmentectomies to the same surgeries performed by thoracotomy or VATS. They reported statistically significant reductions in operative mortality, length of stay, and overall complication rates when RATS was compared to thoracotomy. However, no difference could be found compared to VATS.[40] A higher rate of prolonged postoperative air leak and longer length of hospital stay after anatomical lung resection was reported in the robotic group by Huang et al.[41] In another propensity score-matched analysis, Li et al. found better results for RATS in terms of the number of lymph nodes retrieved, chest tube duration, the volume of chest tube drainage in the first postoperative day, and length of stay in patients with early-stage lung cancer.[42] In recent times, Gonzalez-Rivas et al. have been popularizing uniportal robotic thoracic surgery and have performed several cases of varying complexity.[43,44] This has the potential to further improve the short-term outcomes. However, the data is developing and must be evaluated in prospective studies to assess long-term outcomes.

An extensive review of VATS versus RATS is outside the purview of this chapter. But if one goes through the literature, one can draw the following conclusions. The evidence regarding the superiority of RATS over open techniques in appropriate cases is no longer a debate. Most surgeons accept that the robotic system offers advantages in terms of dexterity, precision, and ability to perform complex maneuvers but feel that the extra cost is not justifiable. This becomes even more relevant in developing nations where cost containment is paramount. It is necessary to consider not only the initial cost of the robot but also the recurring cost of instruments and maintenance. However, some authors argue that mastering the technique leads to better clinical results, shorter length of stay, and lower nursing costs, thereby causing a reduction of costs.[45] Apart from the cost, lack of haptic feedback and bulky system are frequently discussed disadvantages.

With the intuitive surgical patent now gone, several new manufacturers have created their own surgical robots. The prominent ones are the Hugo System by Medtronic, Versius by Cambridge Medical Robotics (CMR) Surgicals, Hinotori by Medicadroid, Senhance Surgical System, Revo-I by Meere Company, and Micro Hand S.[46] We even have our indigenous robotic system, the SSI Mantra, developed and manufactured in India. The developing competition in this area is bound to have an impact on reducing the cost and addressing issues of haptic feedback, closed console model, and portability. Further development in robotic systems will involve the integration of augmented reality and artificial intelligence into the systems. These improvements and the broader availability of robotic systems will lead to widespread use that will help to reduce costs further.

USE OF AUGMENTED REALITY AND ARTIFICIAL INTELLIGENCE IN THORACIC SURGERY

These days, several screen-detected lung nodules are being encountered, many of which will be referred to a thoracic surgeon for resection. Pre- or intraoperative markings are needed in such cases because the nodules are neither visible nor palpable intraoperatively. A group from the Kyoto University has developed a unique preoperative dye-marking system technique using a bronchoscope known as virtual-assisted lung mapping (VAL-MAP).[47] In this technique, a dye called indigo carmine is bronchoscopically injected under the pleura near the tumor before surgery. Surgeons can visualize the dye during VATS, allowing them to localize and resect the lesions completely.

The utilization of hybrid operating rooms equipped with C-arm CT is another novel technique for simultaneous localization and removal of small pulmonary nodules. This method is known as image-guided VATS (iVATS).[48]

Another example of using augmented reality in the field of sublobar lung resections (segmentectomy) is the use of ICG, a dye used to detect organ perfusion. Sublobar resection is emerging as a viable alternative to lobectomy for lesions smaller than 2 cm, which can be resected with an adequate margin. Identification of the correct intersegmental plane has been the bane of this surgery. ICG is injected into a peripheral vein, and the surgical field is then visualized by near-infrared fluorescence imaging using a fluorescence imaging camera (compatible Karl Storz/Stryker camera system). The perfused ICG flows to the vascularized lung, not the devascularized target segment. This causes the remainder of the lung to become fluorescent green while the target segment remains dark. With the help of software integration, the fluorescent green image can be overlaid onto the real-time video during surgery, delineating the intersegmental border between fluorescent and nonfluorescent lung. The plane is marked by electrocautery or a surgical marker, and a precise segmental resection is performed.

THREE-DIMENSIONAL COMPUTED TOMOGRAPHY SIMULATION

Preoperative surgical planning is becoming increasingly relevant in today's thoracic surgical practice evolving from lobar to sublobar resections. An accurate knowledge of the individual anatomy of the pulmonary vasculature and bronchial tree goes a long way in ensuring the safe conduct of surgery based on preoperative identification of any anatomical variation. It also helps in surgical planning based on the required resection margin. Surgeon-friendly 3D-CT image analysis systems have been developed recently and used in thoracic surgery.[49] Synapse Vincent software has been developed by Fuji Film Co., Ltd., Tokyo, Japan. It is widely used to obtain 3D images of pulmonary vessels and the tracheobronchial tree in just a few clicks. Within 10 minutes, a surgeon can get 3D images of bronchovascular structures for surgical planning.[50,51] Even more so, the images are not static but can be freely rotated for visualization from any angle, providing information on the 3D orientation of pulmonary structures. The use of the system and its ability to accurately assess variations in pulmonary vessel branching patterns, leading to satisfactory short-term surgical outcomes, have been reported.[52] Furthermore, these novel dynamic 3D-CT images can be useful for educating surgical residents and medical students.

ISOLATED LUNG PERFUSION: ROLE IN LUNG TRANSPLANTATION AND LUNG TUMORS

Traditionally, isolated lung perfusion (ILP) has been used as an experimental tool to study lung physiology using animal models. Its use has been extrapolated in recent years to salvage marginal donor lungs in lung transplantation by utilizing ex vivo lung perfusion (EVLP) and to deliver high-dose chemotherapy to the lungs, minimizing systemic exposure by selectively delivering agent through the pulmonary artery and selectively diverting venous effluent by a technique called in vivo lung perfusion (IVLP).

Ex Vivo Lung Perfusion in Lung Transplantation

For patients with end-stage lung disease, lung transplantation is currently the only established treatment with the potential to improve survival. However, a severe shortage of donors remains a vexing problem globally. A significant number of patients on the transplant waiting list are unfortunate to never receive an organ in time. The situation in India is even worse with an organ donation rate of 0.4 per million population.[53] On the other hand, the number of brain deaths in India stands at approximately 150,000 each year due to accidents. If even a very small percentage of these unfortunate deaths can be converted to organ donors, the supply of organs can more than meet the demand. Organ donation can be increased by raising awareness at all levels, including community, public/patient, hospital, and government-initiated programs.[54]

While raising awareness is one way to solve the problem, several strategies have been developed to expand the utilization of acceptable lung grafts. These include single lung transplantation, cadaveric and living donor lobar lung transplantations, the use of extended criteria donors (ECDs), and donation after cardiocirculatory death (DCD).[54] EVLP has been developed to increase the utilization of marginal lungs that would otherwise have been rejected.

During brain death and cardiocirculatory death, potential donor lungs are exposed to various insults that include pneumonia, VALI, and neurogenic and hydrostatic pulmonary edema. Grafts from DCD can have additional issues such as aspiration, warm ischemia, hypoxemia, and hypotension (shock lung). These factors increase the chances of primary graft dysfunction (PGD) caused by ischemia-reperfusion injury and additional factors including graft injuries. This negatively impacts the quality of grafts and is a factor that affects short- and long-term morbidity and mortality negatively.[55-58] Transplant centers worldwide are therefore reluctant to accept ECD and DCD lung grafts, compounding the problem of donor shortage.

Ex vivo lung perfusion involves perfusion and ventilation of the donor lungs in an enclosed aseptic controlled unit. The donor lungs are ventilated through an endotracheal tube attached to a ventilator. Perfusion is carried out through a vascular circuit wherein the outflow from the left atrium is passed through a reservoir, pump, oxygenator, heater–cooler unit, and a leukocyte filter and is brought back through the pulmonary artery **(Fig. 3)**. The protocols can vary in perfusate, rate of flow, target left atrial pressure, and ventilatory settings.[59] There are currently three EVLP protocols used globally. These include the Lund protocol, Toronto protocol, and the Organ Care System (OCS) Lung.[60] The original protocol is the Lund protocol that has been further adapted into the Toronto protocol, which is now the most commonly used. The third protocol involves transportable devices that obviate the

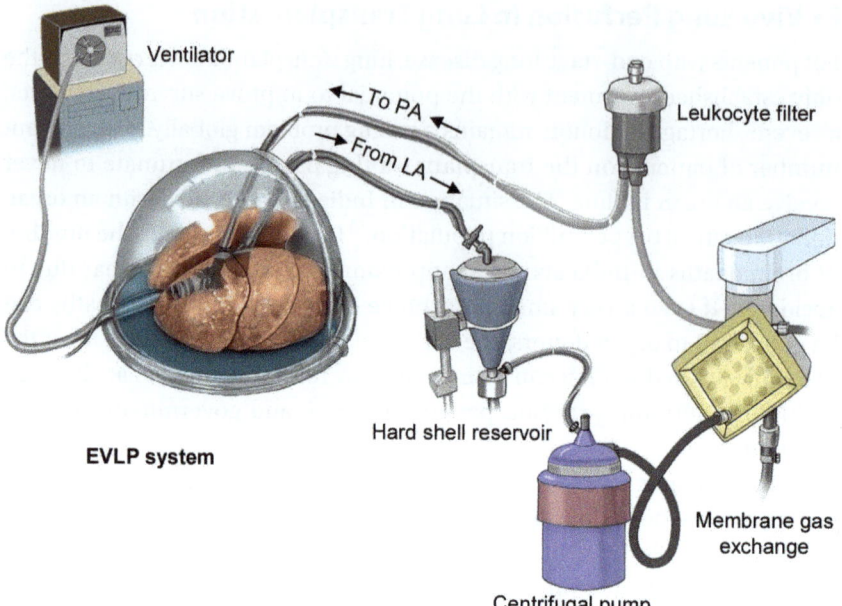

Fig. 3: Ex vivo lung perfusion (EVLP). (LA: left atrium; PA: pulmonary artery)

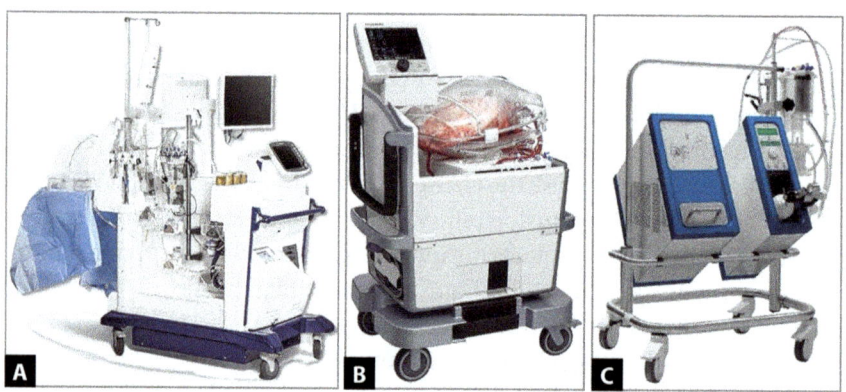

Figs. 4A to C: Commercially available ex vivo lung perfusion (EVLP) systems: (A) XVIVO Perfusion System (XPS)™ by XVIVO® (XVIVO Perfusion AB, Gotberg, Sweden); (B) OCS™ by TransMedics® (Andover, MA, USA); (C) Lung Assist™ by Organ Assist®.

need for keeping the donor lungs in cold storage during transport, thereby reducing the cold ischemia time. Four commercially available EVLP devices are available at present using one or a mix of the three standard protocols: Lung Assist™ by Organ Assist®, XVIVO Perfusion System (XPS)™ by XVIVO®, Vivoline LS1™ by Vivoline Medical®, and OCS™ by Trans Medics® **(Figs. 4A to C)**. The use of portable OCS in lung transplantation has a great potential to improve patient outcomes and is particularly useful in marginal donor lungs, long transportation times, and high-risk recipient or donor/recipient profiles.

These advantages become particularly relevant in the setting of an overall increasing need for suitable donor organs.[61]

By extending the time period of assessment and the potential to optimize the lung grafts from DCD and ECD, EVLP has successfully expanded lung graft pools by reassessing lung grafts from ECD and DCD with comparable short- and long-term outcomes.[62,63]

In Vivo Lung Perfusion in Thoracic Oncology

Pulmonary metastases are a common occurrence in advanced cancers. For patients in whom lung metastases are the only visible disease, pulmonary metastasectomy (PM) has been used to improve survival. However, nearly 50% of the patients who undergo PM will have recurrences.[64] Most recurrences occur in the lungs themselves, suggesting that the lung is the major reservoir of occult metastatic burden. An interesting application of IVLP is to use it to selectively deliver a very high dose of a chemotherapeutic agent into the lung via the pulmonary artery and divert the venous effluent, thereby avoiding systemic distribution. This allows delivery of high drug dose directly to the lung while keeping the systemic toxicity, i.e., hematologic, hepatic, cardiac, and renal, to a minimum.[65] IVLP can be achieved by minimally invasive techniques, such as thoracoscopic lung suffusion.[66] Long-term data is required to substantiate the benefits.

■ LUNG BIOENGINEERING

As we have already discussed, in end-stage lung disease, there is a huge gap between demand and supply of suitable donor lungs for prospective recipients. Among other attempts to address this issue, some revolutionary concepts are being evaluated. These include the use of organs from different species (xenotransplantation) and bioengineering or regenerative medicine. The concept of bioengineering revolves around the creation of a form of tissue scaffold or extracellular matrix (ECM) that is subsequently populated by cells of the desired tissue. The ECM provides mechanical support for the regenerating tissue and establishes the optimal microenvironment for tissue repair and regeneration.[67] Possible sources for creating such scaffolding include human tissue, animal tissue, or synthetic materials. When human or animal tissue is used, it needs to be decellularized to remove antigenic material, which may cause an immune reaction in the recipient. The lung scaffold is then cellularized to create bioengineered lungs, which can then be transplanted into the recipient **(Fig. 5)**. The approach is exciting because of its potential to replace diseased and damaged lungs with biocompatible tissue. However, lung tissue engineering is made more challenging given the multiple cell types involved (e.g., over 40 different cell types in the lung), the need for structural and vascular membrane integrity, and in the case of

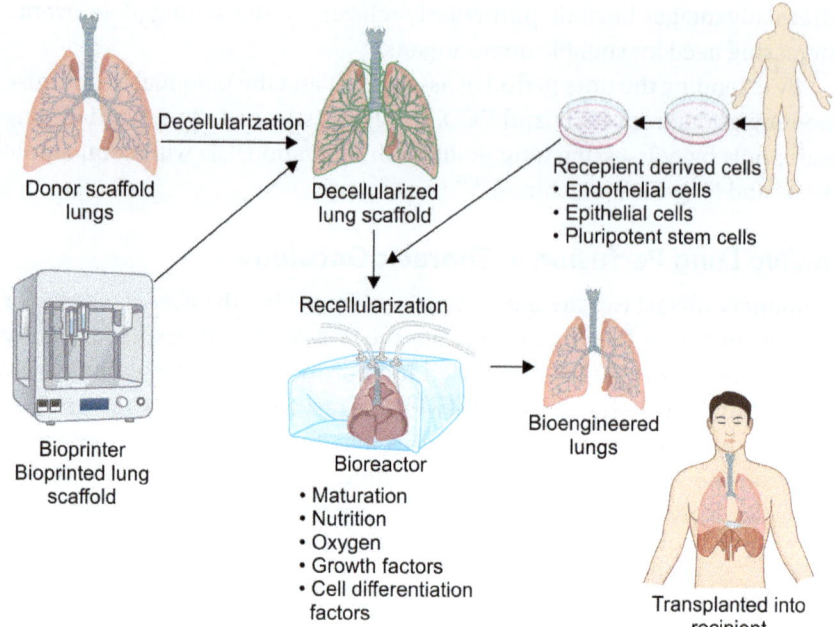

Fig. 5: Schematic representation of process involved in lung bioengineering.

lung tissue, ability to perform adequate gas exchange and the mechanical forces of respiration. The field of bioengineering offers unparalleled potential to drastically extend life expectancy in patients with end-stage lung disease who may otherwise have no options for salvage therapy.

CONCLUSION

Thoracic surgery is constantly evolving, with a huge spectrum from preventive, predictive, diagnostic, and therapeutic interventions to lung transplantation for end-stage lung diseases. From morbid tuberculosis surgery to cutting-edge robotic surgery, there has been a paradigm shift, and the focus has moved from ensuring survival only to improved survival with better quality of life. Ensuring minimal morbidity and early return to normal life has become pivotal in-patient care. Minimally invasive techniques, advanced imaging, early detection programs, improved anesthesia and perioperative care, and the synergy between surgery and medical oncology are driving thoracic surgery into a more patient-centered, precise, and effective future. As newer technology like intraoperative navigation systems, such as electromagnetic navigation and augmented reality guidance, continue to advance, we can expect further refinements in surgical techniques, and the development of even less invasive procedures. These developments will ultimately result in improved outcomes, reduced complications, and enhanced patient quality of life, solidifying the bright future of thoracic surgery in the years to come.

REFERENCES

1. Nakada T, Akiba T, Inagaki T, Morikawa T. Thoracoscopic anatomical subsegmentectomy of the right S2b + S3 using a 3D printing model with rapid prototyping. Interact Cardiovasc Thorac Surg. 2014;19(4):696-8.
2. Desai H, Natt B, Kim S, Bime C. Decreased In-hospital mortality after lobectomy using video-assisted thoracoscopic surgery compared with open thoracotomy. Ann Am Thorac Soc. 2017;14(2):262-266.
3. Zhang R, Ferguson MK. Video-assisted versus open lobectomy in patients with compromised lung function: a literature review and meta-analysis. PLoS One. 2015;10:e0124512.
4. Nath TS, Mohamed N, Gill PK, Khan S. A comparative analysis of video-assisted thoracoscopic surgery and thoracotomy in non-small-cell lung cancer in terms of their oncological efficacy in resection: a systematic review. Cureus. 2022;14(5):e25443.
5. Jutley RS, Khalil MW, Rocco G. Uniportal vs standard three-port VATS technique for spontaneous pneumothorax: comparison of post-operative pain and residual paraesthesia. Eur J Cardiothorac Surg. 2005;28(1):43-6.
6. Rocco G, Khalil M, Jutley R. Uniportal video-assisted thoracoscopic surgery wedge lung biopsy in the diagnosis of interstitial lung diseases. J Thorac Cardiovasc Surg. 2005;129:947-8.
7. Gonzalez D, Paradela M, Garcia J, Dela Torre M. Single-port video-assisted thoracoscopic lobectomy. Interact Cardiovasc Thorac Surg. 2011;12:514-5.
8. Gonzalez-Rivas D, Yang Y, Stupnik T, Sekhniaidze D, Fernandez R, Velasco C, et al. Uniportal video-assisted thoracoscopic bronchovascular, tracheal and carinal sleeve resections. Eur J Cardiothorac Surg. 2016;49(Suppl 1):i6-16.
9. Lyscov A, Obukhova T, Ryabova V, Sekhniaidze D, Zuiev V, Gonzalez-Rivas D. Double-sleeve and carinal resections using the uniportal VATS technique: a single centre experience. J Thorac Dis. 2016;8(Suppl 3):S235-41
10. Wu L, Wang H, Cai H, Fan J, Jiang G, He Y, et al. Comparison of double sleeve lobectomy by uniportal video-assisted thoracic surgery (VATS) and thoracotomy for NSCLC treatment. Cancer Manag Res. 2019;11:10167-74.
11. Fra-Fernández S, Muñoz-Molina GM, Cabañero-Sánchez A, Del Campo-Albendea L, Bolufer-Nadal S, Embún-Flor R, et al. Postoperative morbidity after anatomical lung resections by VATS vs thoracotomy: treatment and intention-to-treat analysis of the Spanish Video-Assisted Thoracic Surgery Group. Cir Esp (Engl Ed). 2023:S2173-5077(23)00122-9.
12. Li WW, Lee TW, Lam SS, Ng CSH, Sihoe ADL, Wan IYP, et al. Quality of life following lung cancer resection: video-assisted thoracic surgery vs thoracotomy. Chest. 2002;122:584-9.
13. Harris CG, James RS, Tian DH, Yan TD, Doyle MP, Gonzalez-Rivas D, et al. Systematic review and meta-analysis of uniportal versus multiportal video-assisted thoracoscopic lobectomy for lung cancer. Ann Cardiothorac Surg. 2016;5(2):76-84.
14. Perna V, Carvajal AF, Torrecilla JA, Gigirey O. Uniportal video-assisted thoracoscopic lobectomy versus other video-assisted thoracoscopic lobectomy techniques: a randomized study. Eur J Cardiothorac Surg. 2016;50:411-5.
15. Szabo Z, Fabo C, Oszlanyi A, Hawchar F, Géczi T, Lantos J, et al. Anesthetic (r)evolution from the conventional concept to the minimally invasive techniques in thoracic surgery—narrative review. J Thorac Dis. 2022;14(8):3045-60.

16. Mineo TC, Tamburrini A, Perroni G, Ambrogi V. 1000 cases of tubeless video-assisted thoracic surgery at the Rome Tor Vergata University. Future Oncol. 2016;12:13-8.
17. Katlic MR. Video-assisted thoracic surgery utilizing local anesthesia and sedation. Eur J Cardiothorac Surg. 2006;30:529-32.
18. Piccioni F, Langer M, Fumagalli L, Haeusler E, Conti B, Previtali P. Thoracic paravertebral anaesthesia for awake video-assisted thoracoscopic surgery daily. Anaesthesia. 2010;65:1221-4.
19. Pompeo E, Mineo D, Rogliani P, Sabato AF, Mineo TC. Feasibility and results of awake thoracoscopic resection of solitary pulmonary nodules. Ann Thorac Surg. 2004;78(5):1761-8.
20. Gonzalez-Rivas D, Fernandez R, de la Torre M, Rodriguez JL, Fontan L, Molina F. Single-port thoracoscopic lobectomy in a nonintubated patient: the least invasive procedure for major lung resection? Interact Cardiovasc Thorac Surg. 2014;19:552-5.
21. Rocco G, La Rocca A, Martucci N, Accardo R. Awake single-access (uniportal) video-assisted thoracoscopic surgery for spontaneous pneumothorax. J Thorac Cardiovasc Surg. 2011;142:944-5.
22. Inoue K, Moriyama K, Takeda J. Remifentanil for awake thoracoscopic bullectomy. J Cardiothorac Vasc Anesth. 2010;24:386-7.
23. Pompeo E, Tacconi F, Mineo D, Mineo TC. The role of awake video-assisted thoracoscopic surgery in spontaneous pneumothorax. J Thorac Cardiovasc Surg. 2007;133:786-90.
24. Noda M, Okada Y, Maeda S, Sado T, Sakurada A, Hoshikawa Y, et al. Is there a benefit of awake thoracoscopic surgery in patients with secondary spontaneous pneumothorax? J Thorac Cardiovasc Surg. 2012;143:613-6.
25. Pompeo E, Dauri M; Awake Thoracic Surgery Research Group. Is there any benefit in using awake anesthesia with thoracic epidural in thoracoscopic talc pleurodesis? J Thorac Cardiovasc Surg. 2013;146:495-7.e491.
26. Tacconi F, Pompeo E, Fabbi E, Mineo TC. Awake video-assisted pleural decortication for empyema thoracis. Eur J Cardiothorac Surg. 2010;37:594-601.
27. Pompeo E, Tacconi F, Mineo TC. Comparative results of non-resectional lung volume reduction performed by awake or non-awake anesthesia. Eur J Cardiothorac Surg. 2011;39:51-8.
28. Gonzalez-Rivas D, Paradela M, Fernandez R, Delgado M, Fieira E, Mendez L, et al. Uniportal video-assisted thoracoscopic lobectomy: two years of experience. Ann Thorac Surg. 2013;95:426-32.
29. Gonzalez Rivas D, Prado RF. (2014). Single port video-assisted thoracoscopic lobectomy under spontaneous ventilation in a high risk patient. CTSNet. [online] Available from: http://www.ctsnet.org/article/single-port-video-assisted-thoracoscopic-lobectomy-under-spontaneous-ventilation-high-risk. [Last accessed November, 2023].
30. Hung MH, Cheng YJ, Hsu HH, Chen JS. Nonintubated uniportal thoracoscopic segmentectomy for lung cancer. J Thorac Cardiovasc Surg. 2014;148:234-5.
31. Pompeo E, Mineo TC. Awake pulmonary metastasectomy. J Thorac Cardiovasc Surg. 2007;133:960-6.
32. Kumar A, Asaf BB, Cerfolio RJ, Sood J, Kumar R. Robotic lobectomy: the first Indian report. J Minim Access Surg. 2015;11(1):94-8.

33. Kumar A, Asaf BB, Pulle MV, Puri HV, Bishnoi S, Gopinath SK. Minimal access surgery for thymoma. Indian J Surg Oncol. 2020;11:625-32.
34. Asaf BB, Kumar A, Vijay CL. Robotic excision of paraesophageal bronchogenic cyst in a 9-year-old child. J Indian Assoc Pediatr Surg. 2015;20(4):191-3.
35. Bin Asaf B, Kodaganur Gopinath S, Kumar A, Puri HV, Pulle MV, Bishnoi S. Robotic diaphragmatic plication for eventration: a retrospective analysis of efficacy, safety, and feasibility. Asian J Endosc Surg. 2021;14(1):70-6.
36. Ashton Jr RC, Connery CP, Swistel DG, DeRose Jr JJ. Robot-assisted lobectomy. J Thorac Cardiovasc Surg. 2003;126:292-3.
37. Huang J, Luo Q, Tan Q, Lin H, Qian L, Lin X. Initial experience of robot-assisted thoracoscopic surgery in China. Int J Med Robot. 2014;10:404-9.
38. Marulli G, Rea F, Melfi F, Schmid TA, Ismail M, Fanucchi O, et al. Robot-aided thoracoscopic thymectomy for early-stage thymoma: a multicenter European study. J Thorac Cardiovasc Surg. 2012;144:1125-30.
39. Park BJ, Melfi F, Mussi A, Maisonneuve P, Spaggiari L, Da Silva RK. Robotic lobectomy for non-small cell lung cancer (NSCLC): long-term oncologic results. J Thorac Cardiovasc Surg. 2012;143:383-9.
40. Kent M, Wang T, Whyte R, Curran T, Flores R, Gangadharan S. Open, video-assisted thoracic surgery, and robotic lobectomy: review of a national database. Ann Thorac Surg. 2014;97:236-44.
41. Huang L, Shen Y, Onaitis M. Comparative study of anatomic lung resection by robotic vs. video-assisted thoracoscopic surgery. J Thorac Dis. 2019;11:1243-50.
42. Li JT, Liu PY, Huang J, Lu PJ, Lin H, Zhou QJ, et al. Perioperative outcomes of radical lobectomies using robotic-assisted thoracoscopic technique vs. video-assisted thoracoscopic technique: retrospective study of 1,075 consecutive p-stage I non-small cell lung cancer cases. J Thorac Dis. 2019;11:882-91.
43. Gonzalez-Rivas D, Ismail M. Subxiphoid or subcostal uniportal robotic-assisted surgery: early experimental experience. J Thorac Dis. 2019;11(1):231-9.
44. Gonzalez-Rivas D, Bosinceanu M, Motas N, Manolache V. Uniportal robotic-assisted thoracic surgery for lung resections. Eur J Cardiothorac Surg. 2022;62(3):ezac410.
45. Dylewski MR, Lazzaro RS. Robotics—the answer to the Achilles' heel of VATS pulmonary resection. Chin J Cancer Res. 2012;24:259-60.
46. Almujalhem A, Rha KH. Surgical robotic systems: what we have now? A urological perspective. BJUI Compass. 2020;1(5):152-9.
47. Sato M, Omasa M, Chen F, Sato T, Sonobe M, Bando T, et al. Use of virtual assisted lung mapping (VAL-MAP), a bronchoscopic multi-spot dye-marking technique using virtual images, for precise navigation of thoracoscopic sublobar lung resection. J Thorac Cardiovasc Surg. 2014;147(6):1813-9.
48. Gill RR, Zheng Y, Barlow JS, Jayender J, Girard EE, Hartigan PM, et al. Image-guided video assisted thoracoscopic surgery (iVATS)—phase I-II clinical trial. J Surg Oncol. 2015;112(1):18-25.
49. Ikeda N, Yoshimura A, Hagiwara M, Akata S, Saji H. Three dimensional computed tomography lung modeling is useful in simulation and navigation of lung cancer surgery. Ann Thorac Cardiovasc Surg. 2013;19(1):1-5.
50. Chen-Yoshikawa TF, Date H. Update on three-dimensional image reconstruction for preoperative simulation in thoracic surgery. J Thorac Dis. 2016;8(Suppl 3):S295-301.

51. Mochizuki K, Takatsuki M, Soyama A, Hidaka M, Obatake M, Eguchi S. The usefulness of a high-speed 3D-image analysis system in pediatric living donor liver transplantation. Ann Transplant. 2012;17(1):31-4.
52. Hagiwara M, Shimada Y, Kato Y, Nawa K, Makino Y, Furumoto H, et al. High-quality 3-dimensional image simulation for pulmonary lobectomy and segmentectomy: results of preoperative assessment of pulmonary vessels and short-term surgical outcomes in consecutive patients undergoing video-assisted thoracic surgery. Eur J Cardiothorac Surg. 2014;46(6):120-6.
53. Deceased organ donation data in India. (2022). [online] Available from: https://www.organindia.org/deceased-organ-donation-data/. [Last accessed November, 2023].
54. Nallusamy S, Shyamalapriya S, Balaji B, Ranjan R, Yogendran. Organ donation—current Indian scenario. J Pract Cardiovasc Sci. 2018;4:177-9.
55. Watanabe T, Cypel M, Keshavjee S. Ex vivo lung perfusion. J Thorac Dis. 2021;13(11):6602-17.
56. Fiser SM, Tribble CG, Long SM, Kaza AK, Kern JA, Jones DR, et al. Ischemia-reperfusion injury after lung transplantation increases risk of late bronchiolitis obliterans syndrome. Ann Thorac Surg. 2002;73:1041-8.
57. Kreisel D, Krupnick AS, Puri V, Guthrie TJ, Trulock EP, Meyers BF, et al. Short- and long-term outcomes of 1000 adult lung transplant recipients at a single center. J Thorac Cardiovasc Surg. 2011;141:215-22.
58. Diamond JM, Lee JC, Kawut SM, Shah RJ, Localio AR, Bellamy SL, et al. Clinical risk factors for primary graft dysfunction after lung transplantation. Am J Respir Crit Care Med. 2013;187:527-34.
59. Schraufnagel DP, Steffen RJ, Vargo PR, Attia T, Elgharably H, Hasan SM, et al. Devices for ex vivo heart and lung perfusion. Expert Rev Med Devices. 2018;15(3):183-91.
60. Nakajima D, Date H. Ex vivo lung perfusion in lung transplantation. Gen Thorac Cardiovasc Surg. 2021;69(4):625-30.
61. Schmack B, Weymann A, Mohite P, Saez DG, Zych B, Sabashnikov A, et al. Contemporary review of the organ care system in lung transplantation: potential advantages of a portable ex-vivo lung perfusion system. Expert Rev Med Devices. 2016;13(11):1035-41.
62. Divithotawela C, Cypel M, Martinu T, Singer LG, Binnie M, Chow CW, et al. Long-term outcomes of lung transplant with ex vivo lung perfusion. JAMA Surg. 2019;154:1143-50.
63. Cypel M, Yeung JC, Liu M, Anraku M, Chen F, Karolak W, et al. Normothermic ex vivo lung perfusion in clinical lung transplantation. N Engl J Med. 2011;364:1431-40.
64. Pastorino U, Buyse M, Friedel G, Ginsberg RJ, Girard P, Goldstraw P, et al. Long-term results of lung metastasectomy: prognostic analyses based on 5206 cases. J Thorac Cardiovasc Surg. 1997;113:37-49.
65. Cypel M, Keshavjee S. Novel technologies for isolated lung perfusion: beyond lung transplant. Thorac Surg Clin. 2016;26(2):139-45.
66. Demmy TL. Thoracoscopic lung suffusion. Thorac Surg Clin. 2016;26(1):109-21.
67. Yi S, Ding F, Gong L, Gu X. Extracellular matrix scaffolds for tissue engineering and regenerative medicine. Curr Stem Cell Res Ther. 2017;12(3):233-46.

CHAPTER 12

Immune Profiling and Therapies in Cancer

Sikhar Kumar, Vanita Noronha, Kumar Prabhash

■ INTRODUCTION

As normal cells evolve into a neoplastic state, they acquire several hallmark capabilities that enable them to become tumorigenic and, ultimately, malignant. The original six hallmarks of cancer were proposed by Hanahan and Weinberg[1] in 2000, to which two more hallmarks were added in 2011, namely "evading immune destruction" and "reprogramming energy metabolism."[2] It was long recognized from clinical epidemiology studies that the immune system plays a key role in the detection and elimination of incipient cancer cells. This hypothesis was strongly reinforced by the demonstration of durable and significant anticancer activity of various immunomodulatory treatment approaches.[3]

Unlike traditional cytotoxic chemotherapy, immunotherapy targets and unleashes the immune system of the patient to generate an antitumor response.[4] The various types of immune therapies such as cancer vaccines and immune checkpoint inhibitors (ICPIs) approved for clinical use have shown remarkable results in various cancers; however, it is also recognized that many patients do not respond to these therapies. Some patients also experience autoimmune toxicities/immune-related adverse events (irAEs), which can occasionally be fatal.[5] Hence, efforts have been made to profile the tumor microenvironment (TME) for biomarker identification and discovery of novel treatment strategies to improve treatment outcomes.[6]

This chapter will first provide a broad overview of various immune cell profiling techniques and their clinical applications. Subsequently, the most common types of immune therapies in clinical practice will be discussed.

■ IMMUNE CELL PROFILING

Immune profiling technologies can be broadly classified into two groups: Transcriptomic-based and proteomic-based **(Box 1)**.

■ TRANSCRIPTOMIC-BASED TECHNOLOGIES

Microarrays

A microarray is an ordered collection of microspots (probes), in which each spot consists of a single species of a nucleic acid and the representative gene

> **BOX 1:** Conventional and high-dimensional technologies for immune cell profiling.
>
> *Transcriptomic based:*
> - Microarrays
> - Bulk RNA sequencing (RNA-Seq)
> - Conventional IHC
> - Fluorescence-based flow cytometry
>
> *Proteomic based:*
> - sc-ATAC-Seq
> - Single-cell RNA sequencing
> - Multiplexed IHC
> - Cytometry by time-of-flight (CyTOF)
>
> (IHC: immunohistochemistry; RNA: ribonucleic acid; sc-ATAC-Seq: single-cell assay for transposase accessible chromatin sequencing)

of interest. First, ribonucleic acid (RNA) targets are obtained from a biological sample by reverse transcription, which are also simultaneously labeled. Deoxyribonucleic acid (DNA) probes are immobilized in a matrix, which are then hybridized with the free labeled targets. A "hybridization signal" is then produced on each probe, which corresponds to the messenger RNA (mRNA) expression level of corresponding gene in the sample. These signals are detected, quantified, and integrated with software tools, which ultimately provide a "gene expression profile" for a given biological sample.[7]

Microarray technology has several limitations. It depends on the quality and amount of RNA extracted from the tissue. Studying rare cell types and differentiating between cells with similar expression patterns are limited. Some other drawbacks include minimal expression of genes due to background hybridization and difficulty in reproducibility between laboratories.[8]

RNA-Sequencing

RNA sequencing (RNA-Seq) overcame one of the major limitations of microarray technology; that is, prior knowledge of the sequences being studied for array design was not mandatory. RNA-Seq enables one to study the transcriptome of the tumor and microenvironment by identifying thousands of genes that are present in a single biological sample. The steps in RNA-Seq include collection of tissue samples and isolating RNA, then sequencing it and preparing a library of complementary DNA (cDNA), sequencing the cDNA fragments and aligning with the reference genome, processing the data followed by quality checking and final data analysis. RNA-Seq has high dynamic range and is useful in identifying single-nucleotide polymorphisms (SNPs). Disadvantages of RNA-Seq include the high cost of processing and the need for complex analysis of sequencing variants.[9]

Conventional Immunohistochemistry

Conventional immunohistochemistry (IHC) or immunofluorescent microscopy allows us to detect cellular antigens within the tissue using enzyme-labeled or fluorochrome-labeled antibodies. This enables cellular-type identification and their spatial location in tissues. A key limitation with this technology is that a maximum of four markers can be used at a single time, as their chromogenic spectra overlap.[10]

■ PROTEOMIC-BASED TECHNOLOGIES

Single-cell RNA Sequencing

This technology overcame the challenges caused by the intratumoral heterogeneity in gene expression as it can dissect phenotypic and functional differences among single cells.[11] This technology is built on the foundation of bulk-RNA Seq, but it has additional steps such as isolating single cells, a powerful amplification process to generate cDNA from small RNA quantities. This enables analysis of the transcriptome at the single-cell level.[12] An advantage of single-cell RNA sequencing (sc-RNA Seq) is its ability to perform single-cell analysis of tumor-infiltrating T-cells. Thus, various T-cell phenotypes such as regulatory, naïve, cytotoxic, and costimulatory T-cells can be identified in a particular sample; hence, it can have a predictive role for various immune therapies.[13]

Cytometry by Time-of-flight

This technology combines mass spectrometry and flow cytometry, thus overcoming the inherent limitations of fluorescence-based cytometry, that is, overlap in emission spectra of individual fluorophores. It uses heavy metal isotopes (lanthanide metals) to label antibodies. The labeled cells are then analyzed at a single-cell level using high throughput spectrometry. Basically, samples are nebulized into single-cell droplets and then vaporized by the high-temperature plasma. This generates an ion cloud with the labeled heavy metal ions, which is then quantified using the mass-to-charge ratio.[14] An advantage of cytometry by time-of-flight (CyTOF) is its requirement of very small cell numbers (1,000–1,000,000), which can be obtained easily from biopsy specimens.[15]

Multiplexed Immunohistochemistry

Multiplexed IHC allows for visualization of multiple markers using fluorescence microscopy. Unlike traditional IHC which can study only one to two markers per tissue section, up to seven fluorescent markers can be studied, allowing evaluation of spatial distribution of various cell types within a tumor.[16]

■ CLINICAL APPLICATIONS OF IMMUNE CELL PROFILING

Researchers now have powerful tools to conduct deep immunophenotyping at the single cell level. Several studies have revealed a complex network of immune cells in the TME in various cancers such as hepatocellular carcinomas, breast carcinomas, and colorectal carcinomas, to name a few.[17-19] Thus, each tumor has been identified to carry its own specific immune signature, which can affect the prognosis independent of its TNM staging. Several studies have attempted to discover biomarkers in cancers such as melanomas, but most of these are yet to be validated and conducted in large, prospective studies.[20] An exception is the Immunoscore, which is validated as a prognostic risk factor in several cancers such as colorectal cancers, breast, and lung cancers and has some predictive value in colorectal cancers.

Immunoscore is a scoring system to summarize the density of CD3+ and CD8+ T-cells within the tumor and its invasive margin. A higher infiltration of immune cells in the tumor was found to correlate with a better prognosis. In an international consortium led by the Society for Immunotherapy in Cancer (STIC), the Immunoscore assay was studied to predict recurrence risk in stage I-III colon cancers. The assay was found to be reproducible and robust, and in a multivariable analysis, its prognostic power was found to be independent of patient age, T stage, N stage, microsatellite instability, and existing prognostic factors.[21] In a pooled analysis of more than 10,000 patients, a lower Immunoscore was associated with poorer overall survival (OS) and disease-specific survival for all cancers.[22] The Immunoscore was also studied as a predictive assay in the IDEA cohort for stage III colon cancers, which evaluated 3 months versus 6 months of adjuvant oxaliplatin-based chemotherapy. A high Immunoscore predicted benefit of 6 months of mFOLFOX6 over 3 months, whereas a low score did not significantly benefit from 6 months of mFOLFOX6.[23]

■ CANCER IMMUNOTHERAPY

Cancer immunotherapy has come a long way, from the late 19th century, when William B Coley, an orthopedic surgeon, first demonstrated the role of the immune system by injecting more than thousands of patients with live and inactivated bacteria such as *Streptococcus pyogenes*, with the aim of inducing sepsis and strong immune responses in patients suffering from inoperable bone sarcomas. He achieved durable and complete remissions in several types of cancers.[24] However, this therapy was not adopted by his contemporaries as they were skeptical of these results. In addition, the development of radiation therapy and chemotherapy, along with further refinement in surgical techniques in the 20th century, resulted in these therapies being established as the mainstay of cancer treatment.

Several decades after Coley's experiments, researchers uncovered the mechanism of action behind Coley's therapies by discovering immune mediators called cytokines.[25] Cytokines encompass a family of signaling chemicals, including chemokines, interferons, interleukins (ILs), adipokines, etc., which are involved in nearly every biological process. IL-2 was used as a single agent to a moderate degree of success in the treatment of metastatic renal cell cancers, where it achieved responses in approximately 20% of patients but was limited by its toxicity profile such as capillary leak syndrome.[26]

The real breakthrough in cancer immunotherapy came in the 21st century with the discovery of T-cell immune checkpoints, such as CTLA-4 (cytotoxic T-lymphocyte antigen 4) and PD-1 (programmed cell death protein 1). These checkpoints prevent autoimmune reactions by playing a negative regulatory role to prevent excessive T-cell activation. But cancer cells can escape immune clearance by suppressing these immune checkpoints. This discovery of the PD-1/L-1 axis, coupled with the development of breakthrough immune checkpoint inhibitor therapies with unprecedented results in melanomas and subsequently other cancers, resulted in the 2018 Nobel Prize in Medicine being awarded to researchers Dr Tasuki Honjo and Dr Allison.

Checkpoint Inhibitor Immunotherapy

PD-1 is expressed on activated T-cells, and its ligand PD-L1 is expressed on tumor cells as well as on tumor-infiltrating immune cells, including APCs (antigen-presenting cells) and B- and T-cells.[27] Both PD-1 and PD-L1 are therapeutic targets, and several monoclonal antibodies have been developed: The anti-PD-1 antibodies nivolumab and pembrolizumab, and the anti-PD-L1 antibodies durvalumab, atezolizumab, and avelumab. CTLA-4 is another identified target for therapeutic blockade, for which there are two approved antibodies in clinical use—ipilimumab and tremelimumab. A select list of labeled indications of these inhibitors is provided in **Table 1**.

Predictive Biomarkers for Checkpoint Inhibitors

PD-1/L-1 remains the most widely used and validated biomarker for ICPIs. PD-L1 is heterogeneously expressed and is a dynamic marker—the threshold between a "positive" and a "negative" report can depend on the type of antibody being used and the type of tissue being studied. That said, most studies have shown a positive correlation between PD-L1 "positive" tumors and clinical efficacy of PD-1 pathway blockers. PD-L1 is an imperfect biomarker though, as high PD-L1 expression does not guarantee tumor response to checkpoint therapy. For example, single agent pembrolizumab in high PD-L1 (>50%) expressors with nonsmall cell lung cancers (NSCLCs) achieves a response rate of approximately 45% only, with early disease

TABLE 1: Select approved indications of immune checkpoint inhibitors.

Agent	Tumor	Indications
Pembrolizumab	Breast cancer	• High-risk early stage [triple negative breast cancer (TNBC)] • Metastatic/unresectable TNBC (PD-L1 CPS ≥10)
	Cervical cancer	Recurrent/metastatic (CPS ≥1)
	Endometrial cancer	Advanced, pretreated, dMMR Advanced, in combination with lenvatinib
	Esophageal cancer	Advanced, squamous, CPS ≥10
	Head and neck cancer	• First-line metastatic/unresectable • Subsequent, postplatinum therapy
	Hodgkin's lymphoma	Relapsed/refractory
	Melanoma	• Adjuvant: Stage IIB, IIC, or III • Unresectable/metastatic
	Nonsmall cell lung cancer	• *Metastatic:* First line, in combination with pemetrexed/platinum, EGFR/ALK negative • *Metastatic:* Second line, TPS ≥1% • *Adjuvant:* Stages IB, II, IIIA
	Renal cell carcinoma	• *Metastatic:* First line, in combination with axitinib/lenvatinib • *Adjuvant:* Intermediate/high risk
	Urothelial carcinoma	• *Advanced/metastatic:* Platinum ineligible • *Advanced/metastatic:* Postplatinum progression
Ipilimumab	Melanoma	*Unresectable/metastatic:* In combination with nivolumab
	Colorectal cancer	*Metastatic, dMMR:* In combination with nivolumab
	Malignant pleural mesothelioma	*Metastatic:* In combination with nivolumab
	Nonsmall cell lung cancer	*Metastatic:* First line, in combination with nivolumab and two cycles of platinum doublet chemotherapy, EGFR/ALK negative
	Renal cell carcinoma	*Metastatic:* Intermediate and poor risk—in combination with nivolumab

(ALK: anaplastic lymphoma kinase; CPS: combined positive score; dMMR: deficient mismatch repair; EGFR: epidermal growth factor receptor; TPS: tumor proportion score) progression noted in approximately 25–30% patients.[28] Conversely, some patients with PD-L1-negative tumors also seem to derive benefit.[29] Several commercial PD-L1 IHC assays are currently in clinical use, such as 22C3, 28-8, SP142, and SP 263—these have shown high concordance and interchangeability in an international harmonizing project.[30] Deficient mismatch repair (dMMR) is another validated predictive biomarker to checkpoint inhibitor therapy. Tumors that lack mismatch repair mechanism are hypermutated than tumors without such defects.[31] These mutations code for mutant proteins, and a minority of these can give rise to neoantigens, which results in greater immunogenicity due to tumor infiltration by CD8+ T-cells. Tumors with dMMR have been noted in 27 different cancer types, 12 of which had a prevalence >1%. The most common cancers with dMMR are endometrial carcinomas (16–27%), colon adenocarcinomas (8–10%), and stomach adenocarcinomas (2–3%).[32] After the demonstration of substantial and durable antitumor responses with pembrolizumab in first-line dMMR solid tumors and colorectal cancers, the United States Food and Drug Administration (US-FDA) granted the first tissue/site agnostic indication to pembrolizumab for unresectable or metastatic dMMR tumors on May 23, 2017.[33] Tumor mutational burden (TMB) is another predictive biomarker. The US FDA has approved pembrolizumab for tumors with a high level of TMB using the FoundationOne CDx assay, and the cutoff point of ≥10 mutations/Mb, as clinical efficacy in this indication was demonstrated in the KEYNOTE-158 trial.[34]

Checkpoint Inhibitor Toxicity

In contrast to cytotoxic chemotherapy, checkpoint inhibitors are generally well tolerated. They have a unique spectrum of side effects known as irAEs. irAEs can include dermatologic, gastrointestinal, hepatic, endocrine, and other less common adverse events. Fatigue is the most common side effect seen in up to 16–24% patients. In general, grade 3/4 irAEs are uncommon with single agent PD-1/L-1 monotherapy but more common with dual CTLA-4/PD-1 therapy. The mainstay of treating irAEs includes withholding the drug, glucocorticoid therapy, and additional immunosuppression in severe/refractory cases.[35]

Chimeric Antigen Receptor T-cell Therapy

Chimeric antigen receptor (CAR) T-cell therapy is labeled as a "next-generation" cellular therapy. They are a form of genetically modified autologous immunotherapy that uses the individual's own T-cells and transduces them with a gene that encodes a CAR to direct the patient's T-cells against the leukemic cells. The T-cells are genetically modified ex vivo, expanded in a production facility, and then infused back into the patient as therapy.

The earliest target studied most extensively has been CD19. This B-cell marker is highly expressed in B-cell acute lymphocytic leukemia and other B-cell malignancies. The clinical results of CAR T-cell therapy in relapsed B-cell leukemias have been very promising, with responses in >80% of patients with acute lymphoblastic leukemia (ALL).[36] These cells persist in the body for >1 year, suggesting long-term uptake. The US-FDA approved anti-CD19 CAR T-cell therapies include tisagenlecleucel and axicabtagene ciloleucel, which are used in relapsed B-cell non-Hodgkin lymphomas as well.[37]

With the impressive results obtained with CAR T-cell therapy in B-cell leukemias, other targets have been extensively studied, with the most progress noted in multiple myeloma. CARs targeting the B-cell maturation antigen (BCMA) (a plasma cell marker) have demonstrated extremely high response rates (80–100%) in refractory multiple myeloma with durable responses, based on which the US-FDA has approved to date two BCMA CAR-T products, idecabtagene vicleucel and ciltacabtagene autoleucel.[38]

A challenge with CAR therapy has been identifying targets in myeloid cancers such as acute myeloid leukemias, as many of the antigens expressed in these malignant cells are also expressed in the bone marrow stem cells, which can result in bone marrow aplasia if treated with CAR therapy. Solid tumors also have shown to be difficult to target with CAR therapy, due to low target expression in tumor cells and fatal side effects in some early studies.[39]

The side effect profile of CAR T-cell therapy includes cytokine release syndrome (CRS), which is observed in nearly all treated patients. CRS is characterized by fever, flu-like symptoms, hypotension, and hypoxia, which can lead to multiorgan damage. Tocilizumab, an IL-6 monoclonal antibody, is recommended for grade ≥2 CRS. The other major side effect of CAR therapy is called ICANS (immune effector cell-associated neurotoxicity syndrome), characterized by confusion, somnolence, and aphasia. Unlike CRS, this toxicity is not only caused by release of cytokines but also due to trafficking of CARs into the central nervous system. Steroids with good intracranial penetration such as dexamethasone are the preferred initial agents for ICANS with seizure prophylaxis and intensive care unit (ICU) care recommended for grade ≥3 toxicity.[40]

■ CANCER VACCINES

Sipuleucel-T is a therapeutic vaccine that is prepared from autologous peripheral blood mononuclear cells obtained by leukapheresis and pulsed ex vivo with a unique fusion protein of granulocyte-macrophage colony-stimulating factor (GM-CSF) and prostatic acid phosphatase (PAP), termed PA2024. GM-CSF was included to strengthen the immune response to PAP alone. Each dose of sipuleucel-T contains a minimum of 50 million autologous CD54+ cells activated with PAP/GM-CSF. Sipuleucel-T was approved by the US-FDA in 2010 for use in metastatic castrate-resistant prostate cancer (asymptomatic or minimally symptomatic) based on data from three randomized trials. The initial two randomized studies had progression-free survival (PFS) as the primary endpoint. Both studies showed a trend toward better time to tumor progression that favored sipuleucel-T (median 11.1 vs. 9.7 months).[41] A subsequent larger phase 3 randomized trial with OS as the primary endpoint showed a clinically meaningful 4.1 months survival benefit (median 25.8 vs. 21.7 months), reflecting a 22% reduction in the risk of death.

ONCOLYTIC VIRUSES

Talimogene laherparepvec (T-VEC) is an oncolytic, genetically modified herpesvirus.[42] It is used as an intralesional therapy that, when injected directly into tumor, results in a direct oncolytic effect from the viral infection and lytic replication, as well as the induction of a systemic immune response. T-VEC was approved by the US-FDA to treat unresectable, injectable cutaneous, subcutaneous, and nodal melanoma with limited visceral disease. This approval was based on a phase 3 trial with a primary endpoint of durable response rate, which was a partial response or complete response occurring at any time during the first 12 months of treatment and lasting for at least 6 months. Durable responses were higher in the T-VEC arm at 16.3% compared with the GM-CSF arm at 2.1%. The overall response rate (ORR) was also significantly increased in the T-VEC arm (26.4%) compared with GM-CSF alone (5.7%), as was the number of complete responders (CRs) (10.8 vs. 1%). T-VEC was well tolerated in this phase III study. The most common toxicities included injection site reactions, fatigue, chills, and fevers.[43]

CONCLUSION

Immunotherapy has revolutionized cancer treatment in the 21st century. ICPIs have now become a standard of care across several solid and lymphoid malignancies, based on large phase 3 randomized trials that have demonstrated superior OS and response rates in a convincing fashion. However, the ideal predictive biomarker for checkpoint therapy is still elusive. PD-L1 IHC remains the most validated and accepted biomarker to date. Immune cell profiling with newer proteomic technologies will open the gateway to better designed and personalized studies in the near future. CAR T-cell therapy has also produced unprecedented response rates and outcomes in relapsed/refractory B-cell malignancies and multiple myelomas. Overcoming resistance to checkpoint inhibitors/CAR T-cell therapy will now become the focus of next-generation studies to further improve outcomes for patients.

■ REFERENCES

1. Hanahan D, Weinberg RA. The hallmarks of cancer. Cell. 2000;100(1):57-70.
2. Hanahan D, Weinberg RA. Hallmarks of cancer: the next generation. Cell. 2011;144(5):646-74.
3. Khalil DN, Smith EL, Brentjens RJ, Wolchok JD. The future of cancer treatment: immunomodulation, CARs and combination immunotherapy. Nat Rev Clin Oncol. 2016;13(5):273-90.
4. Yu Y, Cui J. Present and future of cancer immunotherapy: a tumor microenvironmental perspective. Oncol Lett. 2018;16(4):4105-13.
5. Farkona S, Diamandis EP, Blasutig IM. Cancer immunotherapy: the beginning of the end of cancer? BMC Med. 2016;14:73.
6. Beatty GL, Gladney WL. Immune escape mechanisms as a guide for cancer immunotherapy. Clin Cancer Res. 2015;21(4):687-92.
7. Russo G, Zegar C, Giordano A. Advantages and limitations of microarray technology in human cancer. Oncogene. 2003;22(42):6497-507.
8. Lyons YA, Wu SY, Overwijk WW, Baggerly KA, Sood AK. Immune cell profiling in cancer: molecular approaches to cell-specific identification. NPJ Precis Oncol. 2017;1(1):26.
9. Wang Z, Gerstein M, Snyder M. RNA-Seq: a revolutionary tool for transcriptomics. Nat Rev Genet. 2009;10(1):57-63.
10. Tsurui H, Nishimura H, Hattori S, Hirose S, Okumura K, Shirai T. Seven-color fluorescence imaging of tissue samples based on Fourier spectroscopy and singular value decomposition. J Histochem Cytochem. 2000;48(5):653-62.
11. Potter SS. Single-cell RNA sequencing for the study of development, physiology and disease. Nat Rev Nephrol. 2018;14(8):479-92.
12. Wu AR, Neff NF, Kalisky T, Dalerba P, Treutlein B, Rothenberg ME, et al. Quantitative assessment of single-cell RNA-sequencing methods. Nat Methods. 2014;11(1):41-6.
13. Chung W, Eum HH, Lee HO, Lee KM, Lee HB, Kim KT, et al. Single-cell RNA-seq enables comprehensive tumour and immune cell profiling in primary breast cancer. Nat Commun. 2017;8:15081.
14. Bjornson ZB, Nolan GP, Fantl WJ. Single-cell mass cytometry for analysis of immune system functional states. Curr Opin Immunol. 2013;25(4):484-94.
15. Yao Y, Liu R, Shin MS, Trentalange M, Allore H, Nassar A, et al. CyTOF supports efficient detection of immune cell subsets from small samples. J Immunol Methods. 2014;415:1-5.
16. Tan WCC, Nerurkar SN, Cai HY, Ng HHM, Wu D, Wee YTF, et al. Overview of multiplex immunohistochemistry/immunofluorescence techniques in the era of cancer immunotherapy. Cancer Commun (Lond). 2020;40(4):135-53.
17. Zheng C, Zheng L, Yoo JK, Guo H, Zhang Y, Guo X, et al. Landscape of infiltrating T cells in liver cancer revealed by single-cell sequencing. Cell. 2017;169(7):1342-56.e16.
18. Azizi E, Carr AJ, Plitas G, Cornish AE, Konopacki C, Prabhakaran S, et al. Single-cell map of diverse immune phenotypes in the breast tumor microenvironment. Cell. 2018;174(5):1293-308.e36.
19. Zhang L, Yu X, Zheng L, Zhang Y, Li Y, Fang Q, et al. Lineage tracking reveals dynamic relationships of T cells in colorectal cancer. Nature. 2018;564(7735):268-72.

20. Sade-Feldman M, Yizhak K, Bjorgaard SL, Ray JP, de Boer CG, Jenkins RW, et al. Defining T cell states associated with response to checkpoint immunotherapy in melanoma. Cell. 2018;175(4):998-1013.e20.
21. Pagès F, Mlecnik B, Marliot F, Bindea G, Ou FS, Bifulco C, et al. International validation of the consensus Immunoscore for the classification of colon cancer: a prognostic and accuracy study. Lancet. 2018;391(10135):2128-39.
22. Zhang X, Yang J, Du L, Zhou Y, Li K. The prognostic value of Immunoscore in patients with cancer: a pooled analysis of 10,328 patients. Int J Biol Markers. 2020;35(3):3-13.
23. Pagès F, André T, Taieb J, Vernerey D, Henriques J, Borg C, et al. Prognostic and predictive value of the Immunoscore in stage III colon cancer patients treated with oxaliplatin in the prospective IDEA France PRODIGE-GERCOR cohort study. Ann Oncol. 2020;31(7):921-9.
24. McCarthy EF. The toxins of William B. Coley and the treatment of bone and soft-tissue sarcomas. Iowa Orthop J. 2006;26:154-8.
25. Dinarello CA. Historical insights into cytokines. Eur J Immunol. 2007;37 (Suppl. 1):S34-45.
26. Rosenberg SA. Interleukin 2 for patients with renal cancer. Nat Clin Pract Oncol. 2007;4(9):497.
27. Freeman GJ, Long AJ, Iwai Y, Bourque K, Chernova T, Nishimura H, et al. Engagement of the PD-1 immunoinhibitory receptor by a novel B7 family member leads to negative regulation of lymphocyte activation. J Exp Med. 2000;192(7):1027-34.
28. Reck M, Rodríguez-Abreu D, Robinson AG, Hui R, Csőszi T, Fülöp A, et al. Pembrolizumab versus chemotherapy for PD-L1-positive non-small-cell lung cancer. N Engl J Med. 2016;375(19):1823-33.
29. Wu K, Yi M, Qin S, Chu Q, Zheng X, Wu K. The efficacy and safety of combination of PD-1 and CTLA-4 inhibitors: a meta-analysis. Exp Hematol Oncol. 2019;8:26.
30. Tsao MS, Kerr KM, Kockx M, Beasley MB, Borczuk AC, Botling J, et al. PD-L1 immunohistochemistry comparability study in real-life clinical samples: results of blueprint phase 2 project. J Thorac Oncol. 2018;13(9):1302-11.
31. Le DT, Uram JN, Wang H, Bartlett BB, Kemberling H, Eyring AD, et al. PD-1 blockade in tumors with mismatch-repair deficiency. N Engl J Med. 2015;372(26):2509-20.
32. Bonneville R, Krook MA, Kautto EA, Miya J, Wing MR, Chen HZ, et al. Landscape of microsatellite instability across 39 cancer types. JCO Precis Oncol. 2017;2017:PO.17.00073.
33. Maio M, Ascierto PA, Manzyuk L, Motola-Kuba D, Penel N, Cassier PA, et al. Pembrolizumab in microsatellite instability high or mismatch repair deficient cancers: updated analysis from the phase II KEYNOTE-158 study. Ann Oncol. 2022;33(9):929-38.
34. Marabelle A, Fakih M, Lopez J, Shah M, Shapira-Frommer R, Nakagawa K, et al. Association of tumour mutational burden with outcomes in patients with advanced solid tumours treated with pembrolizumab: prospective biomarker analysis of the multicohort, open-label, phase 2 KEYNOTE-158 study. Lancet Oncol. 2020;21(10):1353-65.
35. Schneider BJ, Naidoo J, Santomasso BD, Lacchetti C, Adkins S, Anadkat M, et al. Management of immune-related adverse events in patients treated with

immune checkpoint inhibitor therapy: ASCO guideline update. J Clin Oncol. 2021;39(36):4073-126.
36. Maude SL, Frey N, Shaw PA, Aplenc R, Barrett DM, Bunin NJ, et al. Chimeric antigen receptor T cells for sustained remissions in leukemia. N Engl J Med. 2014;371(16):1507-17.
37. Fowler NH, Dickinson M, Dreyling M, Martinez-Lopez J, Kolstad A, Butler J, et al. Tisagenlecleucel in adult relapsed or refractory follicular lymphoma: the phase 2 ELARA trial. Nat Med. 2022;28(2):325-32.
38. Berdeja JG, Madduri D, Usmani SZ, Jakubowiak A, Agha M, Cohen AD, et al. Ciltacabtagene autoleucel, a B-cell maturation antigen-directed chimeric antigen receptor T-cell therapy in patients with relapsed or refractory multiple myeloma (CARTITUDE-1): a phase 1b/2 open-label study. Lancet. 2021;398(10297):314-24.
39. Morgan RA, Yang JC, Kitano M, Dudley ME, Laurencot CM, Rosenberg SA. Case report of a serious adverse event following the administration of T cells transduced with a chimeric antigen receptor recognizing ERBB2. Mol Ther. 2010;18(4):843-51.
40. Chou CK, Turtle CJ. Assessment and management of cytokine release syndrome and neurotoxicity following CD19 CAR-T cell therapy. Expert Opin Biol Ther. 2020;20(6):653-64.
41. Higano CS, Schellhammer PF, Small EJ, Burch PA, Nemunaitis J, Yuh L, et al. Integrated data from 2 randomized, double-blind, placebo-controlled, phase 3 trials of active cellular immunotherapy with sipuleucel-T in advanced prostate cancer. Cancer. 2009;115(16):3670-9.
42. Hu JC, Coffin RS, Davis CJ, Graham NJ, Groves N, Guest PJ, et al. A phase I study of OncoVEXGM-CSF, a second-generation oncolytic herpes simplex virus expressing granulocyte macrophage colony-stimulating factor. Clin Cancer Res. 2006;12(22):6737-47.
43. Andtbacka RH, Kaufman HL, Collichio F, Amatruda T, Senzer N, Chesney J, et al. Talimogene Laherparepvec Improves durable response rate in patients with advanced melanoma. J Clin Oncol. 2015;33(25):2780-8.

CHAPTER 13

Venous Ulcer

Rohit Kumar Singh, Ajay K Khanna

■ INTRODUCTION

Ulcers in the lower extremity, particularly venous leg ulcers (VLUs), are the most common chronic ulcers of the lower extremities. These ulcers not only contribute significantly to the socioeconomic challenges within the healthcare system but also exert substantial psychological and physical effects on those individuals who are affected. VLUs frequently manifest in conjunction with post-thrombotic syndrome, progressive chronic venous disease (CVD), varicose veins, and venous hypertension. Various demographic, genetic, and environmental elements have the potential to instigate CVD characterized by venous dilation, valve incompetence, venous reflux, and venous hypertension. The initiation of VLU may be linked to events such as endothelial cell injury, alterations in the glycocalyx, venous shear stress, and changes in adhesion molecules. Heightened endothelial cell permeability, the influx of leukocytes, elevated levels of inflammatory cytokines, matrix metalloproteinases (MMPs), reactive oxygen and nitrogen species, deposition of iron, and tissue metabolites also play a significant role in the development of VLU. The management of VLU involves employing compression and endovenous ablation therapy to address axial reflux. When accompanied by effective wound care and compression therapy, VLU typically exhibits healing within a span of 6 months.[1] The recurrence rate of VLU is notably high, ranging from 50 to 70%. This high recurrence is attributed to factors such as nonadherence to compression therapy, unsuccessful surgical interventions, inaccurate ulcer diagnoses, advancement of venous disease, and a pathophysiology that is not fully comprehended. Chronic venous insufficiency (CVI) causes about 80% of lower leg ulcers, with a prevalence of around 0.3% for venous ulcers and 1% for active or healed ulcers (**Figs. 1A to F**). Approximately 15–30% of VLU patients have concurrent arterial occlusive disease, termed a "mixed ulcer." Additionally, 15% of VLUs do not heal.[2]

■ VENOUS PATHOPHYSIOLOGY

Venous disease arises from three hemodynamic irregularities and their related risk factors:

Venous Ulcer

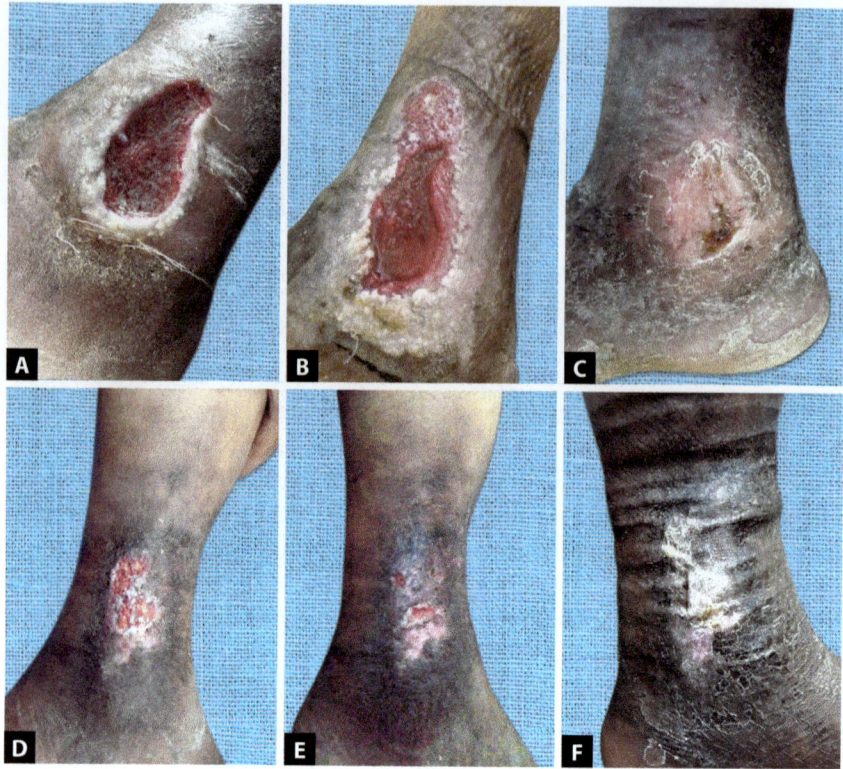

Figs. 1A to F: Active or healed venous ulcers in the lower leg.

1. *Valvular reflux:* Overweight, multiparity, prolonged periods of sitting or standing, and patients who underwent varicose vein surgery contribute to the heightened occurrence of valvular reflux—a common factor in venous-related issues.
2. Venous obstruction in circumstances such as deep vein thrombosis (DVT) and May–Thurner syndrome.
3. The malfunction of the calf-muscle pump, as seen in arthritis, leg surgery, or trauma, and in conditions such as Parkinson's disease, contributes to these issues.[3]

■ RISK FACTORS

- Elderly patients
- Women
- Overweight
- Multiparity
- Prolonged inactivity
- Genetics
- Sedentary profession

- DVT
- Hematological conditions such as factor V mutation, protein C and S deficiency

CLASSIFICATION SYSTEM FOR CHRONIC VENOUS DISEASE

A comprehensive assessment tool for CVD includes a two-part system: A classification and a severity scoring system. The classification, known as CEAP [CEAP: Clinical (C), Etiological (E), Anatomical (A), and Pathophysiological (P)], was established in 1995 after an international consensus conference endorsed by the joint councils of the Society for Vascular Surgery and the North American Chapter of the International Society for Cardiovascular Surgery. The scale has been updated over time and published as the revised CEAP classification and the 2020 update of the CEAP classification system[4] **(Fig. 2 and Tables 1 & 2)**

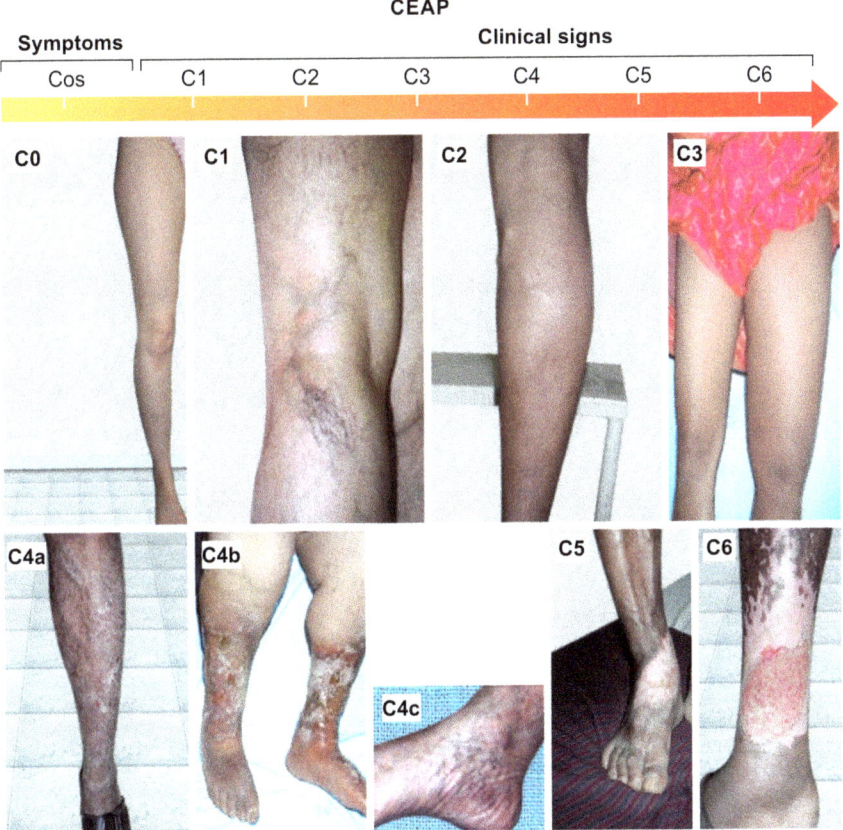

Fig. 2: Clinical photographs of patients arranged according to CEAP (Clinical Etiological Anatomical Pathophysiological) classification.

TABLE 1: The 2020 update of the CEAP (Clinical Etiological Anatomical Pathophysiological) classification.

Class	Description
Clinical (C) class:	
C0	No visible or palpable signs of venous disease
C1	Telangiectasia or reticular veins
C2	Varicose veins
C2r	Recurrent varicose veins
C3	Edema
C4	Changes in skin and subcutaneous tissue secondary to chronic venous disease (CVD)
C4a	Pigmentation or eczema
C4b	Lipodermatosclerosis or atrophie blanche
C4c	Corona phlebectatica
C5	Healed ulcer
C6	Active venous ulcer
C6r	Recurrent venous ulceration
Symptomatic or not: Subscript "S" or subscript "A"	S: Symptomatic, including ache, pain, tightness, skin irritation, heaviness, and muscle cramps, and other complaints attributable to venous dysfunction A: Asymptomatic
Etiological (E) class:	
Ep	Primary
Es	Secondary
Esi	Secondary—intravenous
Ese	Secondary—extravenous
Ec	Congenital
En	None identified
Anatomical (A) class:	
As	Superficial
Ad	Deep
Ap	Perforators
An	No identifiable venous location
Pathophysiological (P) class:	
Pr	Reflux
Po	Obstruction
Pr,o	Reflux and obstruction
Pn	No pathophysiology identified

Note: Reporting of pathophysiological class must be accompanied by the relevant anatomical location.
Source: Lurie et al.[4]

TABLE 2: The 2020 update of CEAP (Clinical Etiological Anatomical Pathophysiological): Summary of anatomical classification.

Anatomical classification	Segment number*	New anatomical site†	Description
As (superficial)	1	Tel	Telangiectasia
	1	Ret	Reticular veins
	2	GSVa	Great saphenous vein, above knee
	3	GSVb	Great saphenous vein, below knee
	4	SSV	Small saphenous vein
	–	AASV	Anterior accessory saphenous vein
	5	NSV	Nonsaphenous vein
Ad (deep)	6	IVC	Inferior vena cava
	7	CIV	Common iliac vein
	8	IIV	Internal iliac vein
	9	EIV	External iliac vein
	10	PELV	Pelvic vein
	11	CFV	Common femoral vein
	12	DFV	Deep femoral vein
	13	FV	Femoral vein
	14	POPV	Popliteal vein
	15	TIBV	Crural (tibial) vein
	15	PRV	Peroneal vein
	15	ATV	Anterior vein
	15	PTV	Posterior tibial vein
	16	MUSV	Muscular vein
	16	GAV	Gastrocnemius vein
	16	SOV	Soleal vein
Ap (perforator)	17	TPV	Thigh perforator vein
	18	CPV	Calf perforator vein
An (no venous anatomic location identified)			

*Numbers of anatomical segments used in the 2004 revision of the CEAP classification.
†New specific anatomical location(s) to be reported under each Pathophysiological (P) class to identify anatomical location(s) corresponding to P class.
Source: Lurie et al.[4]

CLINICAL EXAMINATION OF ULCER

Venous ulcers typically manifest in the Gaiter region, primarily anterior to the medial malleolus, pretibial area, and the lower third of the leg **(Figs. 3A to E)**. Characterized by painless, shallow depth, irregular edges, and distinct margins, these ulcers exhibit yellow or white exudate. Pain, if present, intensifies toward the day's end and alleviates with leg elevation. Measurement of the ulcer surface area serves as a reliable prognosis and healing indicator. Associated skin changes include venous dilation, telangiectasias, varicose veins, and edema. The revised Venous Severity Score (r-VCSS) provides a quantitative measure for patients with venous ulcers, aiding assessment.[5-7]

Evaluation of Lower Leg Ulcer

Following a comprehensive clinical history, examination, and biochemical investigations, specific diagnostic steps are taken. Venous duplex plays a crucial role, providing insights into superficial veins, perforators, and detecting DVT. Ankle–brachial pressure index (ABPI) is measured to guide compression stocking pressure, a key aspect of venous ulcer treatment. Computed tomography venography (CTV)/magnetic resonance venography (MRV) is employed for recurrent ulcerations or suspected deep vein incompetence. Endovenous imaging [intravascular ultrasound (IVUS)/venography] and air plethysmography assess deep venous abnormalities and venous volume, respectively. In cases of prolonged nonhealing ulcers, a biopsy may be necessary due to the potential risk of malignant transformation (Marjolin's ulcer).[8]

Screening for Calf Muscle Pump

Assessing the calf-muscle pump is crucial in evaluating individuals at risk of venous insufficiency, a major contributor to chronic venous issues. The

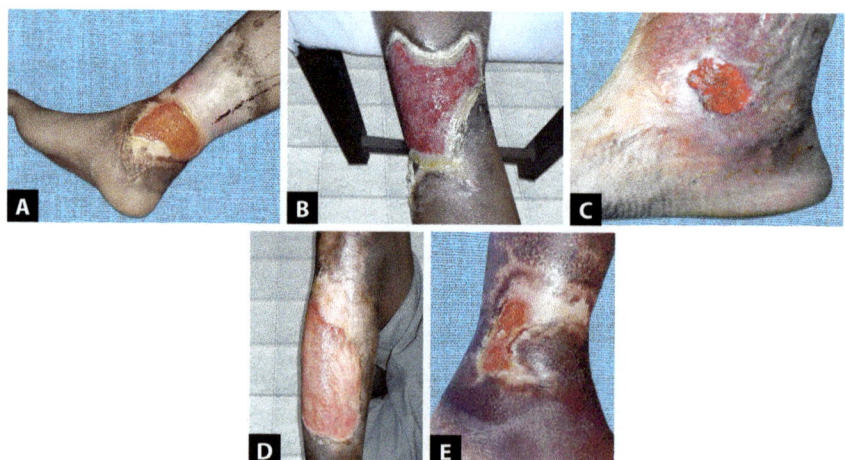

Figs. 3A to E: Typical location of venous ulcers in the Gaiter region.

evaluation includes ankle joint motion, calf muscle strength, and gait pattern. An effective calf-muscle pump demands a mobile ankle with dorsiflexion beyond 90°. Proper gait activation involves going up and down on toes while standing. Individuals with venous disease often exhibit a "shuffling gait," indicating compromised calf-muscle pump function.[9]

Ankle–Brachial Pressure Index

The ankle-brachial index (ABI) stands as the simplest noninvasive technique to ascertain associated lower extremity arterial occlusive disease **(Table 3)**. A cuff is positioned just above the ankle, inflated beyond systolic pressure, and slowly deflated with a Doppler probe placed over the posterior tibial or dorsalis pedis artery. The ankle pressure, the highest return Doppler signal, is recorded, while the brachial pressure, measured at the distal brachial or radial artery, is the denominator for ABI calculation. The highest ankle pressures divided by the higher brachial pressures determine the ABI, offering a more consistent measure with significance at measurements exceeding two standard deviations. ABPI also aids in guiding venous ulcer management.[10]

Toe Pressure

Digital pressure measurement mirrors arm and ankle methods, using a minicuff at the digit's base connected to a standard manometer. Flow return during cuff deflation is detected by devices such as photoplethysmography (PPG) probes or continuous-wave Doppler flow detectors. Toe pressures, particularly useful in patients prone to arterial calcification, such as diabetics and those with chronic kidney disease, provide insights, with waveform analysis or transcutaneous oxygen tension ($tcPO_2$) as alternatives when digital arteries are calcified.

Venous Duplex

Duplex ultrasound serves as the principal diagnostic tool for investigating suspected DVT, CVI, and other venous disorders. Combining imaging with

TABLE 3: Relation of ABPI with severity of disease.

ABPI	Inference
>1.30	Noncompressible
1.00–1.29	Normal
0.91–0.99	Borderline (equivocal)
0.41–0.90	Mild–moderate PAD
<0.4	Severe PAD

(ABPI: ankle–brachial pressure index; PAD: peripheral arterial disease)

Doppler-derived data enhances examination accuracy by revealing venous flow characteristics. Augmentation maneuvers, such as the calf pump and manual distal compression, aid in demonstrating flow. CVI results from elevated venous pressure due to outflow obstruction, pathological reflux, or both, often linked to valvular incompetence. Duplex scans directly assess for obstruction, evaluating vein appearance, compressibility, and flow patterns. Testing for reflux involves upright patient positioning, with venous flow parameters indicating abnormality if exceeding specified durations. For suprainguinal venous obstruction suspicion, comprehensive leg duplex assessment and abdominal/pelvic vein ultrasound are recommended as part of the initial evaluation.[11]

Role of Computed Tomography/Magnetic Resonance Venography

The Duplex scan has limitations in evaluating the deep veins of the abdomen and pelvis, necessitating cross-sectional imaging for precise assessment during interventions. CTV offers less-invasive yet accurate imaging with 96% sensitivity and 95% specificity for proximal DVT. It excels in detecting extrinsic compression syndromes. MRV, an ionizing radiation-free alternative, boasts 92% sensitivity and 95% specificity for DVT. Gadolinium-based contrast agents enhance vessel visualization, accuracy, and differentiation of thrombi age and hasten acquisition times. Assessing thrombus structure, direct thrombus imaging provides insights into composition changes, crucial for intervention decisions. Indirect signs on MRV, such as vein distension and enhanced vein wall, suggest acute thrombosis. This methodological approach ensures comprehensive evaluation and consideration of thrombus composition before interventions, offering a nuanced understanding of thrombus dynamics.

The triggered angiography noncontrast-enhanced (TRANCE) magnetic resonance imaging (MRI) technique captures vascular signal intensity variations throughout the cardiac cycle, allowing image subtraction for venograms and arteriograms without contrast agents. Utilizing three-dimensional turbo spin-echo (3D TSE) sequences with cardiac triggering, TRANCE-MRI provides high-resolution vessel images by subtracting sequential images. It excels in assessing varicose veins in lower extremities and deep veins in the pelvis and abdomen, offering a comprehensive view of venous status. In patients with venous ulcers and DVT, higher H_2O levels at 10-mm depth indicate increased subcutaneous water. Non-DVT venous ulcer patients, as per near-infrared spectroscopy (NIRS), show worse fluid retention at the 5-mm (dermis) level, showcasing H_2O value variations between DVT- and non-DVT-associated venous ulcers.[4,11]

Endovenous Imaging

Traditionally, angiography has been the gold standard for diagnosing vascular issues, but it lacks validation for CVD. With endovascular treatment options, IVUS has become a strong contender, though no imaging method is validated for clinical CVI.

Venography

Traditional ascending venography, employing foot vein access and contrast injection, is obsolete as it offers no additional benefits over Doppler ultrasound for deep venous obstruction screening. Venography through popliteal vein (POPV), femoral vein (FV), or common femoral vein (CFV) access was once utilized for suprainguinal venous obstruction evaluation, revealing collaterals and flattened common iliac vein (CIV) (pancaking) to indirectly diagnose left CIV obstruction.[12]

Intravascular Ultrasound

Intravascular ultrasound stands out as a valuable tool in delving into deep venous pathologies. In a manner akin to CTV and MRV, IVUS provides accurate assessments of both the cross-luminal diameter and the surface area of deep veins. Its distinctive feature lies in its capability to uncover subtle intraluminal changes and abnormalities in the vein wall, proving more adept than venography in detecting lesions in deep veins as demonstrated in the VIDIO (venogram versus intravascular ultrasound for diagnosing and treating iliofemoral vein obstruction) trial. Despite its invasive nature, the use of IVUS could play a role in selecting patients for venous stenting, contingent upon successfully navigating the lesion with a guidewire.[12,13]

Plethysmography

Air plethysmography quantifies the overall volume change (in mL/s) within the calf area encircled by the cuff, noting the response to gravity-dependent filling (venous filling index) and leg elevation-induced drainage (venous drainage index). Swift filling and sluggish elevation drainage signify generalized venous insufficiency and blockage. This differs from ultrasound flow assessments focused on specific vein segments during squeezing and releasing actions.

■ FACTORS PROLONGING VENOUS LEG ULCER HEALING

Venous ulcers experience prolonged healing due to challenges in transitioning from the inflammatory to the proliferative phase, untreated ambulatory venous hypertension, difficulty in reducing interstitial fluid, inflammation, biofilm, and controlling drainage or infection. Additionally, the absence of local growth factors contributes to the delayed healing.

■ BIOFILM IN VENOUS ULCER

Chronic wounds' failure to heal, despite proper care, is attributed to the presence of bacterial biofilm. The dense extracellular matrix (ECM), associated with bacterial cells such as *Staphylococcus aureus*, *Pseudomonas aeruginosa*, *Proteus mirabilis*, and *Escherichia coli*, contains polysaccharides, proteins, and deoxyribonucleic acid (DNA). This matrix offers structural protection, enhancing bacterial resistance to antibodies, inflammatory cells, antibiotics, and antiseptics. The presence of cell septum formation indicates bacterial cell division, leading to colonization in wounds.[14-16]

■ GENE EXPRESSION IN NONHEALING VENOUS LEG ULCER

Gene Expression of Epidermal Wound Bed

Distinct gene expression in keratinocytes at the edge of nonhealing venous ulcers reveals key insights. The prominently upregulated genes include secreted frizzled-related protein 4 (*SFRP4*), a mediator of Wnt signaling crucial for embryogenesis, carcinogenesis, angiogenesis, and epidermal cell mobility. *SFRP4* is strongly linked to cell apoptosis. Another upregulated gene, branched-chain aminotransferase 1 (*BCAT1*), influences cell growth and apoptosis. Conversely, the most downregulated gene group codes for keratin 16 and others essential for epidermal maintenance, impairing timely repair associated with epidermal injury in nonhealing venous ulcers.

Elevated gene expression in nonhealing venous wounds involves proteins linked to tissue injury, ECM formation, and wound healing. Properdin, vital for tissue inflammation, aids in assembling C3Bb on the surface. Dermatopontin, an ECM protein crucial for cell–matrix interactions and collagen assembly, shows increased expression, potentially influenced by transforming growth factor-beta 1 (TGF-β1) in wound healing. Heparin-binding epidermal growth factor (HB-EGF), essential for epithelization, experiences downregulation. This EGF-like growth factor's mitogenic and migratory effects on keratinocytes and fibroblasts support dermal repair and angiogenesis, presenting a noteworthy aspect in nonhealing venous ulcers.[17]

■ VARIOUS PREDICTORS OF VENOUS WOUND HEALING

Laser Speckle Imaging

The wound healing can be assessed by several methods. Laser speckle imaging (LSI) is a noninvasive method for evaluating tissue blood flow, including cutaneous wounds. Utilizing near-infrared laser speckle contrast analysis, systems such as Moor FLPI-2 illuminate tissue up to 1 mm in depth, creating a 16-color-coded perfusion image. This image represents the interaction between photons and Doppler-shifted red cells, forming a dynamic speckle pattern. High perfusion results in rapid variation, seen as low area contrast, while low perfusion yields high contrast. LSI proves clinically useful for venous ulcer assessment, demonstrating acceptable sensitivity and specificity, especially at the wound edge, and predicting healing outcomes.

Transcutaneous Measurement of Oxygen Partial Pressure

Transcutaneous measurement of oxygen partial pressure ($TcPO_2$), a polarographic technique, gauges skin surface partial pressure of oxygen (pO_2) to evaluate microvascular circulation. Measured at 43-45°C with skin sensors, it is accurate in noncompressible arteries and applicable in diabetic and renal patients. Acute wounds exhibit around 60 mm Hg pO_2, while chronic wounds average 35 mm Hg. $TcPO_2$ levels below 20 or 30 mm Hg are independent predictors of complications in chronic wound healing.

Skin Perfusion Pressure

Various techniques evaluate skin perfusion pressure (SPP), a measure of microvascular circulation. These include radioisotope clearance, PPG, and laser Doppler. Laser Doppler, known for its speed, effectiveness, and ease of operation, is the most commonly employed method for SPP measurement. An SPP increase exceeding 20 mm Hg is indicative of favorable wound healing outcomes.[18]

Oxygen-to-see Method

The optical measurement technique combines white light spectrometry and laser Doppler flowmetry to generate a comprehensive map detailing oxygen saturation, relative hemoglobin levels, and blood flow in specific tissues.

Indocyanine Green Fluorescence Imaging

Indocyanine green fluorescence imaging (ICG-FI) visualizes foot perfusion and measures the washout of ICG in peripheral tissues. Utilizing time–intensity curves from the ICG-FI record allows for quantitative perfusion assessment. This innovative technique proves valuable in evaluating alterations in foot perfusion, offering insights into potential outcomes for wound healing.

pH Assessment

During the process of functional wound healing, the pH undergoes a gradual reduction from initial alkaline values (around pH 8-8.5) to the pH levels characteristic of intact skin (5.5-6). If the pH remains elevated, it results in a slowdown or cessation of wound healing as evidenced by diminished cell proliferation and migration in chronic wounds. Chronic wounds further exhibit a centripetal increase in pH, leading to intensified hydrogen-ion extrusion and peripheral acidification of the wound. This decreased pH acts as an impediment to keratinocyte migration, proliferation, and viability, thereby contributing to the challenges encountered in the healing of chronic wounds.[13-19]

ASSOCIATION OF CYTOKINE CONCENTRATIONS AND WOUND HEALING IN VENOUS ULCER

When leg ulcers happen on the lower limbs, it is usually because of ongoing issues with blood flow called chronic venous hypertension. The healing of these sores involves a complex process, and it is guided by special substances called cytokines and growth factors that are present in the wound. Markers such as tumor necrosis factor-alpha (TNF-α), interleukin-1β (IL-1β) (inflammation), beta (β)-fibroblast growth factor (βFGF), vascular endothelial growth factor (VEGF) (angiogenesis), TGF-β1 (fibrogenesis/fibroblast proliferation), and matrix metallopeptidase 2 (MMP2) and MMP9 (proteolysis) can gauge wound biological activity. A prospective observational study by Manjit et al. established a positive and linear relationship between the initial βFGF levels in wound fluid and ulcer size in chronic venous ulceration.[18] VEGF concentrations inversely correlated with patient age, while TGF-1 levels increased during venous ulcer healing, indicating enhanced fibrogenesis, matrix deposition, and proliferation in the healing wound.

TREATMENT OF VENOUS ULCER

The primary objective of treatment is the healing of ulcers, with secondary goals encompassing edema reduction, pain management, and recurrence prevention. Treatment modalities for venous ulcers encompass conservative approaches involving mechanical methods, medications, advanced wound therapy, and surgical options.[20]

General Principles

At the heart of CVD, active VLUs stand out as a severe manifestation, falling under the clinical class C6 in the CEAP classification.[4] The development of VLUs is closely linked to chronic venous hypertension, influenced by factors such as venous reflux, blockages in blood flow, weak calf muscles, and overweight. This condition places a notable economic strain on healthcare, affecting nearly 1% of the population and rising to 3% in individuals aged 80 years and above. While a significant percentage of VLUs heal within a year, there is a persistent 7% that remains unhealed after 5 years, coupled with a concerning recurrence rate of up to 70% within 3 months postwound closure. The integration of a multidisciplinary approach and adherence to the TIME (Tissue, Infection/inflammation, Moisture balance, and Edge of the wound) concept have advanced diagnostic procedures and clinical outcomes in the realm of chronic wound care. Despite the absence of randomized controlled trials (RCTs), the TIME principles are widely embraced in the treatment of VLUs.

Pain Control

Addressing pain is a significant concern for individuals with VLUs, encompassing both persistent pains linked to the wound and discomfort experienced during dressing changes. A thorough pain assessment involves considering factors such as site, intensity, attributes, recurrence, and temporal aspects while also identifying triggers and effective relievers. Although various tools are available for pain assessment, the visual analog scale (VAS) is commonly used. A meta-analysis found an 80% incidence of pain associated with the wound,[21] with an average intensity score of 4 on a 0-10 VAS scale. It is worth noting that there is a lack of trials examining interventions for persistent pain in VLU patients. Nevertheless, the World Health Organization's endorsed three-step analgesic ladder is deemed as an efficacious strategy for addressing chronic pain in these instances.

Antibiotics and Antiseptics

In the realm of VLUs, bacterial colonization is a common occurrence, though often deemed clinically inconsequential. The impact of infection on ulcer healing is a noted concern. Despite the common practice of prescribing systemic antibiotics or topical agents, evidence from a Cochrane review challenges the routine use of systemic antimicrobials for VLUs. Moreover, there is scant support for the efficacy of topical antibiotics. Notably, topical cadexomer iodine, an antiseptic, exhibits promise in enhancing VLU healing compared to standard care. Similarly, silver dressings, acknowledged for their antimicrobial effects, may elevate the probability of VLU healing, necessitating further investigation into time-to-healing outcomes.

Mobilization and Physical Therapy

The primary objective of mobilization and rehabilitation for VLUs is to mitigate venous hypertension and edema. Achieving this involves activating the calf muscle venous pump through particular physical activities or biomechanical interventions. Despite the theoretical benefits, empirical evidence demonstrating enhanced VLU healing or reduced recurrence rates from physical activities or targeted therapeutic interventions remains scarce. Given the common occurrence of comorbidities in elderly VLU patients, addressing issues such as ankle stiffness, inadequacy of the calf muscle venous pump, and overweight is crucial for optimizing wound healing. Assessing arterial status through techniques such as CW Doppler and measuring ankle pressure and ABI is essential, particularly in patients with peripheral artery disease in the lower extremities. An ABI exceeding 0.8 may be deemed normal, allowing the initiation of comprehensive compression therapy. In cases involving diabetes and arteries that are resistant to compression, an arterial Doppler ultrasound or toe pressure assessment may be necessary to rule out arterial disease.[22]

Wound Care

Specialized care for chronic wounds demands the expertise of well-trained nurses or wound care professionals, ideally integrated into a multidisciplinary team. A comprehensive assessment of VLUs should encompass considerations such as site, ulcer extents, exudate quantity and category (mild/moderate/severe), wound bed appearance (irregular shape), condition of the wound edge (attached, rolled), presence of clinical infection signs, and alterations in the surrounding skin. The pivotal goal of wound bed preparation is to transform the biological milieu of a long-lasting wound into that resembling an acutely healing wound.

Debridement

Wound debridement involves eliminating necrotic tissue, debris, or foreign matter from a wound, following the prior step of wound cleansing, which focuses on removing surface contaminants, bacteria, and remnants of past dressings from the wound and its adjacent skin. Techniques for wound debridement comprise surgical/sharp debridement, mechanical debridement, enzymatic debridement, autolytic debridement, and biosurgical debridement using sterile larvae.[20-23]

Dressings and Topical Agents

Numerous wound dressings are utilized for VLUs, but a recent Cochrane review highlighted the need for further research to assess the efficacy of specific dressings or topical agents in improving VLU healing. Another review on protease-modulating matrix treatment also emphasized the low-quality evidence on its influence on ulcer healing or adverse events. Although certain dressings may be beneficial for managing wounds with disproportionate exudate, the evidence supporting hyperbaric oxygen therapy for VLU healing remains unreliable.

Compression Therapy

At the core of conservative approaches to treat VLUs is compression therapy, playing a pivotal role in the treatment strategy demonstrating effectiveness in compressing leg veins and soft tissues. It improves venous hemodynamics, alleviating the effects of venous hypertension. Numerous studies unequivocally support the role of compression therapy in enhancing VLU healing compared to cases without compression, contributing to pain reduction as well.[23]

Compression Materials

Commencing VLU treatment through various compression methods involves elastic compression stockings (ECS), superimposed ECS, elastic bandages, inelastic bandages (IB), adjustable compression garments (ACG), and intermittent pneumatic compression (IPC). Ideal for smaller VLUs, superimposed ECS utilizes an inner stocking with sustained 20 mm Hg pressure, worn day and night for effective healing. The second stocking, applying 20–25 mm Hg during the day, complements the process. Multicomponent, multilayer inelastic bandages, such as IB, demonstrate their efficacy through the "static stiffness index" (SSI). IB, with an SSI >10 mm Hg, rivals the SSI of "four-layer" bandages, supporting their comparable healing potential **(Figs. 4A to E)**. This variety in compression methods allows tailored approaches for VLU management.[23-26]

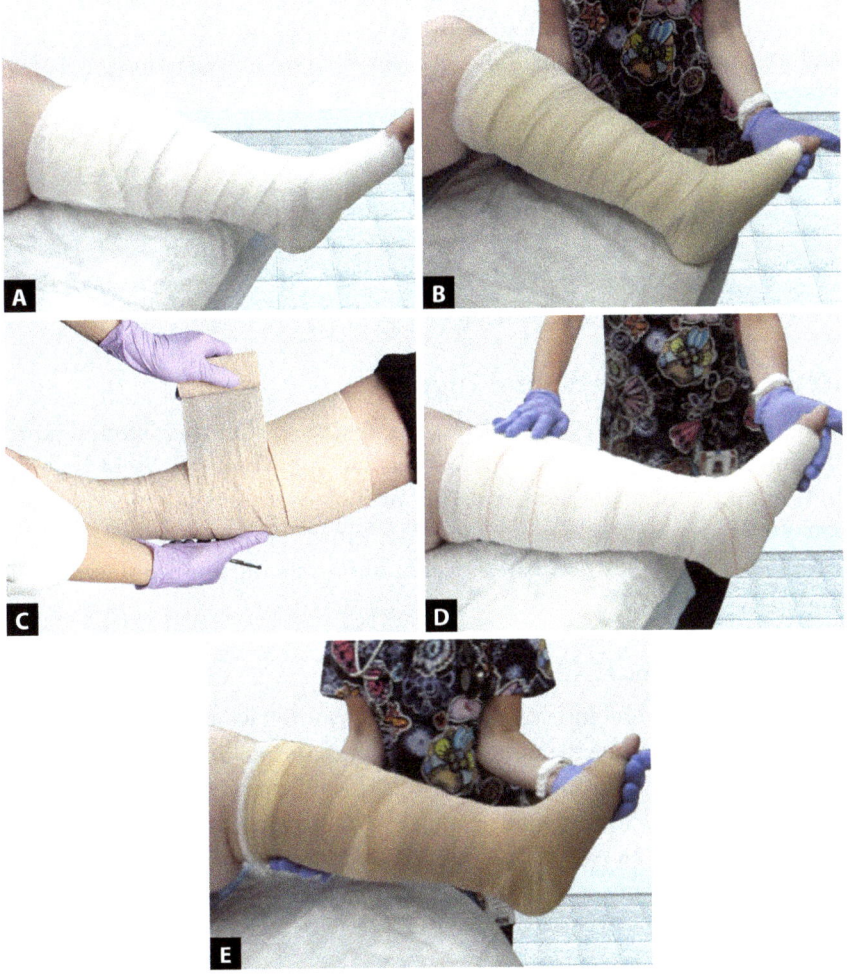

Figs. 4A to E: Four-layer bandage applied in patients with chronic venous ulcer.

Compression Stockings

Compression stockings serve as maintenance therapy post-VLU healing, with specific recommendations for various conditions. For CVD (CEAP C4b), below-knee ECS at 20–40 mm Hg alleviates skin induration. Post-thrombotic syndrome patients benefit from similar stockings to reduce severity, considering IPC for additional relief. Addressing superficial and deep venous issues is essential to determining the recurrence of VLUs.[23-27] Alternatively, conservative below-knee ECS therapy helps prevent recurrence, with higher pressure correlating with lower recurrence rates, albeit with a trade-off in compliance. Optimal results emerge when patients maintain hosiery compliance, irrespective of compression level.

■ OTHER WOUND THERAPIES

Therapeutic Ultrasound

The effectiveness of therapeutic ultrasound in promoting VLU healing is still unclear. Review authors indicate a potential small effect, but conclusive evidence is lacking.

Electromagnetic Therapy

In three RCTs involving 94 patients, electromagnetic therapy (EMT) effects on VLU were explored. All trials compared EMT with sham EMT. Due to heterogeneity, a meta-analysis was not feasible, leaving the effects of EMT undetermined pending high-quality RCTs.

Negative Pressure Wound Therapy

Randomized controlled trial data supporting vacuum-assisted closure therapy as a main treatment for VLUs is lacking. However, there is some indication that it might accelerate the healing process when incorporated into a management regimen that includes punch skin graft transplantation. However, the specific context of evaluation limits the applicability of this finding.[26]

■ GROWTH FACTORS

Utilizing intralesional injection, granulocyte–monocyte colony-stimulating factor (GM-CSF) has been employed to enhance the healing process of VLUs. Various other mechanisms for delivering growth factors, such as autologous platelet-rich plasma, autologous platelet-rich fibrin matrix membrane, basic fibroblast growth factor, vitronectin:growth factor, platelet-derived growth factor, calcitonin gene-related peptide, and vasoactive intestinal polypeptide, currently are either in the experimental phase or lack conclusive evidence from RCTs.

HUMAN AMNIOTIC MEMBRANE ALLOGRAFTS IN VENOUS LEG ULCERS

Approximately 80 amniotic products are currently in developmental stages, each claiming unique structural characteristics relevant to ulcer healing. Various forms of amniotic membrane allograft, including fresh, lyophilized, cryopreserved, and dehydrated types, have demonstrated comparable results, albeit at a low evidence level, mainly supported by case series, retrospective studies, registries, and medium-sized industry-sponsored efficacy studies. The wound healing effects of amniotic membranes on chronic wounds primarily stem from their ability to coordinate ECM remodeling, provide a range of growth factors, stimulate wound fibroblasts and keratinocytes through paracrine mechanisms, and downregulate inflammation by suppressing pro-inflammatory molecules. Amniotic membranes are available in various forms, such as fresh, cryopreserved, dehydrated, and lyophilized (dehydration with freeze-drying).[27]

FLAP RECONSTRUCTION

Free Tissue Transfer

Initiating the process of harvesting a free flap for ulcer repair involves thoughtful consideration of various factors. For addressing large defects, the latissimus dorsi muscle becomes a significant choice, while moderately sized wounds may find a solution in the rectus abdominis or split latissimus dorsi. Smaller ulcers can be effectively managed with the serratus or gracilis muscle. The selection of arterial inflow is a strategic decision based on factors such as lesion location and arterial condition. Typically, the posterior tibial artery is preferred, considering its lower potential for spasm. However, adjustments may be made if arterial abnormalities or specific ulcer locations necessitate alternative choices.[25-29]

Distally-based Sural Fasciocutaneous Flap

Based on the sural nerve as its base, this flap derives its blood supply from the vascular network alongside the sural nerve. Arising from either the popliteal artery or a sural artery, the superficial sural artery follows a subfascial course in the proximal calf. Effective in covering sizable venous ulcers, it does present side effects such as donor site pain and numbness at the lateral aspect of the foot.

Other Options

Cross-leg Flaps

Immobilization-requiring methods such as muscle or fasciocutaneous flaps are unsuitable, especially for the elderly. Local cutaneous flaps are ineffective for significant venous ulcer defects. Moreover, the presence of lipodermatosclerotic skin around the ulcer hinders the use of local flaps for coverage.[30]

■ MEDICAL MANAGEMENT
Micronized Purified Flavonoid Fraction

Micronized purified flavonoid fraction (MPFF) is a widely utilized venoactive drug (VAD) for treating CVD. MPFF exhibits various pharmacologic actions, including reducing endothelial cell activation, serum concentrations of adhesion molecules and growth factors, leukocyte adhesion, venous valve deterioration, and pro-inflammatory mediator production. These properties lead to improved venous tone, reduced venous distension, enhanced lymphatic drainage, and clinical benefits, alleviating symptoms of CVD, such as edema, skin changes, and aiding VLU healing. The recommended dose of Daflon (MPFF) is 1,000 mg once daily for 6 months, with infrequent and minor side effects.[31]

In addition to compression therapy, two non-VADs, pentoxifylline and sulodexide, enhance VLU healing. Pentoxifylline, a methylxanthine, serves as a nonselective phosphodiesterase inhibitor with antioxidant and anti-inflammatory properties, reducing blood viscosity and clot formation. The usual dose is 400 mg thrice daily. Sulodexide, a low-molecular-weight heparin and dermatan sulfate combination, offers antithrombotic, profibrinolytic, and anti-inflammatory effects. The dose is 25 mg twice daily. Aspirin, *Ruscus* extract, MPFF, calcium dobesilate, horse chestnut extract, hydroxyethylrutoside, and red vine leaf extract are also employed for symptomatic relief in conjunction with compression therapy.

■ ROLE OF SURGERY IN VENOUS ULCER

Indications for varicose vein surgery encompass symptomatic veins, duplex evidence of reflux over 1 second, ineffective compression stocking trial (6 weeks to 3 months), venous ulcer, lipodermatosclerosis, recurring minor or significant hemorrhage, and nonhealing chronic venous ulcer. Surgical options include open surgery, endovenous techniques such as radiofrequency ablation (RFA), endovenous laser ablation (EVLA), endovenous steam ablation (EVSA), and endovenous microwave ablation (EVMA). Nonthermal/nontumescent options involve sclerotherapy, mechanochemical ablation (MOCA), adhesive glue [*n*-butyl cyanoacrylate (nBCA)], and high-intensity focused ultrasound (HIFU) to prevent venous ulcer recurrence.[32]

High Ligation of the Great Saphenous Vein

Approaching the great saphenous vein (GSV) is facilitated by a 2.5-cm oblique incision below and lateral to the pubic tubercle, ensuring reliable access to the saphenofemoral junction. Preoperative ultrasound-guided marking enhances precision, allowing a minimal incision and subcutaneous dissection. Identification of the GSV's main trunk and six tributaries, which vary in number and position, requires careful dissection of the FV. High ligation of the GSV is then performed near the FV, often employing a double ligation on a proximal stump, with the second ligation using a suture ligature.

Great Saphenous Vein Stripping

Central to the classic varicose veins operation, GSV stripping significantly reduces recurrence rates when combined with high ligation. Following flush ligation, a transverse venotomy is created, and a stripper, often wire or disposable plastic, is passed distally. Reflux facilitates smooth stripper passage, typically reaching the knee level. A secondary incision near the knee aids in palpable stripper exposure. Optimal GSV stripping involves a downward direction, enhancing tributary avulsion and minimizing saphenous nerve injuries.[33]

Operative Technique for Small Saphenous Vein Procedures

Following anesthesia induction, patients are placed prone, with cautious padding of bony areas. A small transverse skin incision, guided by preoperative ultrasound marking, is made just distal to the saphenopopliteal junction. Incision length is tailored to subcutaneous tissue thickness. The fascia is opened along the incision, revealing the small saphenous vein (SSV). Tracing the SSV distally, between fascia and calf muscles, requires Doppler assurance due to its artery-like appearance. The SSV is divided between clamps, with care to dissect in the perivenous plane and avoid injuring the sural nerve usually adherent to the SSV's distal third, making stripping generally unnecessary.

Excision of Local Varicosities (Mini-Phlebectomy)

Incorporating a range of incision orientations, the surgical procedure involves using specialized instruments such as hooks, iris forceps, and fine-pointed clamps for vein retrieval. Small dermal varicosities are meticulously avulsed, while larger veins are carefully grasped and brought through corresponding incisions. These vein loops are prepared by removing excess fat, followed by double clamping and division. A preventive measure involves rolling the vein onto the clamp to avoid premature avulsion. The surgical goal is the complete removal of varicose segments; if a vein breaks during the process, it can be reacquired through the creation of a new incision.[29]

Transilluminated Powered Phlebectomy

TriVex employs tumescent dissection, transillumination, and powered phlebectomy for ambulatory phlebectomy. It eliminates the need for general or regional anesthesia due to tumescent anesthesia. The device, akin to those for subcutaneous fat removal, is inserted through a small incision. By transilluminating veins and performing phlebectomy, it disrupts and removes varicosities across a broad area.

Subfascial Endoscopic Perforator Surgery

Subfascial endoscopic perforator surgery (SEPS) utilizes endoscopic tools for minimally invasive interruption of incompetent perforators in CVI. Introduced by Hauer in 1980, it became a widely accepted and safe surgical method due to its minimally invasive approach. SEPS involves one or two endoscopic ports, exsanguination, thigh tourniquet, and balloon dissection for subfascial space widening. The procedure is performed with a camera port and a distal port under video control, exploring the subfascial space and dividing perforators using endoscopic scissors or harmonic scalpel after clip placement. However, this technique is not very popular now-a-days because of the technical problems and associated complications.

■ OTHER WOUND THERAPIES

The efficacy of therapeutic ultrasound in improving VLU healing is uncertain, with potential effects considered small. EMT's impact on VLU was explored in three RCTs involving 94 patients, comparing it with sham EMT. Meta-analysis was hindered by heterogeneity, leaving effects unestablished. Regarding negative-pressure wound therapy, there is no RCT evidence supporting its primary use for VLU treatment, but it might reduce healing time within specific contexts, such as a treatment regimen involving punch skin graft transplantation.[32]

Endovenous Technique for Varicose Veins

In patients undergoing endovenous thermal ablation for superficial venous incompetence, it is advisable to use ultrasound-guided tumescent anesthesia. Buffered solutions can mitigate periprocedural pain.

Radiofrequency Ablation

Mechanism of Action

Destruction of the endothelium, collagen contraction, and thrombus formation result in fibrosis within the vein during endovenous thermal ablation. Duplex ultrasonography guides the procedure, ensuring access—

10 cm below the popliteal area. Local anesthesia is administered, a sheath is inserted, and the closure FAST catheter is advanced. Perivenous tumescent anesthesia, a mixture of lidocaine, epinephrine, and saline, protects surrounding tissues. Segments of the vein are treated independently for 20-second intervals, with compression recommended postoperatively.[33]

Endovenous Laser Ablation

Endovenous laser ablation, akin to RFA, uses laser energy, specifically wavelengths such as 810, 980, 1,470, or 1,940 nm, delivered via bare or jacket-tipped fibers to induce fibrosis and vein occlusion. GSV access is near the popliteal area, and treatment energy averages 50–80 J/cm. Continuous pullback is used during the procedure, and early endovenous ablation is recommended for patients with active venous leg ulceration. Managing incompetent veins is recommended for individuals with healed ulcers and superficial venous incompetence, minimizing the risk of recurrence. Ultrasound-guided foam sclerotherapy (UGFS) is a viable option for ablating the subulcer venous plexus in patients with active venous leg ulceration.[26-30]

Endovenous Steam Ablation

Endovenous steam ablation employs steam to heat veins to 120°C, causing endothelial destruction and fibrosis. Done under local tumescent anesthesia, a 16-gauge needle punctures the vein under ultrasound. The steam catheter releases controlled steam puffs and is retracted stepwise. A trial comparing EVLA with EVSA found noninferiority in truncal occlusion and better postprocedural pain and satisfaction with EVSA.

Sclerotherapy

Sclerotherapy effectively treats various vein types and sizes, focusing on smaller vessels such as reticular veins and telangiectasias. The procedure involves introducing a chemical into the vein, causing endothelial damage, thrombosis, and subsequent fibrosis. Sclerotherapy, a versatile treatment for various veins, introduces a chemical into the vein to induce endothelial damage, leading to thrombosis and fibrosis. Absolute contraindications include a patent foramen ovale, allergy to the sclerosant, acute cellulitis, and pregnancy. Relative contraindications involve asthma, hypercoagulable state, and advanced arterial disease. Liquid sclerotherapy treats smaller veins, while foam sclerotherapy, creating a foam-like consistency, enhances contact with the vein wall. The primary limitation is vein diameter, requiring contact for effective treatment. The qualities of an ideal sclerosing agent include efficiently damaging the endothelium, having a low incidence of adverse events, and causing minimal pain during injection. Sodium tetradecyl sulfate boasts an extensive track record of safety and effectiveness in addressing telangiectasias, reticular veins, and varicose veins, making it the most commonly utilized detergent sclerosant. Conversely, sodium morrhuate is not favored due to its elevated risk of skin necrosis and anaphylaxis. Similarly, ethanolamine oleate, a viscous solution challenging to inject, sees limited use. In the liquid sclerotherapy approach, after dilution, multiple syringes with 30-gauge needles are filled and assembled. Treatment begins with the largest veins, proceeding in a central-to-peripheral direction. Sclerosant quantity varies based on vein size; larger varicose veins typically receive 1 mL or less per site, while reticular veins and smaller telangiectasias may require 0.25–0.5 and 0.1–0.2 mL per injection, respectively. Injections are administered at 2- to 3-cm intervals until the entire target vessel length is treated. Bleeding is minimized by placing a gauze sponge over each site, securing it with tape. Graduated compression hoses are worn for 1–3 days post-treatment to reduce thrombus formation.[27-29]

Ultrasound-guided foam sclerotherapy utilizes a three-way stopcock connected to two syringes, following Tessari's (1999) method.[34] The effective foam criteria include bubble size (100 µm or less) and a specific air-to-liquid ratio. The foam amount is determined by the $V = \pi \times (D/2) \times L$ formula. The procedure involves ultrasound-guided foam creation, needle placement confirmation, and controlled foam injection. Graduated compression stockings (30–40 mm Hg) are worn post-treatment for 24 hours (reticular veins and telangiectasias) or 7–10 days (varicose veins and perforators).

Mechanicochemical Ablation (MOCA)

Foam sclerotherapy offers advantages for treating truncal reflux, notably obviating the need for tumescent anesthesia. Ongoing evaluations explore treatments that eliminate tumescent anesthesia. MOCA with the ClariVein device is a novel, minimally invasive approach. The catheter, featuring a rotating wire causing mechanical damage and vein wall spasm, administers a liquid sclerosant, typically sodium tetradecyl sulfate. MOCA, compared to RFA, exhibits less pain, faster recovery, and earlier return to work. Trials report closure rates of 87–97%, with a 2-year study noting a 96% occlusion rate. An RCT demonstrates similar occlusion rates between MOCA and RFA at 92% after 4 weeks.[31]

Adhesive Closure/Cyanoacrylate Embolization/VenaSeal Sapheno Closure System

The VenaSeal Closure System (Medtronic, Minneapolis, Minnesota), utilizing nBCA glue through a catheter, eliminates the need for tumescent anesthesia. Upon contact with ionic compounds in the blood, the glue polymerizes, forming a flexible adhesive end product. Comprising an introducer sheath, infusion catheter, dispenser gun, and proprietary cyanoacrylate adhesive, the system accesses the refluxing truncal vein. Ultrasound-guided injections of glue are made centrally, followed by single injections at 3-cm intervals as the catheter is withdrawn, delivering 0.1 mL of adhesive every 3 cm along the treated vein. Treatment concludes 5 cm cranial from the access site.[31-33]

High-intensity Focused Ultrasound (HIFU)

High-intensity focused ultrasound is entirely noninvasive, employing ultrasound energy directed from a transducer onto the skin above the vein. The device applies gentle pressure, closing the vein without the risk of thrombosis or excess heat. Focused therapeutic ultrasound, using a linear ultrasound array for real-time imaging, targets the specific vein. The Sonovein machine, designed for HIFU, automatically gauges vein depth, adjusting energy delivery to safeguard the skin. Precise heat is generated by focused ultrasound, guided by real-time imaging, resulting in ablation of a rice-sized tissue volume at 85–90°C. HIFU achieves permanent vein closure through fibrosis without requiring vein cannulation or any insertion into the target vein.

■ MEASURES TAKEN TO PREVENT RECURRENCE OF ULCER

The recurrence of venous ulcers is notably high, reaching up to 70%. Key strategies for preventing recurrence involve venous intervention, prolonged use of compression stockings, and the beneficial combination of leg elevation with compression stockings. Lifestyle modifications such as diet adjustments, nutritional supplements, smoking cessation, weight management, maintaining cardiac health, and robust psychosocial support contribute to ulcer prevention. Elevating the lower limb for at least 1 h/day, 6 days a week, is recommended for reducing recurrence. Progressive resistance exercise to enhance calf muscle pump function and continued compression therapy are viable measures. Surgical correction of superficial venous reflux at an early date, coupled with long-term compression bandaging, significantly reduces ulcer recurrence rates. Additionally, sclerotherapy demonstrates potential in lowering the risk of venous ulcer recurrence.

■ CONCLUSION

Addressing chronic venous ulcers poses a therapeutic challenge, emphasizing the need for a comprehensive diagnostic assessment from the outset of treatment. Beyond conservative methods, it is crucial to alleviate venous hypertension, with compression therapy playing a central role. Novel local management techniques are currently undergoing trials. For nonhealing venous ulcer patients, especially after compression therapy and in the absence of deep vein incompetence, considerations include superficial venous surgery, foam sclerotherapy, or ligation of affected veins as integral components of the overall treatment strategy. To prevent recurrences, regular clinical evaluations and patient education on skin care, elevation, exercise, and lifelong compression therapy along with an early superficial venous intervention are strongly emphasized.

REFERENCES

1. Khanna AK, Kumar S. Venous scenario in India. Indian J Surg. 2023;85(Suppl. 1):S1-6.
2. Prakash S, Tiwary SK, Mishra M, Khanna AK. Venous ulcer. Surg Sci. 2013;4(2):144-50.
3. Khanna AK, Katiyar A, Khanna S, Nath G, Kumar P, Tiwary SK. Bacteriological study of varicose vein specimens. Indian J Surg. 2023;85(Suppl 1):93-9.
4. Lurie F, Passman M, Meisner M, Dalsing M, Masuda E, Welch H, et al. The 2020 update of the CEAP classification system and reporting standards. J Vasc Surg Venous Lymphat Disord. 2020;8:342-52.
5. Stana J, Maver U, Potočnik U. Genetic biases related to chronic venous ulceration. J Wound Care. 2019;28(2):59-65.
6. Agale SV. Chronic leg ulcers: epidemiology, aetiopathogenesis, and management. Ulcers. 2013;2013:1-9.
7. Nelzen O. Prevalence of venous leg ulcer: the importance of the data collection method. Phlebolymphology. 2008;15(4):143-50.
8. Varghese R, Patel M, Rajarshi M, Khanna AK. Varicose veins—how to investigate. Indian J Surg. 2021;85(4):15-21.
9. Tiwary SK, Ajaya A, Kumar S, Kumar P, Khanna AK. Role of neutrophil to lymphocyte ratio and IL-6 as novel prognostic markers in varicose veins. Indian J Surg. 2023;2:1-6.
10. Obermayer A, Aubry JF, Barnat N. Extracorporeal treatment with high intensity focused ultrasound of an incompetent perforating vein in a patient with active venous ulcers. EJVES Vasc Forum. 2021;50:1-5.
11. Chen CW, Tseng YH, Wong MY, Wu CM, Lin BS, Huang YK. Stasis leg ulcers: venous system revises by triggered angiography non-contrast-enhanced sequence magnetic resonance imaging. Diagnostics (Basel). 2020;10:707.
12. Cavezzi A, Labropoulos N, Partsch H, Ricci S, Caggiati A, Myers K, et al. Duplex ultrasound investigation of the veins in chronic venous disease of the lower limbs—UIP consensus document. Part II. Anatomy. Eur J Vasc Endovasc Surg. 2006;31:288-99.
13. De Maeseneer M, Pichot O, Cavezzi A, Earnshaw J, van Rij A, Lurie F, et al. Duplex ultrasound investigation of the veins of the lower limbs after treatment for varicose veins—UIP consensus document. Eur J Vasc Endovasc Surg. 2011;42:89-102.
14. Metzger PB, Rossi FH, Kambara AM, Izukawa NM, Saleh MH, Pinto IM, et al. Criteria for detecting significant chronic iliac venous obstructions with duplex ultrasound. J Vasc Surg Venous Lymphat Disord. 2016;4:18-27.

15. Coleridge-Smith P, Labropoulos N, Partsch H, Myers K, Nicolaides A, Cavezzi A. Duplex ultrasound investigation of the veins in chronic venous disease of the lower limbs—UIP consensus document. Part I. Basic principles. Eur J Vasc Endovasc Surg. 2006;31:83-92.
16. Arnoldussen CW, de Graaf R, Wittens CH, de Haan MW. Value of magnetic resonance venography and computed tomographic venography in lower extremity chronic venous disease. Phlebology. 2013;28(Suppl 1):169-75.
17. Harris C, Duong R, Vanderheyden G, Byrnes B, Cattryse R, Orr A, et al. Evaluation of a muscle pump-activating device for non-healing venous leg ulcers. Int Wound J. 2017;14(6):1189-98.
18. Manjit SG, Heatley F, Liu X, Bradbury A, Bulbulia R, Cullum N, et al. A randomized trial of early endovenous ablation in venous ulceration. N Engl J Med. 2018;378:2105-14.
19. Rasmussen L, Lawaetz M, Serup J, Bjoern L, Vennits B, Blemings A, et al. Randomized clinical trial comparing endovenous laser ablation, radiofrequency ablation, foam sclerotherapy, and surgical stripping for great saphenous varicose veins with 3-year follow-up. J Vasc Surg Venous Lymphat Disord. 2013;1:349-56.
20. Singer AJ, Tassiopoulos A, Kirsner RS. Evaluation and management of lower-extremity ulcers. N Engl J Med. 2017;377:1559-67.
21. Leren L, Johansen E, Eide H, Falk RS, Juvet LK, Ljoså TM. Pain in persons with chronic venous leg ulcers: a systematic review and meta-analysis. Int Wound J. 2020;17(2):466-84.
22. Bernatchez SF, Eysaman-Walker J, Weir D. Venous leg ulcers: a review of published assessment and treatment algorithms. Adv Wound Care (New Rochelle). 2021;11:28-41.
23. Milic DJ, Zivic SS, Bogdanovic DC, Karanovic ND, Golubovic ZV. Risk factors related to the failure of venous leg ulcers to heal with compression treatment. J Vasc Surg. 2009;49(5):1242-7.
24. Coleridge-Smith P, Lok C, Ramelet AA. Venous leg ulcer: a meta-analysis of adjunctive therapy with micronized purified flavonoid fraction. Eur J Vasc Endovasc Surg. 2005;30(2):198-208.
25. Coelho A, O'Sullivan G. Usefulness of direct computed tomography venography in predicting inflow for venous reconstruction in chronic post-thrombotic syndrome. Cardiovasc Intervent Radiol. 2019;42:677-84.
26. Nicolaides AN. The most severe stage of chronic venous disease: an update on the management of patients with venous leg ulcers. Adv Ther. 2020;37:S19-24.
27. Bianchi C, Cazzell S, Vayser D, Reyzelman AM, Dosluoglu H, Tovmassian G, et al. A multicentre randomised controlled trial evaluating the efficacy of dehydrated human amnion/chorion membrane (EpiFix) allograft for the treatment of venous leg ulcers. Int Wound J. 2018;15(1):114-22.
28. Noda K, Kawai K, Matsuura Y, Ito-Ihara T, Amino Y, Ushimaru M, et al. Safety of silk-elastin sponges in patients with chronic skin ulcers: a phase I/II, single-center, open-label, single-arm clinical trial. Plast Reconstr Surg Glob Open. 2021;9:35-56.
29. Tiwary SK, Choubey KK, Nath G, Kumar P, Khanna AK. Effect of four-layer dressing on the microbiological profile of venous leg ulcer. J Wound Care. 2023;32(Sup3):S22-30.

30. Tiwary SK, Shukla D, Tripathi AK, Agrawal S, Singh MK, Shukla VK. Effect of placental-extract gel and cream on non-healing wounds. J Wound Care. 2006;15(7):325-8.
31. Tiwary SK, Kumar A, Mishra SP, Kumar P, Khanna AK. Study of association of varicose veins and inflammation by inflammatory markers. Phlebology. 2020;35(9):679-85.
32. De Maeseneer MG, Kakkos SK, Aherne T, Baekgaard N, Black S, Blomgren L, et al. Editor's choice—European Society for Vascular Surgery (ESVS) 2022 clinical practice guidelines on the management of chronic venous disease of the lower limbs. Eur J Vasc Endovasc Surg. 2022;63(2):184-267.
33. Jindal R, Dekiwadia DB, Krishna PR, Khanna AK, Patel MD, Padaria S, et al. Evidence-based clinical practice points for the management of venous ulcers. Indian J Surg. 2018;80(2):171-82.
34. Darke SG, Baker SJA. Ultrasound-guided foam sclerotherapy for the treatment of varicose veins. Br J Surg. 2006;93(8):969-74.

CHAPTER 14

Paget's Disease of Breast

Vani Parmar, Bhavika Kothari, Basila Ameer Ali

■ INTRODUCTION

Paget's disease (PD) of the breast, a disorder of the nipple–areola complex, was first described by Sir James Paget in 1874[1] and is an uncommon disease. It accounts for 1–3% of all breast malignancies.[2,3] It is an eczematous lesion of nipple **(Fig. 1)** and is associated with in situ carcinoma or invasive carcinoma in the underlying tissue. It may also develop in ectopic breast and accessory nipples. The average age at diagnosis is 57 years, but the disease has also been found in adolescents and in people in their late 80s.[4,5]

■ PATHOLOGY

Paget's disease is a rare cutaneous intraepithelial malignancy, which is characterized by the presence of round malignant glandular cells, which are large, foamy cells (called *Paget cells*) that may contain mucin within the squamous epithelium of nipple and may also extend in the areola and adjacent breast skin. These *Paget cells* are large with clear cytoplasm and atypical nuclei. *Paget cells* are more often located in the basal region of the epidermis, either as a single layer or as clusters of cells forming gland-like structures or nests.[6] They show a classical intraductal extension through lactiferous ducts onto the surface of the nipple, known as the

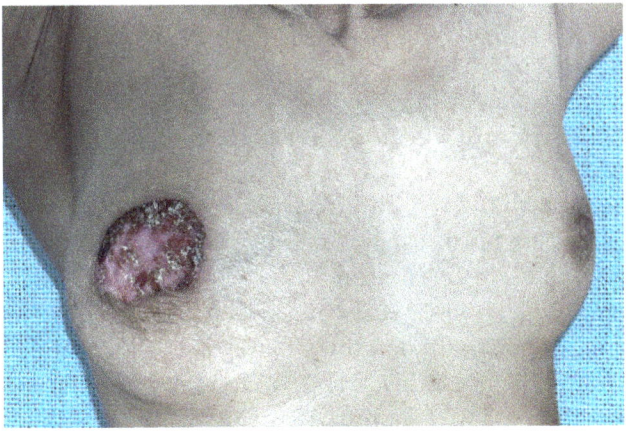

Fig. 1: Clinical presentation of Paget's disease of nipple.

"*Pagetoid spread*." However, there is uncertainty regarding the origin of PD, and there are two theories regarding the origin: The epidermotropic theory and intraepidermal origin theory.

The first theory, "*epidermotropic theory*," suggests that Paget's cells arise in the ductal cells and spread along the basement membrane to the nipple.[7,8] This theory is supported by the presence of underlying ductal carcinoma in situ (DCIS) with PD. The expression of a high level of HER2/neu oncogene in Paget cells, at the same level as in underlying DCIS, also supports epidermotropic theory.

The second theory, "*intraepidermal theory*," suggests that in situ neoplastic transformation occurs in pre-existing benign intraepidermal clear cells of the nipple-areolar complex (Toker cells) and is not associated with any coexisting neoplastic process in the affected breast. Further support for this theory has come from ultrastructural studies demonstrating microvilli and desmosomal attachments between the keratinocytes and Paget cells, findings which mitigate against the migratory nature of the Paget cell and suggest an intraepidermal origin.[9,10] A hybrid theory has also been proposed as Paget cells can originate either epidermotropically or intraepidermally, as per circumstances and local conditions prevail.

Paget cells' expression patterns on immunohistochemical staining are similar to those of underlying breast cancer cells, such as epithelial membrane antigen, carcinoembryonic antigen (CEA), and mucins. Paget cells may also show HER2/neu positivity; however, estrogen and progesterone antigens' expressions are usually absent.

■ PRESENTATION

Paget's disease constitutes around 1-3% of all primary breast cancers. The underlying breast cancer is present in between 93 and 100%, usually associated with central and multifocal tumors located near the areola. PD is divided into three different subtypes based on the presence or extent of associated disease:
1. PD of nipple without DCIS
2. PD of nipple with DCIS in the underlying lactiferous ducts within 2 cm of the nipple
3. PD of nipple with DCIS in the underlying lactiferous ducts and associated DCIS or invasive breast cancer elsewhere in the breast extending ≥2 cm from the nipple-areolar complex

The majority of PD (>90%) is associated with underlying DCIS or invasive ductal carcinoma (IDC). In one study, only 7% of patients with PD of the nipple have no evidence of invasive or noninvasive disease. In PD, nearly 60% of cases with underlying invasive tumors are of high grade with poor prognosis, and also majority of the underlying DCIS (>95%) is of high nuclear grade, predisposing for greater risk of developing high-grade invasive disease. The high expression of HER2/neu is also a factor for higher nuclear grade and poor prognosis in patients with invasive carcinoma. In <10% of cases, PD has an associated palpable mass. In PD of breast, multifocality and multicentricity are reported at a high rate (40 and 35%, respectively).

Clinical Presentation

Symptoms of PD of the breast develop insidiously and may present for months and years and may also extend from nipple into areola (centrifugal growth pattern). In a more advanced lesion, it may also involve the periareolar skin or even result in complete destruction of the nipple **(Figs. 2A and B)**. The lesion includes flaking, crusty, thickened skin on or around the nipple, itching or burning sensation, irritation, redness, nipple erosion, nipple flattening, and nipple inversion. A breast lump may also be palpable with yellowish or blood-stained discharge. The lesions are usually unilateral and very rarely bilateral. There are no clinical and epidemiologic factors known that predispose PD.

In the early stage, the nipple appears normal and the only symptom may be nipple pruritus. The lesion first affects the nipple, areola, and later involves the adjacent skin of breast. These are often mistaken for those of some benign skin conditions, such as dermatitis, eczema, or psoriasis.[9-11] The inflammatory component may be improved by topical treatment, a result that masks the underlying condition, and this may cause a delay in diagnosis.[12] As PD is rare, it may be misdiagnosed at first, and symptoms often persist for several months before being correctly diagnosed with a more serious underlying condition, such as breast cancer. PD is rarely bilateral, one of the distinguishing factors from eczema. Rarely, the lesion may be hyperpigmented, similar to superficial spreading melanoma. Sometimes,

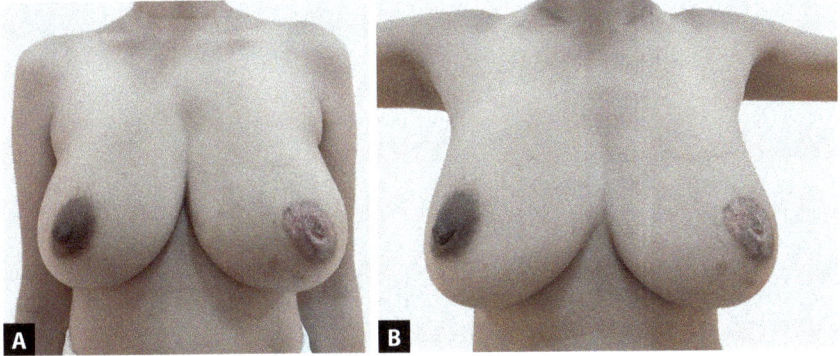

Figs. 2A and B: Left breast Paget's disease with multicentric DCIS. Left breast biopsy showed DCIS high-grade ER/PgR negative, HER2neu 3+. (DCIS: ductal carcinoma in situ; ER: estrogen receptor; PgR: progesterone receptor)

males may also be affected with similar characteristics, but they have poor prognosis compared to females.[13,14]

■ INVESTIGATION

The workup for patients with PD includes radiological investigation as well as pathology.

Traditional imaging modalities, such as mammography, may depict a mass or calcification or architectural distortion, which represents invasive cancer or in situ carcinoma, although not always. Mammography is the initial investigation of choice, having a high sensitivity, especially in cases where a palpable mass is present.[15] However, there are reports of negative mammograms with underlying cancer. Bilateral mammogram is still required for assessment of contralateral breast and also for follow-up in patients with conservative surgery.

Mammographic findings in PD may include skin thickening of the nipple–areolar region, nipple retraction, discrete mass, asymmetric density, suspicious microcalcifications, or may even be normal **(Figs. 3A to C)**. In PD of breast, with a clinically palpable mass lesion, mammography is 97% sensitive; however, with no palpable lesion, it detects the underlying malignancy in 50% of patients. Mammography cannot discriminate between DCIS and invasive disease, nor can it predict their subtype. Thus, it has limited use in planning the extent of the surgical procedure.

Ultrasound (US) examination may be helpful and should be considered as a part of the initial evaluation, especially when mammography is negative. The US findings may include mass, thickening of the nipple–areolar complex and/or flattening, sometimes microcalcifications, ductal ectasia, and asymmetry. It is also used for the assessment of the axillary nodes.

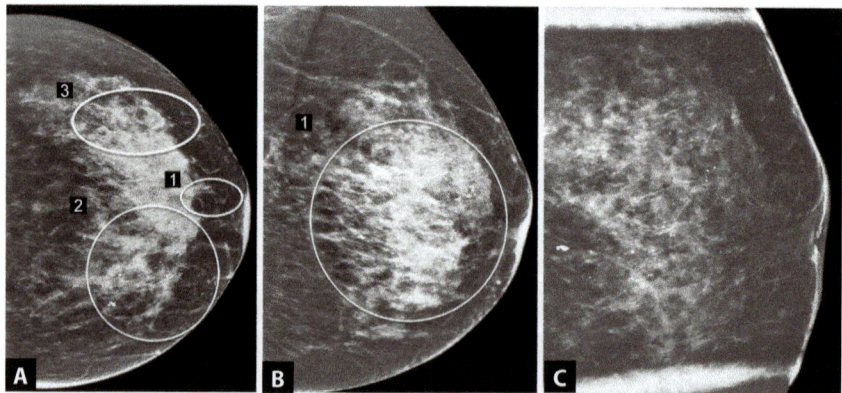

Figs. 3A to C: Mammogram showing multicentric microcalcification (encircled). (A) Left craniocaudal (CC) view; (B) Left mediolateral oblique (MLO) view; (C) Left breast magnification view showing microcalcification.

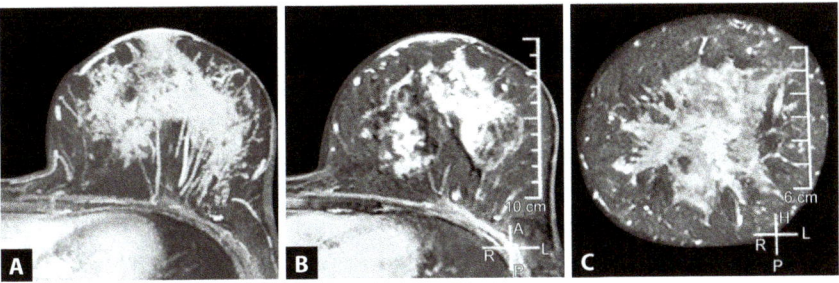

Figs. 4A to C: Magnetic resonance imaging (MRI) confirming multicentric disease in the left breast. (A) Left postcontrast axial maximum intensity projection (MIP); (B) Left postcontrast axial; (C) Left postcontrast coronal.

As mammography and US have their own limitations in evaluating patients with PD, additional evaluation with magnetic resonance imaging (MRI) can help detect underlying invasive cancer and DCIS. Contrast-enhanced MRI of breast is known to be highly sensitive and effective diagnostic modality for detection of clinically and mammographically occult cancer, multifocal, or multicentric lesions and in evaluation of patients with PD preoperatively before considering breast conservation surgery **(Figs. 4A to C)**.[16] Contrast-enhanced breast mammograms have also been used in certain cases as an alternative to MRI for detecting occult cancers, multifocal, and multicentric disease in breast.

There are various forms of biopsy available, such as punch biopsy, wedge biopsy, or superficial shave biopsy of epidermis to prove PD. However, wedge biopsy has proven to be the most useful method, as adequate representative material for biopsy is possible and likely to include a part of the underlying lactiferous duct. In patients with suspected PD of breast, full-thickness biopsy of the nipple or areolar (2–4 mm diameter) is recommended. The biopsy is done as punch or full-thickness incisional biopsy or wedge-shaped full-thickness incisional biopsy.

The immunohistochemical staining for CEA, mucin, or Her-2 oncoprotein may be helpful in making diagnosis; however, negative result does not exclude PD of breast.

▪ TREATMENT

Mastectomy has long been regarded as the standard therapy for PD, even in the absence of other clinical signs of malignancy. Patients undergoing mastectomy should be offered sentinel lymph node biopsy, and if found positive, then axillary lymph node dissection is needed.[17,18] However, with improvements in imaging, breast-conserving therapy may be used in patients with unifocal disease, which is limited to the nipple–areolar region. Breast-conserving surgery, including removal of the nipple and areola followed by whole-breast radiation therapy, is a safe option for people with PD of the breast.[14,19] Breast-conserving therapy has shown to be equally efficient in local control and survival in early invasive breast cancer as compared to mastectomy.[20] However, in patients with PD undergoing breast conservation surgery, the entire nipple–areolar complex with a cone of underlying retroareolar tissue should be excised and should include any other abnormal radiological finding. If conservation surgery is done, then axilla should be addressed with limited axillary evaluation (sentinel node biopsy or low axillary sampling), especially if an invasive component is present or suspected.

Better aesthetic results can be obtained with oncoplastic surgical techniques combined with contralateral mammaplasty or mastopexy if required for breast symmetry. Skin-saving mastectomy is feasible when disease is limited to the nipple and areola. An immediate or delayed nipple–areolar reconstruction, with or without tattooing, may be done for symmetrical, color-matched nipple–areolar complex **(Figs. 5A and B)**. If breast-conservative therapy is used, patients are followed up with regular mammography. However, mastectomy should be performed if relapse occurs. If the underlying mass has invasive cancer with a high risk of axillary node metastases, the appropriate therapy is based on the pathologic findings of the mass and axillary staging. In some cases where there is significant invasive component and axillary nodes, neoadjuvant chemotherapy may need to be started first, followed by assessment and surgery, mostly mastectomy in view of advanced disease status or multicentricity, with axillary clearance. If the disease has been confirmed prechemotherapy as limited to a single focus, breast conservation may be offered safely even after neoadjuvant chemotherapy.

Radiation therapy in PD treated with mastectomy depends on the associated invasive cancer, presence of nodal disease, or skin involvement (similar to any postmastectomy radiation indicators). Breast conservation surgery for PD should be combined with radiation therapy, as the local recurrence rate is as high as 40% in patients undergoing only central quadrant lumpectomy, despite adequate negative surgical margins. European Organisation for Research and Treatment of Cancer (EORTC) conducted a single-arm prospective trial in patients with PD of the nipple, where the patients were treated with excision of the nipple–areolar component and the underlying retroareolar tissue to achieve negative margins followed by whole breast radiation therapy. They reported a 5-year local recurrence rate of 5.2%, which is significantly better than the outcomes reported with lumpectomy alone.[11]

Adjuvant chemotherapy and hormonal therapy are recommended based on pathological factors, such as the presence or absence of lymph

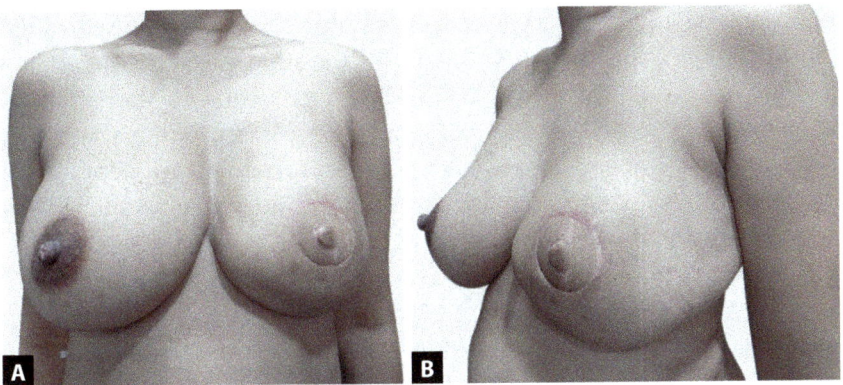

Figs. 5A and B: Left breast skin-saving mastectomy and whole breast reconstruction using LD flap with 340 cc silicone implant and primary nipple reconstruction.

node involvement, estrogen and progesterone receptors, and HER2 protein overexpression in the invasive cancer cell. Prognosis is determined primarily by the presence or absence of an invasive component,[21,22] and recommendations for systemic therapy have been suggested accordingly.

Limited reports are available on the treatment of PD with radiation alone in selected patients with lesions confined to the nipple without detectable breast tumor. This is not an accepted standard. It has been reported to have a local recurrence rate of 0–17%; however, the numbers are very small. Hence, this approach needs further evaluation and can only be offered to patients with minimal disease who cannot undergo surgery.[11]

■ PROGNOSIS

As PD is often associated with DCIS or invasive cancer in the breast parenchyma, prognosis is determined by the stage of the underlying malignancy if present. Unfavorable prognostic factors include palpable breast tumor, enlarged lymph node, histological type of breast cancer, and younger age group.

According to the National Cancer Institute's (NCI) Surveillance, Epidemiology, and End Results program, for women with both PD of the breast and invasive cancer in the same breast, the 5-year relative survival declined with increasing stage of the cancer (stage I, 95.8%; stage II, 77.7%; stage III, 46.3%; stage IV, 14.3%).[14,19,23,24] Presence of Paget's disease itself does not have any impact on the disease outcomes, but only on the kind of surgery offered.

■ CONCLUSION

Paget's disease of breast continues to be considered an indicator of underlying malignancy, the extent of which decides its treatment and outcomes.

It presents as an ulcer or erythema of the nipple and is diagnosed with a full-thickness wedge or punch biopsy of the nipple. As the underlying malignancies in PD of breast may be multifocal and multicentric, mammography is not sufficient. MRI may be necessary for the evaluation. Total mastectomy and breast-conservative procedures are appropriate depending on the findings and multifocality/multicentricity, followed by appropriate adjuvant therapy. Invasive cancers associated with PD of the breast tend to be more aggressive, mostly hormone receptor negative and HER2 positive, some even HER2 positive, and are treated accordingly. The prognosis and survival of patients with PD depend on the associated invasive or in situ component and depend on the stage at presentation and tumor biology.

■ REFERENCES

1. Paget J. On the disease of the mammary areola preceding cancer of the mammary gland. St Bartholomew's Hosp Rep. 1874;10:87-9.
2. The World Organization. The World Health Organization histological typing of breast tumors—second edition. Am J Clin Pathol. 1982;78:806-16.
3. Bulens P, Vanuytsel L, Rijnders A, van der Schueren E. Breast conserving treatment of Paget's disease. Radiother Oncol. 1990;17:305-9. doi: 10.1016/0167-8140(90)90004-G.
4. Caliskan M, Gatti G, Sosnovskikh I, Rotmensz N, Botteri E, Musmeci S, et al. Paget's disease of the breast: the experience of the European Institute of Oncology and review of the literature. Breast Cancer Res Treat. 2008;112(3):513-21.
5. Kanitakis J. Mammary and extramammary Paget's disease. J Eur Acad Dermatol Venereol. 2007;21(5):581-90.
6. Karakas C. Paget's disease of the breast. J Carcinog. 2011;10:31.
7. Muir R. The pathogenesis of Paget's disease of the nipple and associated lesions. Br J Surg. 1935;22:728-37.
8. Muir R. Further observations on Paget's disease of the nipple and associated lesions. J Pathol. 1939;49:299-312.
9. Sagami S. Electron microscopic studies in Paget's disease. Med J Osaka Univ. 1963;14:173-88.
10. Jahn H, Osther PJ, Nielsen EH, Rasmussen G, Andersen J. An electron microscopic study of clinical Paget's disease of the nipple. APMIS. 1995;103:628-34.
11. Harris JR, Lippman ME, Morrow M, Osborne CK (Eds). Diseases of the Breast, 4th edition. Philadelphia: Lippincott Williams & Wilkins; 2009.
12. Sakorafas GH, Blanchard K, Sarr MG, Farley DR. Paget's disease of the breast. Cancer Treat Rev. 2001;27:9-18.
13. Ashikari R, Park K, Huvos AG, Urban JA. Paget's disease of the breast. Cancer. 1970;26:680-5.
14. Kawase K, DiMaio DJ, Tucker SL, Buchholz TA, Ross MI, Feig BW, et al. Paget's disease of the breast: there is a role for breast-conserving therapy. Ann Surg Oncol. 2005;12:391-7.

15. Sripathi S, Ayachit A, Kadavigere R, Kumar S, Eleti A, Sraj A. Spectrum of imaging findings in Paget's disease of the breast—a pictorial review. Insights Imaging. 2015;6(4):419-29.
16. Amano G, Yajima M, Moroboshi Y, Kuriya Y, Ohuchi N. MRI accurately depicts underlying DCIS in a patient with Paget's disease of the breast without palpable mass and mammography findings. Jpn J Clin Oncol. 2005;35(3):149-53.
17. Sukumvanich P, Bentrem DJ, Cody 3rd HS, Brogi E, Fey JV, Borgen PI, et al. The role of sentinel lymph node biopsy in Paget's disease of the breast. Ann Surg Oncol. 2007;14(3):1020-3.
18. Laronga C, Hasson D, Hoover S, Cox J, Cantor A, Cox C, et al. Paget's disease in the era of sentinel lymph node biopsy. Am J Surg. 2006;192(4):481-3.
19. Marshall JK, Griffith KA, Haffty BG, Solin LJ, Vicini FA, McCormick B, et al. Conservative management of Paget disease of the breast with radiotherapy: 10- and 15-year results. Cancer. 2003;97(9):2142-9.
20. Dalberg K, Hellborg H, Wärnberg F. Paget's disease of the nipple in a population based cohort. Breast Cancer Res Treat. 2008;111(2):313-9.
21. Dixon AR, Galea MH, Ellis IO, Elston CW, Blamey RW. Paget's disease of the nipple. Br J Surg. 1991;78:722-3.
22. Chaudary MA, Millis RR, Lane EB, Miller NA. Paget's disease of the nipple: a ten year review including clinical, pathological and immunohistochemical findings. Breast Cancer Res Treat. 1986;8:139-46.
23. Ries LAG, Eisner MP. Cancer of the female breast. In: Ries LAG, Young JL, Keel GE, Eisner MP, Dan Lin Y, Horner MJD (Eds). SEER Survival Monograph: Cancer Survival Among Adults: U.S. SEER Program, 1988-2001, Patient and Tumor Characteristics. Bethesda, MD: National Cancer Institute, SEER Program; 2007.
24. Chen CY, Sun LM, Anderson BO. Paget disease of the breast: changing patterns of incidence, clinical presentation, and treatment in the U.S. Cancer. 2006;107(7):1448-58.

CHAPTER 15

Management of Testicular Tumors

Sameer Trivedi, Koti Sridhar Reddy

■ INTRODUCTION

Testicular tumors, although uncommon overall, are the predominant malignant tumors in young men and their incidence is increasing globally. Testicular tumors most commonly arise from germ cells, whereas other non-germ cell tumors (GCTs) and sex cord–stromal tumors are rarely reported.[1] The precancerous lesion for malignant testicular GCTs, initially described as carcinoma in situ, is currently called germ cell neoplasia in situ (GCNIS). In the current era, GCTs have an excellent prognosis with an overall cure rate of >95% and a cure rate of around 90% in those with metastatic disease.[2] This rise in cure rate from <30% in the 1950s is mainly attributed to the sensitivity of GCTs toward systemic therapy and use of a multidisciplinary treatment approach.[1] This chapter focuses on the recent advances in the management of testicular tumors, with brief discussion on epidemiology, tumor types, risk factors, clinical presentation, and diagnosis.

■ EPIDEMIOLOGY

In the industrialized world, men between 14 and 44 years have the highest incidence of testicular cancer.[3] This accounts for around 1% of all newly diagnosed male cancers. They are more common in some regions than others; for example, the rate is 9.9/100,000 in Norway, 9.4 in Denmark, and 9.2 in Switzerland, but only 1/100,000 in Africa and Asia.[4] In the United States, white men (6.9/100,000 males) are more likely to develop testicular cancer than black men (1.2/100,000 males).[1] In certain nations in northern Europe, the prevalence has doubled in the last two decades. The cost of GCT in the United States is predicted to rise by 23.9% between 2020 and 2026. Seminomas (SEMs) comprise around 50% of testicular tumor burden, while the remaining burden is due to various types of non-SEM or mixed testicular GCTs. About 70% of individuals have stage I disease at diagnosis, whereas another 30% have metastasized disease. Overall, patients have a 95% chance of surviving 5 years after their diagnosis, and those with stage I testicular tumors have a 99% chance of surviving 15 years after their first diagnosis.[1]

■ TUMOR TYPES

The World Health Organization has classified testicular tumors as GCNIS-related testicular GCTs, GCNIS-unrelated testicular GCTs, testicular adnexal tumors, and testicular sex cord–stromal tumors **(Box 1)**. Testicular GCTs have diagnostic biomarkers and histological variations that are consistent with the abnormal maturation of the physiological germ cell toward full spermatogenesis. Some testicular GCTs are linked to GCNIS, including SEMs and nonseminomatous germ cell tumors (NSGCTs) including embryonal carcinoma, postpubertal yolk sac tumor, choriocarcinoma, placental site trophoblastic tumor, and postpubertal teratomas, with or without malignant transformation. Testicular GCTs that are not produced by GCNIS include prepubertal teratomas, tumors of the yolk sac, and spermatocytic tumors (which include cells identical to secondary spermatocytes and are frequently encountered in the elderly). The malignant testicular tumors are more common and are usually categorized as SEM (originating from germinal epithelium of the seminiferous tubules) and non-SEM (containing pure or combined elements of choriocarcinoma, embryonal carcinoma, yolk sac tumor, teratoma, with or without seminomatous components).[5]

BOX 1: Classification of testicular tumors.[5,6]

Germ cell tumors (95% of all testicular cancers):
- Derived from germ cell neoplasia in situ:
    - Seminoma
    - Nonseminoma (nonseminomatous germ cell tumors)
- Embryonal carcinoma
- Yolk sac tumor (postpubertal)
- Trophoblastic tumors (e.g., choriocarcinoma, placental site trophoblastic tumor)
- Teratoma (postpubertal) with or without malignant transformation

Mixed and unclassified germ cell tumors:
- Not derived from germ cell neoplasia in situ:
    - Spermatocytic tumor
    - Teratoma (prepubertal)
    - Yolk sac tumor (prepubertal)

Sex cord–stromal tumors (<5% of all testicular cancers):
- Leydig cell tumor
- Sertoli cell tumor
- Granulosa cell tumor
- Mixed and unclassified sex cord–stromal tumors

Mixed germ cell and stromal tumors (proportion of all testicular cancers not well defined):
- Gonadoblastoma

Miscellaneous tumors (proportion of all testicular cancers not well defined)
- Ovarian epithelial-type tumors
- Hemangioma
- Hematolymphoid tumors

Tumors of the collecting duct and rete testis (adenocarcinoma)

RISK FACTORS

Cryptorchidism is most consistently associated with testicular tumor and its presence leads to five-times increased risk.[7] Other risk factors include low sperm count and hypospadias. The disruption of endogenous hormone signaling by xenobiotics during the perinatal period is thought to play a role in the development of cryptorchidism, low sperm count, hypospadias, and testicular cancers. According to the available literature, the growth of testicular cancers can be affected by postnatal environmental or lifestyle variables such as food or exposure to endocrine-disrupting substances.[8] However, the primary mutational driver of testicular cancers remains unidentified.[1] More than 40% of testicular tumors have a hereditary component. While those with a positive family history have a far higher risk, >90% of patients have no such history.[9] Testicular cancer has also been associated with male infertility, both in the affected person and in first-degree relatives. In addition, 5–6% of patients with testicular tumor have GCNIS in their contralateral testis, and the chance of developing testicular tumor of the opposite testis is increased in men with testicular tumor. There is proven evidence that within 15 years of diagnosis, a 2% probability of acquiring testicular malignancy in the contralateral testis exists.[1] Epidemiological studies have shown that the rate of testicular tumors peaks between the ages of 25 and 29 years for non-SEM and between the ages of 35 and 39 years for SEM, with a secondary, lesser peak after the age of 80 years. Sex hormone activity is primarily responsible for this age distribution. Moreover, the rate varies by race: 2.08/100,000 for Caucasians, 1.19/100,000 for Hispanics, 0.60/100,000 for Asians, and 0.36/100,000 for African-Americans.[10,11]

CLINICAL FEATURES

A patient with testicular tumor may present with a painless scrotal swelling, an incidental finding on imaging, post-traumatic symptom, or scrotal pain. Rarely, it may present as a locally advanced fungating lesion. Less frequently, patient presentation may suggest retroperitoneal (RP) lymphadenopathy or metastatic disease (hemoptysis, cachexia, and breathlessness) **(Table 1)**.[1,11]

Testicular changes may be noticed by the patient or a sex partner. Epididymitis is an important differential diagnosis of a scrotal swelling. Further evaluation is required if tenderness, swelling, or abnormalities noticed on examination persist even after antibiotic treatment. An alternative diagnosis needs to be confirmed to exclude testicular tumor in patients presenting with a scrotal swelling.[11]

DIAGNOSTIC WORK-UP

Trans-scrotal ultrasonography (USG) is the principal diagnostic imaging investigation for a male with a testicular mass. The diagnosis is typically confirmed with a high inguinal orchiectomy if the USG findings indicate testicular tumor. With the increasing utility of USG, ambiguous or impalpable tumors are identified and treated. In patients with small testicular lesions, located away from the testicular hilum, partial orchiectomy can be offered, particularly in patients who have already had a contralateral orchiectomy.[1]

A metastatic lesion biopsy is recommended for patients with metastatic disease. Para-aortic nodes, the primary lymphatic drainage pathway of the testes, cannot be identified without further radiological investigations, such as computed tomography (CT) or magnetic resonance imaging (MRI) of the abdomen and chest **(Figs. 1 and 2)**. Serum tumor marker (STM) levels are measured to aid in the diagnosis and management of testicular cancer **(Table 2)**. Since raised alpha-fetoprotein (AFP) and/or beta-human chorionic gonadotropin (β-hCG) levels are also seen in hepatocellular carcinoma, gastric carcinoma, and other malignancies, patients with raised STMs should have histological confirmation.[1]

TABLE 1: Signs and symptoms of testicular tumor.[11]

Local	Metastases
Intratesticular mass	Gastrointestinal symptoms
Firmness and heaviness of the testicle	Gynecomastia
Painless swelling and redness	Lumbar back pain
Acute pain in the testicle or scrotum	Neck mass
Dull ache in the scrotum or abdomen	Respiratory symptoms

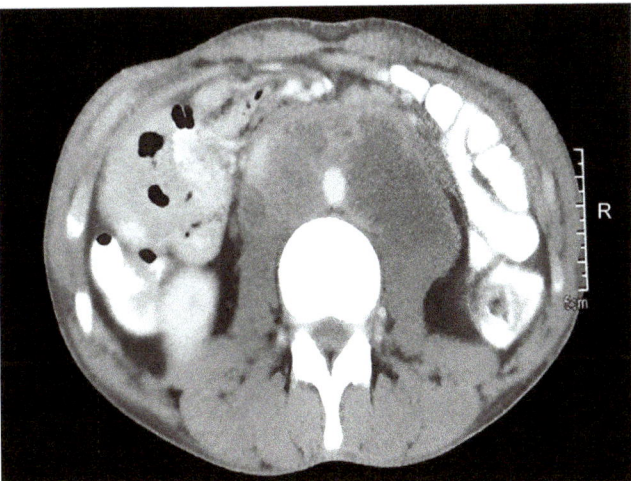

Fig. 1: Axial cut section [contrast-enhanced computed tomography (CECT) Whole Abdomen)] showing conglomerated mass of lymph node (LN).

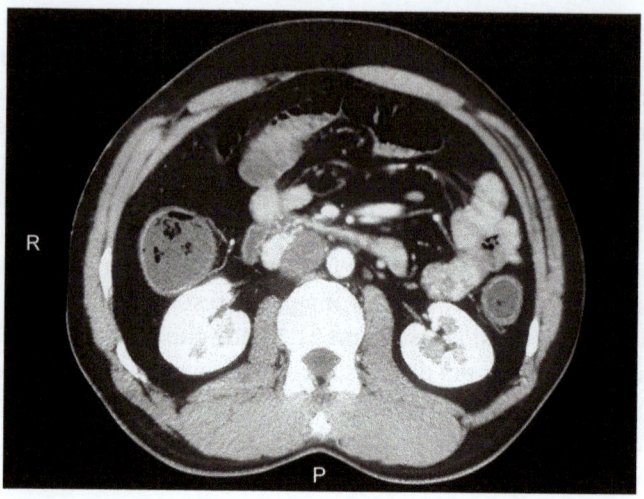

Fig. 2: Axial cut section [contrast-enhanced computed tomography (CECT) Whole Abdomen] showing interaortocaval lymph node (LN) group.

TABLE 2: Characteristics of serum tumor markers in testicular tumor.

Serum tumor markers	Molecular mass (Da)	Half-life	Tumor type	False-positive results
AFP	70,000	5–7 days	• NSGCT [50–70% low stage (I, IIA, IIB) and NSGCT 60–80% high stage (IIC, III) NSGCT] • Embryonal, teratoma, yolk sac	• Malignancies of liver, biliary tract, pancreas, stomach, and lung • Liver diseases—infection, alcohol induced, autoimmune
β-hCG	38,000	24–36 hours	• NSGCT (20–40% low-stage NSGCT and 40–60% high-stage GCT) • Choriocarcinoma, embryonal *seminomas* (15%)	• Marijuana use • Malignancies of liver, biliary tract, pancreas, kidney, bladder, stomach, and lung
LDH	134,000	24 hours	Nonspecific (20% of low-stage GCT and 20–60% of high-stage GCT)	Lymphoma

(AFP: alpha-fetoprotein; β-hCG: beta-human chorionic gonadotropin; GCT: germ cell tumor; LDH: lactate dehydrogenase; NSGCT: nonseminomatous germ cell tumor)

■ DIAGNOSTIC IMAGING

Role of Magnetic Resonance Imaging

An alternative imaging technique to the traditional CT is MRI. With a sensitivity of 94% for MRI and 98.4% for CT, MRI is said to be comparable to CT.

Due to its expense, MRI is typically not advised for use in staging and tracking therapy response. MRI with lymphotropic nanoparticles shows improved sensitivity and specificity. The sensitivity was increased from 70.5 to 88.2% and the specificity from 68 to 92% by the use of nanoparticles as they are trapped in lymph nodes (LNs) harboring metastases (Mets).[2]

According to the current recommendations, MRI is the technique of choice for diagnosing brain Mets. Brain Mets are identified in 2–3% of patients with Mets and are almost solely found in patients with non-SEM. Brain MRI should always be done after clinical suspicion of brain Mets or β-hCG >5,000. Although guidelines appropriately support routine brain MRI in patients in the International Germ Cell Cancer Collaborative Group (IGCCCG) poor-risk category, there is no clear consensus on whether asymptomatic patients should get brain MRI.[2]

Role of Positron Emission Tomography/ Computed Tomography

When conducting a diagnostic investigation, lesions can be accurately identified, thanks to the certain path of metastatic spread in GCTs. The gold standard in this field is still conventional CT, though fluorodeoxyglucose (FDG) positron emission tomography (PET)/CT is frequently used in clinical settings without any supporting data for staging and managing testicular tumors. There is not enough sensitivity to recognize patients who are at risk of relapsing. The sensitivity, specificity, positive predictive value (PPV), and negative predictive value (NPV) of PET/CT for assessing RPLNs in non-SEM following chemotherapy are 59, 92, 91, and 62%, respectively. However, during conventional PET imaging, teratoma, necrotic tissue, and scar have low FDG uptake values, making it challenging to distinguish between these tissue types. It is not advised to manage postchemotherapy residual non-SEM with conventional PET/CT. Removing an RP mass surgically is frequently associated with severe morbidity and may call for multiple visceral and multiple vascular resections. The PPV and NPV of studies using FDG PET/CT are 23–50% and 94–96%, respectively, in patients with >3 cm residual SEM. PET/CT is only recommended for patients with residual SEM lesions >3 cm by the National Comprehensive Cancer Network (NCCN), European Society for Medical Oncology (ESMO), and European Association of Urology (EAU) guidelines.

■ HISTOPATHOLOGY AND DIFFERENTIAL DIAGNOSIS

Differentiation of SEMs from non-SEMs in testicular GCTs is of critical importance as their treatment algorithm differs significantly after orchiectomy. SEMs do not result in elevated serum AFP levels; histopathological examination (HPE) is the main diagnostic method; however, spermatocytic tumors, malignant Sertoli cell tumors, and lymphomas may mimic SEM. β-hCG and AFP are able to identify choriocarcinoma and yolk sac tumors, respectively, but they are not sensitive or specific enough.[1]

Non-SEM testicular GCTs tend to affect younger patients (median age of diagnosis is lower) and are more often a heterogeneous collection of non-SEM tumor subtypes than SEM tumors. They tend to spread further and more quickly than others. Though majority of testicular GCTs are diagnosed based on routine morphology and STMs, immunochemistry (IHC) is important in difficult cases and includes KIT (positive in SEM and negative in non-SEM) and OCT4 (sensitive and specific for embryonal carcinoma and SEM).[1]

Diagnosis becomes cumbersome in the presence of metastatic testicular GCT, especially if located in unusual locations and in the absence of distinct primary tumor (such as a regressed testicular GCT). In such patients, IHC for selected markers may be useful. Less commonly, the diagnosis may be confounded by malignant transformation of a teratoma. Tumors of germ cell origin can be distinguished with the aid of fluorescence in situ hybridization for i(12p) in certain patients.[1]

■ STAGING AND PROGNOSIS

The American Joint Committee on Cancer (AJCC)-recommended tumor, lymph node, and metastasis (TNM) classification system is used to stage testicular germ cell cancers. However, staging also includes levels of lactate dehydrogenase (LDH), AFP, and β-hCG following orchidectomy, collectively termed S stage **(Table 3)**. These serum markers' concentrations provide insight into the extent to which metastatic disease produces markers and aids in prognostication. Among patients receiving chemotherapy for metastatic GCTs, the S stage is determined according to the levels of serum markers on the first day of the first chemotherapy cycle.[1]

Testicular tumor has three stages. If a testicular tumor is diagnosed at stage I, it will be contained within the testes and epididymis (though it may have invaded the spermatic cord or scrotum). If it is diagnosed at stage II, it will have spread to the regional (RP) LNs, and if it is diagnosed at stage III, it will have progressed beyond the RPLNs. NSGCTs with RPLN Mets are often classed as stage II; however, this changes to stage III if postorchiectomy STMs are highly high (S2 and S3). Pelvic LN Mets are regarded as distant Mets in testicular tumors because the testicular lymphatic drainage is to the RPLNs.[12] The levels of postorchiectomy STMs are estimated for staging. The markers are regarded as normal for staging if they are elevated before orchiectomy and return to normal afterward. AFP and β-hCG each has a biological half-life of <7 and 3 days, respectively. Patients taking chemotherapy should have their STM levels measured on day 1 of the first cycle to be used for staging and risk assessment.[13] In the staging, risk stratification, diagnosis, and surveillance of GCTs, the STMs AFP, β-hCG, and LDH are crucial. These STMs are neither sensitive nor specific, since approximately 25% of stage I NSGCTs and 18% of stage I SEMs recur while having normal STMs before relapse, and a large number of patients have normal STMs when metastatic disease is discovered. These limitations have prompted the quest for other biomarkers, and microRNAs (miRNAs) present an exciting possibility. Cancer patients may experience dysregulation of miRNAs, which play a role in regulating gene expression.[14] Excellent specificity and PPV for miR-371a-3p was demonstrated in diagnosing active

TABLE 3: The American Joint Committee on Cancer (AJCC) prognostic stage grouping system for testicular germ cell tumors (2017).[17]

Stage	Tumor (T)	Node (N)	Metastasis (M)	S stage (S)
Stage 0	pTis	N0	M0	S0
Stage I				
Stage I	pT1–4	N0	M0	SX
Stage IA	pT1	N0	M0	S0
Stage IB	pT2	N0	M0	S0
	pT3	N0	M0	S0
	pT4	N0	M0	S0
Stage IS	Any pT/TX	N0	M0	S1–3
Stage II				
Stage II	Any pT/TX	N1–3	M0	SX
Stage IIA	Any pT/TX	N1	M0	S0
	Any pT/TX	N1	M0	S1
Stage IIB	Any pT/TX	N2	M0	S0
	Any pT/TX	N2	M0	S1
Stage IIC	Any pT/TX	N3	M0	S0
	Any pT/TX	N3	M0	S1
Stage III				
Stage III	Any pT/TX	Any N	M1	SX
Stage IIIA	Any pT/TX	Any N	M1a	S0
	Any pT/TX	Any N	M1a	S1
Stage IIIB	Any pT/TX	N1–3	M0	S2
	Any pT/TX	Any N	M1a	S2
Stage IIIC	Any pT/TX	N1–3	M0	S3
	Any pT/TX	Any N	M1a	S3
	Any pT/TX	Any N	M1b	Any S

TABLE 4: The International Germ Cell Cancer Collaborative Group prognostic grouping.[18]

	Prognosis grouping (risk status)					
	Good		Intermediate		Poor	
	NSGCT	SEM	NSGCT	SEM	NSGCT	SEM[ǁ]
Nonpulmonary visceral metastases or mediastinal primary metastases	No	No	No	Yes	Yes	NA
AFP*	<1,000	Normal	1,000–10,000	Normal	>10,000	NA
β-hCG*	<5,000	Any	5,000–50,000	Any	>50,000	NA
LDH*	<1.5 × ULN	Any	1.5–10.0 × ULN	Any	>10 × ULN	NA
5-year PFS	89[†] (90[‡])	82[†] (87[‡])	75[†] (76[‡])	67[§]	41[†] (55[‡])	NA
5-year OS	92[†] (95[‡])	86[†] (93[‡])	80[†] (85[‡])	72[§]	48[†] (64[‡])	NA

(AFP: alpha-fetoprotein in ng/mL; β-hCG: beta-human chorionic gonadotropin in IU/L; IU: international units; LDH: lactate dehydrogenase; NA: not applicable; NSGCT: nonseminomatous germ cell tumor; OS: overall survival; PFS: progression-free survival; SEM: seminoma; ULN: upper limit of normal)
*Markers for risk classification following orchiectomy.
[†]Based on a study by the International Germ Cell Cancer Collaborative Group (IGCCCG).[11]
[‡]Based on a study by Kier et al.[19]
[§]Based on only a few patients.
[ǁ]No seminoma cases classified as poor prognosis.

germ cell malignancy in patients with GCTs. Serum levels of miRNA-371a-3p by polymerase chain reaction testing were shown to have sensitivity of 90.1% and specificity of 94% for the primary diagnosis of GCT in a prospective trial, significantly outperforming conventional cancer markers.[15] Notably, miR-371a-3p was associated with tumor size and stage, and it was modified by treatment outcomes.[16]

The use of adjuvant chemotherapy (for SEMs or non-SEMs in testicular GCTs), radiotherapy (RT) (for SEM), and RPLN dissection (for non-SEMs in testicular GCTs) after orchiectomy in these patients is debatable because irrespective of the treatment method used, >95% with stage I SEM and non-SEMs are cured. The IGCCCG prognostic system considers whether metastatic spread consists of mediastinal primary Mets or nonpulmonary visceral Mets, as well as postorchiectomy STM levels **(Table 4)**, but it is difficult to conduct studies with sufficient power due to the high cure rate of stage I GCTs. Thus, most prognostic studies have revealed pathological risk factors and biomarkers that predict relapse after orchiectomy.[1]

According to a number of studies, a larger tumor size—specifically, one that is at least 3-4 cm in diameter—predicts recurrence for SEMs. In some studies, but not in others, it has also been demonstrated that lymphovascular invasion (LVI) and rete testis invasion are predictors of the recurrence of testicular GCTs. Vascular invasion has been demonstrated in numerous studies to predict relapse in non-SEM testicular GCTs. A higher risk of relapse is also linked to a higher percentage of embryonal carcinoma in GCTs that are not SEMs. Finally, it has been tentatively demonstrated that the existence of novel biomarker, CXC-chemokine ligand 12 (CXCL12), in non-SEM GCTs can independently predict recurrence.[1]

MANAGEMENT OF GERM CELL TUMORS

Germ Cell Neoplasia in Situ

Most GCNIS will progress to testicular GCTs if left untreated for >7 years. The contralateral testis also contains GCNIS in about 2.5-5.0% of patients with testicular GCTs. Only people with risk factors for testicular GCTs, such as a history of a maldescended testis, with a testicular capacity of <12 mL and age <40 years, should be screened for contralateral GCNIS. These patients have a 30% chance of acquiring GCNIS. Patients with GCNIS of the testis are candidates for either radiation to the testis or orchiectomy. Surveillance with routine USG is preferred for male persons who desire to father children; however, biopsy of the contralateral testis can be offered and the same treatments given to all other patients.[1]

Stage I

For stage I testicular tumors, accepted management options include active surveillance, adjuvant chemotherapy with a single cycle of carboplatin for SEM and active surveillance, adjuvant chemotherapy with a single cycle of bleomycin, etoposide, and cisplatin (BEP), or primary retroperitoneal lymph node dissection (RPLND) for non-SEM[2] **(Flowcharts 1 and 3)**.

Orchiectomy alone is effective in curing clinical stage I SEM in the vast majority of individuals. In between 10% and 20% of patients, the illness recurs. Variables for assessing the likelihood of recurrence include tumor size and rete testis infiltration rate. Large tumors (>4 cm in diameter) that have spread into the rete testis are more likely to spread and relapse. The likelihood of relapse within 5 years is 15.9% for those with one risk factor and 31.5% for those with two. The 5-year relapsing rate (RR) for tumors without risk factors was 4%.[2] Adjuvant therapy may lessen the risk of relapse. RRs range from 0.5 to 5% after adjuvant RT of 20 Gy to the RPLNs. Adjuvant radiation is associated with a high risk of developing a second malignancy. Two-to-sixfold increased risk of acquiring a second cancer

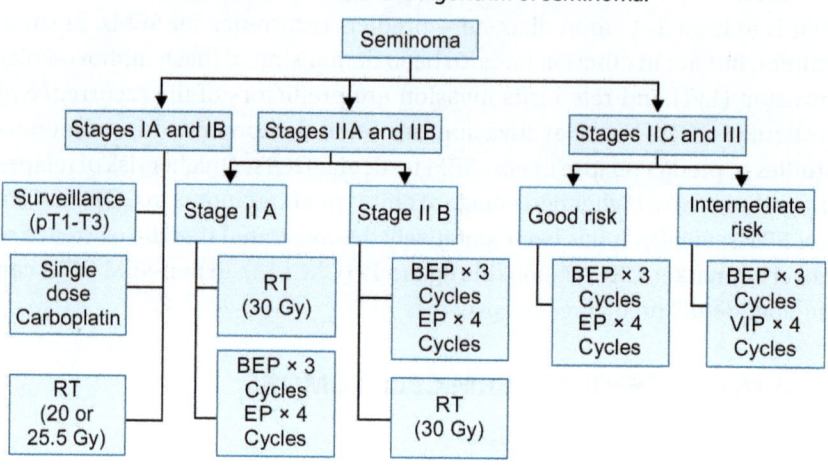

Flowchart 1: Treatment algorithm of seminoma.

relates to radiation therapy. Due to the significant risk of fatal late effects, adjuvant radiation is no longer recommended for the treatment of stage I SEM unless in exceptional patients. It has also been reported that a single cycle of adjuvant carboplatin had an RR of 2–9%, depending on the existence of risk factors. Two cycles of carboplatin, as were formerly used as adjuvant treatment, are not necessary; a single cycle is sufficient (5-year relapse-free rates of 94.7 and 96% for one vs. two cycles). The vast majority of authoritative organizations and guidelines around the world advocates for the use of active surveillance. Therefore, the general strategy is to treat relapsed patients with systemic chemotherapy while sparing the majority of patients from needless toxicity.[2]

Nonseminoma (Flowchart 3)

Histological subtypes of stage I non-SEM include embryonal carcinoma, yolk sac tumor, choriocarcinoma, teratoma, and mixed tumors of any category, including SEM.[2] Occult Mets were found in 47.5% of patients with LVI positivity and 16.9% of patients with LVI negativity, according to a meta-analysis. The combined rates of occult Mets for embryonal carcinoma presence and absence were 33.2 and 16.2%, respectively.[20] In 50-80% of cases of stage I non-SEM, orchiectomy alone is the cure. Treatment options for clinical stage I non-SEM include active surveillance, one round of BEP, and primary RPLND. Regardless of LVI, single-cycle BEP will reduce the RR to 0–6.5%. In 8–18% of patients who experience primary RPLND, relapse will occur. Although RPLND is sometimes necessary, it should only be performed by highly trained surgeons who have a track record of reviving antegrade ejaculation in >99% of patients using nerve-spring operations. Although relapses are more common in clinical stage I non-SEM, all relapses are still

Flowchart 2: Treatment algorithm of residual mass after chemotherapy in seminoma.

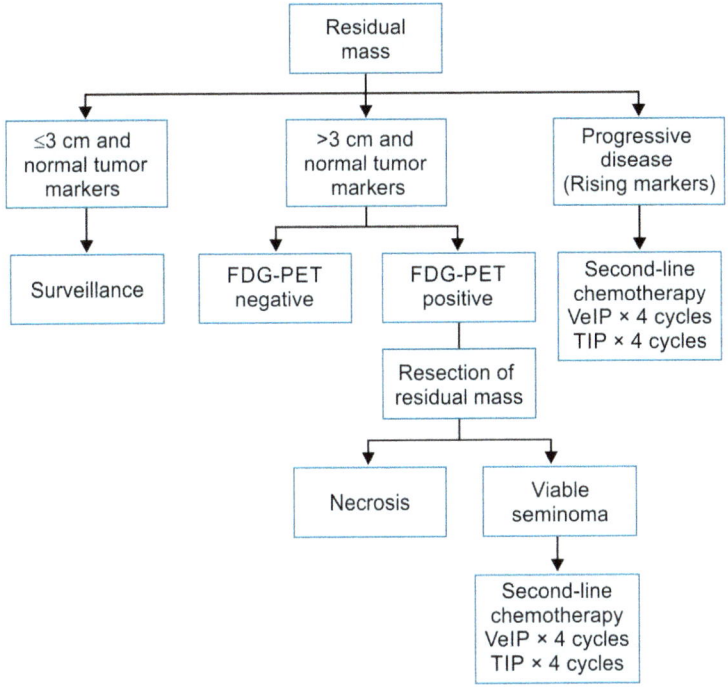

(BEP: bleomycin, etoposide, cisplatin; EP: etoposide, cisplatin; FDG: fluorodeoxyglucose; PET: positron emission tomography; RT: radiotherapy; TIP: paclitaxel, ifosfamide, cisplatin; VeIP: vinblastin, ifosfamide, cisplatin; VIP: etoposide, ifosfamide, and cisplatin)

considered to be in the good risk category by the IGCCCG, and cure rates remain between 99 and 100%.

Stage IIA and IIB Seminomas

In patients in clinical stage IIA SEM with low-volume metastatic disease and infradiaphragmatic Mets <2 cm, RT is advised. Following RT, the RR is moderate (5%), and the overall survival (OS) is nearly 100%. For these patients, chemotherapy is a respectable substitute for RT. Clinical stage IIB SEM cases that have infradiaphragmatic Mets between 2 and 5 cm are advised to undergo chemotherapy using either four cycles of etoposide and cisplatin (EP) or three cycles of BEP.[1]

Stages IIA and IIB Nonseminomatous Tumors

Treatment should consist of either three cycles of BEP or four cycles of EP for patients with non-SEM tumors that are clinical stage IIA or stage IIB. The patient has clinical stage III disease and an intermediate to poor

Management of Testicular Tumors

Flowchart 3: Treatment algorithm of nonseminomatous germ cell tumor (NSGCT).

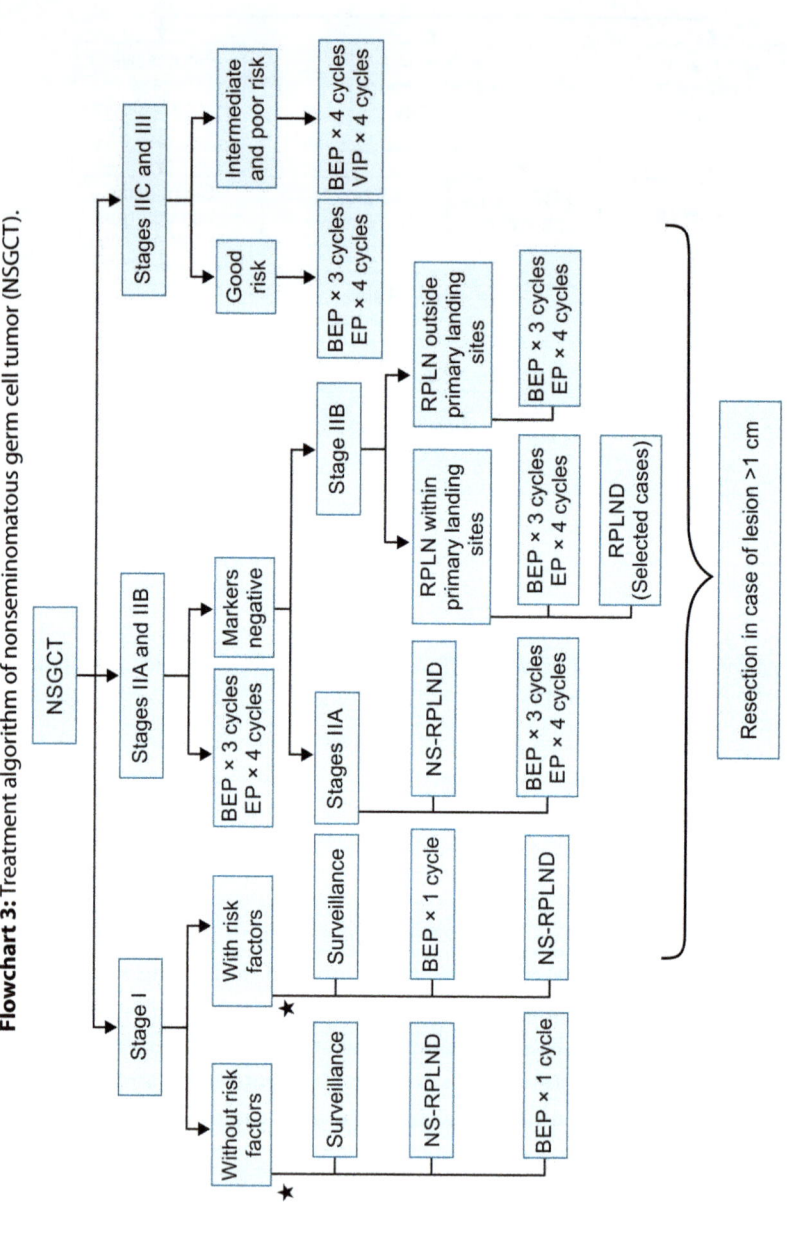

*Stage II tumor
(BEP: bleomycin, etoposide, cisplatin; EP: etoposide, cisplatin; NS-RPLND: nerve-sparing retro-peritoneal lymph node dissection; RPLN: retroperitoneal lymph node; VIP: etoposide, ifosfamide, and cisplatin)

prognosis, though, if any of the STM levels are classified as S2 or S3. Four cycles of BEP or four cycles of etoposide, ifosfamide, and cisplatin (VIP) should be administered to such patients. After receiving chemotherapy, patients with a residual RP tumor >1 cm must have excision of tumor.[21] The surgical area must be narrowed to the left or right side of the body to protect the nerves that control antegrade ejaculation. Three cycles of BEP, four cycles of EP, or primary RPLND can be used for nerve-sparing operations in the treatment of stage IIA and stage IIB non-SEM tumors without high STMs **(Figs. 3A and B)**. However, RPLND is normally not recommended for stage IIB disease. For pathological stage N1, surveillance is the recommended treatment

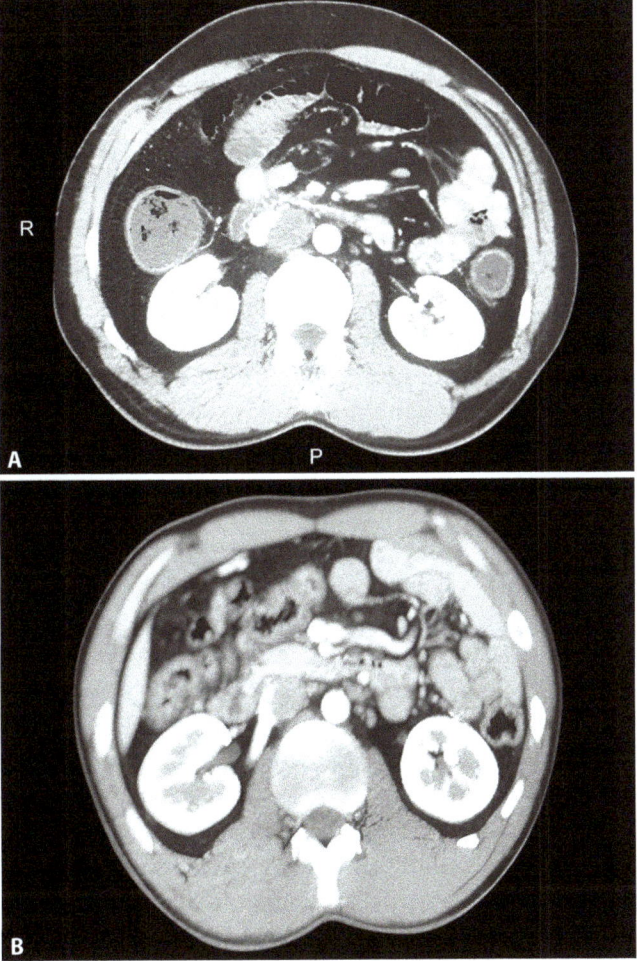

Figs. 3A and B: (A) Axial cut section [contrast-enhanced computed tomography (CECT) W/A] showing interaortocaval lymph node (LN) group in the prechemotherapy stage; (B) Axial cut section (CECT W/A) showing interaortocaval LN group in the postchemotherapy stage with partial remission.

because the relapse rate is <20%. In most cases, postoperative surveillance is all that is required when a teratoma of pathological stage N2 or N3 has been completely excised. In the case of rapidly progressing lesions with rising STM levels, RPLND should not be performed; instead, primary chemotherapy must be administered. After chemotherapy, if there are any lesions >1 cm, RPLND should be performed. If a chemo patient develops a tumor despite stable or decreasing STM, further testing is warranted to rule out the possibility of a teratoma or an undifferentiated malignant tumor.[1]

Stage IIC and Stage III Seminoma and Nonseminomatous Tumors

According to the IGCCCG risk classification, chemotherapy with BEP, EP, or cisplatin, etoposide, and ifosfamide (PEI) remains the standard treatment for advanced testicular GCTs. Three BEP cycles or four EP cycles are recommended for patients with a good prognosis. For patients with a poor prognosis, four cycles of BEP or VIP are required. Granulocyte colony-stimulating factor can be used as a primary preventative measure for complications associated with neutropenia. Prophylactic antibiotic treatment may help reduce the severity of febrile neutropenia in some patients with advanced or metastatic testicular GCTs.[1] Measuring STM levels after the first cycle of chemotherapy is necessary for monitoring treatment response and identifying individuals with inadequate marker decline who may benefit from dose-intensified chemotherapy. In extremely rare cases, the tumor size may rise despite a drop in STM count, a phenomenon typical of the expanding teratoma syndrome; imaging is typically used to diagnose these patients as having growing teratoma syndrome. Once chemotherapy has been finished, the teratoma can be removed surgically. One in two persons with testicular germ cell cancers will develop brain Mets. All patients with brain Mets need to be treated, although the best way to do so (which could involve chemotherapy, RT, and/or surgery) is still being debated.[1] Patients with recurrent brain Mets should be treated with a multimodal strategy; a combination of systemic chemotherapy and cranial radiation improved survival in a multivariate analysis. Finally, it is worth noting that in the later stages of testicular GCTs, patients may be harmed if they undergo whole brain RT in conjunction with chemotherapy.[21] This is because it can cause central nervous system toxicity, such as progressive multifocal leukoencephalopathy or cerebral atrophy. This has led to the rise in popularity of stereotactic radiosurgery as a viable alternative for the radiation therapy of oligometastases, or solitary brain Mets. The need for further neurosurgical excision of a single residual mass following the first chemotherapy and radiation therapy is unknown.[1]

SALVAGE TREATMENT

About 20–30% of patients recur after initial treatment, despite their unusual sensitivity to cisplatin-based chemotherapy. Salvage chemotherapy is necessary for these patients. Only a small subset of patients may be candidates for salvage surgery if the relapse is localized to a single spot, such as the retroperitoneum. About 20% of relapsed patients can be cured with this method.[2] If STMs are normal, then RPLND may be an option for patients with stage I illness who have experienced a relapse in the RP but have no bulky disease (LNs <2 cm). However, chemotherapy is the typical management for those with recurrent illness. Factors such as prior chemotherapy, medical comorbidities, and contraindications to particular medication are to be taken into consideration to choose the appropriate regimen. Risk stratification criteria for de novo stage III disease (e.g., good-risk: BEP 3 or EP 4, intermediate- or poor-risk: BEP 4 or VIP 4) should be used to determine chemotherapy selection for patients who are chemotherapy-naive or whose only prior chemotherapy was only carboplatin (for stage I SEM). Due to the possibility of pulmonary side effects, we try to refrain from administering patients more than four cycles of chemotherapy that contains bleomycin.[12] Patients with severe illness who relapse after receiving first-line chemotherapy have the choice of receiving either conventional dosage chemotherapy (CDCT) or high-dose chemotherapy (HDCT) plus autologous stem cell transplantation.[22] Carboplatin with etoposide is the most often used HDCT, whereas paclitaxel, ifosfamide, and cisplatin (TIP)[23] and vinblastine, ifosfamide, and cisplatin (VeIP)[22] are suitable choices for CDCT.[24]

An ongoing problem arises when HDCT is used instead of CDCT. While some facilities recommend HDCT for all recurrent patients, others claim that some individuals are overtreated. Salvage treatment options include both CDCT and HDCT.[25-27] To identify patients for HDCT in a safe manner, a more accurate predictive model is needed. Third and fourth lines of therapy have a chance of saving patients, but they are also far more toxic and have lower cure rates. If the patient relapses again after receiving salvage chemotherapy, there is no hope. Regimens such as gemcitabine, oxaliplatin with or without paclitaxel, or epirubicin and cisplatin have shown limited efficacy and very infrequent cures.[2]

POSTCHEMOTHERAPY SURGERY

All lesions should be surgically removed if any metastatic locations are found following the last round of chemotherapy (initial or salvage). The retroperitoneum is the area where the tumor is most likely to linger after treatment. Without raised STMs, postchemotherapy RPLND is necessary in non-SEM with residual LNs >1 cm **(Figs. 4A and B)**. Despite the infrequent occurrence of active malignancy (4%) and teratoma (24%), specialists

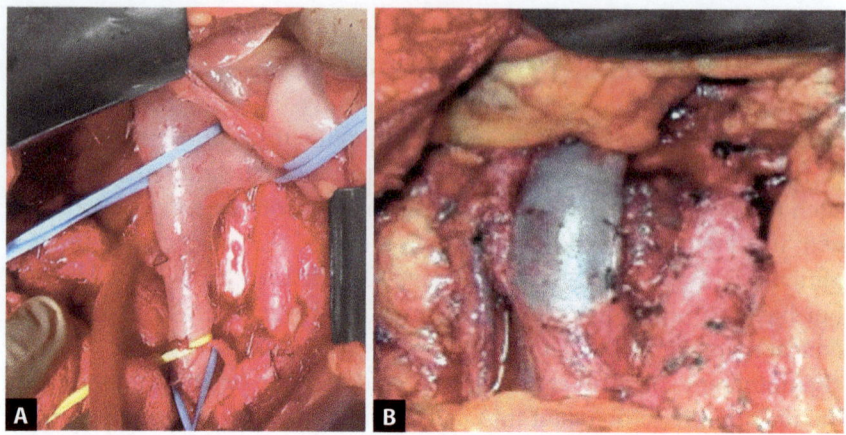

Figs. 4A and B: (A) Intraoperative photograph of retroperitoneal lymph node dissection (RPLND) with dissection of interaortocaval, precaval, paracaval, and preaortic group of lymph node (LN); (B) Intraoperative photograph of RPLND with dissection of interaortocaval group of LN.

are divided over surgical removal of LNs smaller than 1 cm. Histological examination of tissue from patients with LNs larger than 1 cm revealed teratoma in 30–80% and viable GCT in 10–15%. The surgical management of persistent SEM is complicated. These patients should be watched because, as indicated before, viable malignancy is extremely rare in residual RP disease <3 cm. A PET/CT-negative residual mass >3 cm is unlikely to contain viable cancer and is therefore not a candidate for postchemotherapy RPLND. One of the trickiest decision-making scenarios is presented by RPLNs >3 cm that are positive on PET/CT. If the risk of morbidity is modest, postchemotherapy RPLND can be administered to these patients. If the risk of morbidity is too great, patients should be observed and given salvage treatment only if they relapse. When a tumor is expanding, it is advised to administer salvage chemotherapy.[25]

PLATINUM-RESISTANT DISEASE AND EMERGING TREATMENTS

In testicular GCTs, platinum-resistant disease continues to be a management challenge, and the best salvage therapy to achieve disease remission is still up for debate.[28] It has been established that cisplatin-induced deoxyribonucleic acid (DNA) damage, unaltered p53 signaling, and a heightened chemotherapy-induced apoptotic response because of mitochondrial priming are all important determinants of platinum sensitivity.[29] Regardless of the IGCCCG risk class, p53 mutations and MDM2 amplifications have been reported to be strongly related to poor outcomes in platinum-resistant testicular GCTs. Recent whole-exome sequencing of platinum-resistant testicular GCTs has revealed several hallmarks of platinum-resistant disease, including increasing copy number and structural aberrations, and an increased frequency of mutations affecting KIT, p53, and WNT/CTNNB1 signaling genes, as well as loss of pluripotency genes and hypermethylation. However, it is unknown how exactly these changes will affect mitochondrial priming.

Results from a study including the potent MET inhibitor cabozantinib are expected in December 2025 (NCT04876456).[30] Only one of nine patients given the anti-CD30 medication brentuximab vedotin achieved a complete response (CR) and another had a partial response (PR).[31] Two CRs and three PRs were seen in 14 patients with refractory disease after treatment with the demethylating medication guadecitabin coupled with cisplatin.[32] By 2035, researchers hope to know the effectiveness of BEP 1 as an adjuvant treatment for patients with risk factors associated with stage I SEM in the SWENOTECA-ABC study (NCT02341989).[33] The goal of the SAKK 01/18 research (NCT03937843) is to use a single cycle of carboplatin followed by involved-node RT in place of three to four cycles of cisplatin-based chemotherapy in stage II SEMs.[34] In good-risk metastatic SEMs, the SEMITEP trial (NCT01887340) aims to reduce treatment intensity based on the PET/CT results following two cycles of chemotherapy.[35] The "Tiger" phase 3 randomized trial (NCT02375204), which compares the conventional dose salvage regimen of TIP 4 and HDCT with TI-CE 3, is one of the most significant studies, and its results are likely to be announced in 2024.[36] The results of a randomized phase 2 trial testing oral etoposide as maintenance therapy after HDCT are expected in 2026.[37]

■ BEYOND CONVENTIONAL MEDICINE

Like many other areas of study and development, modern medicine has seen the rise of artificial intelligence (AI). A small testicular lesion-predicting model was developed using machine learning (ML) in a recent retrospective radiomics study. Using a linear model and linear support vector machine methods, a computer was trained to evaluate 42 patients on testicular MRI scans for classification between GCT and non-GCT as well as SEM and non-SEM. In both cases, acquired accuracy was 89 and 86%.[38] Deep-learning technology was used in a retrospective study to look for tumor-infiltrating lymphocytes (TILs) in GCT tissue. When researchers compared the human tally to the algorithm used by computers, they found a correlation coefficient of 0.89. When comparing the agreement between the algorithm and experts, as well as between the experts themselves, there was a higher level of agreement with the algorithm, suggesting a fair level of consensus.[39] A study involving histological samples from 80 individuals with postchemotherapy RPLND also uses ML to try to predict the histology. Trained machines showed 88% specificity, 72% sensitivity, and 88% NPV in distinguishing between benign (necrosis/fibrosis) and malignant (viable cancer/teratoma) tissue.[40] Finding teratoma and active malignancy in postchemotherapy residual mass is one of the most difficult challenges in the clinical management of GCTs;[28] consequently, this work is helping to plug a painful information gap. Researchers in Denmark employed ML algorithms to analyze genomic markers in saliva DNA to foretell cisplatin-induced nephrotoxicity.[29] Nephrotoxicity-related genetic markers were located in the *NAT1* and *NAT2* genes, as well as the intergenic space between the *CNTN6* and *CNTN4* genes. A receiver operating characteristic curve of 0.731 was achieved by combining these with previously identified indicators at ERCC1, ERCC2, and SLC22A2, as well as clinical features. With further testing, AI has the potential to become a useful tool for enhancing medical diagnoses and treatments.[2]

■ CONCLUSION

Over the past three decades, the cure rates of testicular tumors have improved. However, the treatment and cure of cisplatin-resistant cases are still challenging, and their optimal treatment is still unknown. In this group of patients, further research is warranted to enhance the current therapeutic options and to attain better outcomes. A review of currently evolving research suggests various promising novel molecules being investigated and once the positive findings of this research are out, the management of patients with testicular tumor will further evolve. Additionally, the use of AI and ML shows a way toward a promising future.

■ REFERENCES

1. Cheng L, Albers P, Berney DM, Feldman DR, Daugaard G, Gilligan T, et al. Testicular cancer. Nat Rev Dis Primers. 2018;4(1):29.
2. Chovanec M, Cheng L. Advances in diagnosis and treatment of testicular cancer. BMJ. 2022;379:e070499.
3. De Toni L, Šabovic I, Cosci I, Ghezzi M, Foresta C, Garolla A. Testicular cancer: genes, environment, hormones. Front Endocrinol (Lausanne). 2019;10:408.
4. Znaor A, Lortet-Tieulent J, Jemal A, Bray F. International variations and trends in testicular cancer incidence and mortality. Eur Urol. 2014;65(6):1095-106.
5. Moch H, Cubilla AL, Humphrey PA, Reuter VE, Ulbright TM. The 2016 WHO classification of tumours of the urinary system and male genital organs—part a: renal, penile, and testicular tumours. Eur Urol. 2016;70(1):93-105.
6. Moch H, Amin MB, Berney DM, Compérat EM, Gill AJ, Hartmann A, et al. The 2022 World Health Organization classification of tumours of the urinary system and male genital organs-part a: renal, penile, and testicular tumours. Eur Urol. 2022;82(5):458-68.
7. Ferguson L, Agoulnik AI. Testicular cancer and cryptorchidism. Front Endocrinol (Lausanne). 2013;4:32.
8. Faja F, Esteves S, Pallotti F, Cicolani G, Di Chiano S, Delli Paoli E, et al. Environmental disruptors and testicular cancer. Endocrine. 2022;78(3):429-35.

9. Yazici S, Del Biondo D, Napodano G, Grillo M, Calace FP, Prezioso D, et al. Risk factors for testicular cancer: environment, genes and infections—is it all? Medicina (Kaunas). 2023;59(4):724.
10. Li Y, Lu Q, Wang Y, Ma S. Racial differences in testicular cancer in the United States: descriptive epidemiology. BMC Cancer. 2020;20(1):284.
11. Shaw J. Diagnosis and treatment of testicular cancer. Am Fam Physician. 2008;77(4):469-74.
12. Wee CE, Gilligan TD. Management of testicular germ cell tumors. Clin Adv Hematol Oncol. 2023;21(4):179-88.
13. Gilligan TD, Seidenfeld J, Basch EM, Einhorn LH, Fancher T, Smith DC, et al. American Society of Clinical Oncology Clinical Practice Guideline on uses of serum tumor markers in adult males with germ cell tumors. J Clin Oncol. 2010;28(20):3388-404.
14. Peng Y, Croce CM. The role of microRNAs in human cancer. Signal Transduct Target Ther. 2016;1(1):15004.
15. Nappi L, Thi M, Lum A, Huntsman D, Eigl BJ, Martin C, et al. Developing a highly specific biomarker for germ cell malignancies: plasma miR371 expression across the germ cell malignancy spectrum. J Clin Oncol. 2019;37(33):3090-8.
16. Dieckmann KP, Simonsen-Richter H, Kulejewski M, Anheuser P, Zecha H, Isbarn H, et al. Serum tumour markers in testicular germ cell tumours: frequencies of elevated levels and extents of marker elevation are significantly associated with clinical parameters and with response to treatment. BioMed Res Int. 2019;2019:e5030349.
17. Amin MB, Greene FL, Edge SB, Compton CC, Gershenwald JE, Brookland RK, et al. The Eighth Edition AJCC Cancer Staging Manual: continuing to build a bridge from a population-based to a more "personalized" approach to cancer staging. CA Cancer J Clin. 2017;67(2):93-9.
18. Mead GM, Stenning SP. The International Germ Cell Consensus Classification: a new prognostic factor-based staging classification for metastatic germ cell tumours. Clin Oncol (R Coll Radiol). 1997;9(4):207-9.
19. Kier MG, Lauritsen J, Mortensen MS, Bandak M, Andersen KK, Hansen MK, et al. Prognostic factors and treatment results after bleomycin, etoposide, and cisplatin in germ cell cancer: a population-based study. European Urology. 2017;71(2):290-8.
20. Blok JM, Pluim I, Daugaard G, Wagner T, Jóźwiak K, Wilthagen EA, et al. Lymphovascular invasion and presence of embryonal carcinoma as risk factors for occult metastatic disease in clinical stage I nonseminomatous germ cell tumour: a systematic review and meta-analysis. BJU Int. 2020;125(3):355-68.
21. Feldman DR, Lorch A, Kramar A, Albany C, Einhorn LH, Giannatempo P, et al. Brain metastases in patients with germ cell tumors: prognostic factors and treatment options—an analysis from the Global Germ Cell Cancer Group. J Clin Oncol. 2016;34(4):345-51.
22. Kondagunta GV, Bacik J, Donadio A, Bajorin D, Marion S, Sheinfeld J, et al. Combination of paclitaxel, ifosfamide, and cisplatin is an effective second-line therapy for patients with relapsed testicular germ cell tumors. J Clin Oncol. 2005;23(27):6549-55.

23. Loehrer PJ, Gonin R, Nichols CR, Weathers T, Einhorn LH. Vinblastine plus ifosfamide plus cisplatin as initial salvage therapy in recurrent germ cell tumor. J Clin Oncol. 1998;16(7):2500-4.
24. Adra N, Abonour R, Althouse SK, Albany C, Hanna NH, Einhorn LH. High-dose chemotherapy and autologous peripheral-blood stem-cell transplantation for relapsed metastatic germ cell tumors: the Indiana University experience. J Clin Oncol. 2017;35(10):1096-102.
25. Laguna MP, Pizzocaro G, Klepp O, Algaba F, Kisbenedek L, Leiva O, et al. EAU guidelines on testicular cancer. Eur Urol. 2001;40(2):102-10.
26. Gilligan T, Lin DW, Aggarwal R, Chism D, Cost N, Derweesh IH, et al. Testicular cancer, version 2.2020, NCCN Clinical Practice Guidelines in Oncology. J Natl Compr Canc Netw. 2019;17(12):1529-54.
27. Oldenburg J, Berney DM, Bokemeyer C, Climent MA, Daugaard G, Gietema JA, et al. Testicular seminoma and non-seminoma: ESMO-EURACAN clinical practice guideline for diagnosis, treatment and follow-up. Ann Oncol. 2022;33(4):362-75.
28. Heidenreich A, Paffenholz P, Nestler T, Pfister D. Management of residual masses in testicular germ cell tumors. Expert Rev Anticancer Ther. 2019;19(4):291-300.
29. Mele T, Reid A, Huddart R. Recent advances in testicular germ cell tumours. Fac Rev. 2021;10:67.
30. King J. (2023). A phase II trial evaluating the efficacy of cabozantinib in the treatment of incurable patients with refractory germ cell tumors. clinicaltrials.gov. Report No.: NCT04876456. [online] Available from https://clinicaltrials.gov/study/NCT04876456. [Last accessed November, 2023].
31. Necchi A, Anichini A, Raggi D, Giannatempo P, Magazzù D, Nicolai N, et al. Brentuximab vedotin in CD30-expressing germ cell tumors after chemotherapy failure. Clin Genitourin Cancer. 2016;14(4):261-4.e4.
32. Albany C, Fazal Z, Singh R, Bikorimana E, Adra N, Hanna NH, et al. A phase 1 study of combined guadecitabine and cisplatin in platinum refractory germ cell cancer. Cancer Med. 2021;10(1):156-63.
33. St Olavs Hospital. (2023). A randomized phase III study comparing one course of adjuvant bleomycin, etoposide and cisplatin (BEP) and one course of carboplatin AUC7 in clinical stage I seminomatous testicular cancer. clinicaltrials.gov. Report No.: NCT02341989. [online] Available from https://clinicaltrials.gov/study/NCT02341989. [Last accessed November, 2023].
34. Swiss Group for Clinical Cancer Research. (2023). Reduced intensity radio-chemotherapy for stage IIA/B seminoma. A multicenter, open label phase II trial with two cohorts. clinicaltrials.gov. Report No.: NCT03937843. [online] Available from https://clinicaltrials.gov/study/NCT03937843. [Last accessed November, 2023].
35. Gustave Roussy, Cancer Campus, Grand Paris. (2016). Therapeutic strategy guided by PET-TDM for patients with grade I or metastatic seminoma. clinicaltrials.gov. Report No.: NCT01887340. [online] Available from https://clinicaltrials.gov/study/NCT01887340. [Last accessed November, 2023].
36. Alliance for Clinical Trials in Oncology. (2023). A randomized phase III trial comparing conventional-dose chemotherapy using paclitaxel, ifosfamide, and cisplatin (TIP) with high-dose chemotherapy using mobilizing paclitaxel plus ifosfamide followed by high-dose carboplatin and etoposide (TI-CE) as first

salvage treatment in relapsed or refractory germ cell tumors. clinicaltrials.gov. Report No.: NCT02375204. [online] Available from https://clinicaltrials.gov/study/NCT02375204. [Last accessed November, 2023].
37. Adra N. (2023). Randomized phase 2 trial of maintenance oral etoposide or observation following high-dose chemotherapy for relapsed metastatic germ-cell tumor. clinicaltrials.gov. Report No.: NCT04804007. [online] Available from https://clinicaltrials.gov/study/NCT04804007. [Last accessed November, 2023].
38. Feliciani G, Mellini L, Carnevale A, Sarnelli A, Menghi E, Piccinini F, et al. The potential role of MR based radiomic biomarkers in the characterization of focal testicular lesions. Sci Rep. 2021;11(1):3456.
39. Linder N, Taylor JC, Colling R, Pell R, Alveyn E, Joseph J, et al. Deep learning for detecting tumour-infiltrating lymphocytes in testicular germ cell tumours. J Clin Pathol. 2019;72(2):157-64.
40. Baessler B, Nestler T, Pinto Dos Santos D, Paffenholz P, Zeuch V, Pfister D, et al. Radiomics allows for detection of benign and malignant histopathology in patients with metastatic testicular germ cell tumors prior to post-chemotherapy retroperitoneal lymph node dissection. Eur Radiol. 2020;30(4):2334-45.

INDEX

Page numbers followed by *b* refer to box, *f* refer to figure, *fc* refer to flowchart, and *t* refer to table.

A

Abdomen 81*f*
   acute 186
   lower 106
   ultrasonography of 61, 63*t*
   upper 106
Abdominal drains 178
   usage of 178
Abdominal surgery, elective 180
Abdominal wall, layers of 100
Ablative therapies 168
Abortion 59
Abscess 61, 68, 69
   intra-abdominal 67
Absorption 18*f*
Acetaminophen 177
Achalasia 43, 44*f*
   cardia 43, 44*f*
   diagnosis of 43
Achlorhydria 77
Acute abdominal decision making model 11
Acute appendicitis 53, 54, 58, 63, 63*t*, 68*t*, 71
   diagnosis of 53, 61
   intraoperative grading of 67
Adenocarcinoma 137
   staging system of 77
Adenomas
   adrenal 152
   non-functional 153
Adenoneuroendocrine carcinoma, mixed 77
Adjuvant chemotherapy 185, 254
   use of 266
Adrenal adenoma, contrast-enhanced computed tomography of 158*f*
Adrenal gland, hypersecreting 161
Adrenal hyperplasia, bilateral 164
Adrenal incidentaloma 151-153, 155*t*, 159*b*
   differential diagnosis of 152, 153*f*
   majority of 152
   management of 151, 160
Adrenal masses, malignant 158*t*
Adrenal tumors, nonfunctional benign 166
Adrenalectomy 162*f*
   laparoscopic 161, 165

Adrenaline 151, 174
Adrenocortical carcinoma 153-155
   contrast-enhanced computed tomography of 158*f*
   management of 166
Adrenocorticotropic hormone 155, 174
   confirmation of 156
Adult appendicitis score 54, 56-58, 62
Advanced vessel sealing devices 67
Adverse allergic reactions 19
Albumin 19
   ischemia-modified 60
Aldosterone 153
   hypersecretion 154
   secreting lesions 164
   serum 156
   simultaneous hypersecretion of 156
Aldosteronism 156
   subclinical primary 164
   surgical outcome, primary 165
Aldosteronomas 164
Alkaline phosphate 115
Allergy 198
Alpha-blockers 156
Alpha-fetoprotein 261, 262, 266
Alvarado scoring method 54
Alvimopan 179
American Association for Surgery of Trauma 68
American College of Gastroenterology 136, 142
American College of Surgeons National Surgical Quality Improvement Program 7, 66
American Joint Committee on Cancer 264
   Tumor 75
American Society of Anesthesiologists 176, 181, 198
   classification 7
Amniotic membrane 239
   allograft 239
Analgesia
   multimodal 181, 187
   patient-controlled 179
Analgesics 176
   drugs, usage of 178
Anaplastic lymphoma kinase 216

Anastomotic biliary stricture 127
Androgen
  excess 155
  hypersecretion, majority of 156
Androstenedione 156
Anesthesia 7, 181
  local 198
  monitoring depth of 7
  regional 198
  thoracic epidural 198
Anesthetic gases, humidification of 178
Angiodysplasia 137, 138, 140, 142
Angioectasia 138
Angioembolization 142*f*
Angiography 35, 146
Angiomatous malformations 138*f*, 143
  diagnosis of 141
Angiotensin-converting enzyme
      inhibitors 156
Angiotensin-receptor blockers 156
Ankle-brachial pressure index 229
Anomalous biliary anatomy, suspicion
      of 26
Antibiotics 235
  prophylaxis 187
Antiemetics, different class of 177
Antigen, carcinoembryonic 250
Anti-hypertensive medication 156, 165
Antimicrobial prophylaxis 181
Antiseptics 235
Anxiety 154, 175
Anxiousness 90
Aortoenteric fistula 138
Apfel score 177
Aphasia 218
Appendectomy 64, 69
  laparoscopic 67, 70
  timing of 66
Appendiceal neuroendocrine tumors 95
Appendicectomy, incidental 53
Appendicitis 61, 63, 70
  acuta multicenter 64
  acute 53, 54, 58, 63, 63*t*, 68*t*, 71
  complicated 67, 70
  inflammatory response 54, 56, 57, 62
      score 57
  perforated 69
  uncomplicated 64-67, 71
  urinary biomarker 60
Appendix 68
  region of 61
Areola, removal of 253
Argentaffinomas 74
Armamentarium 82
Arrhythmias 154

Arterial blood gas 187
Arterial disease, peripheral 229
Arterial reconstruction, benefit of 119
Arteriovenous malformations 141
  surgery 33
Artery, pulmonary 203, 204*f*
Artificial intelligence 1-9, 10*f*, 11-13, 201
  applications of 3
  limitations of 11
  role of 5, 7, 11,
  tools, Gartner hype cycle for 4*f*
  use of 5*f*
Artificial neural networks 2
Aspirin 240
Asthma 176
Atezolizumab 215
Atherosclerosis 33
Atrophie blanche 226
Atrophy-hypertrophy complex 26
Autoimmune disorders 131
Autoimmune inflammatory disease 131
Autologous peripheral blood mononuclear
      cells 218
Autologous stem cell transplantation 273
Autonomic nervous system 174
Autonomous cortisol secretion 155
  mild 162
Avelumab 215
Axicabtagene ciloleucel 218
Axillary nodes, assessment of 252

B

Balloon
  dilatation 130
  serial inflation of 144
B-cell
  acute lymphocytic leukemia 218
  malignancy 218
  maturation antigen 218
Benign biliary stricture 113, 113*t*, 118*t*,
      126, 126*f*, 128, 129
  management of 113
  repair 26
Beta-human chorionic gonadotropin 261,
      262, 266
Beta-lipoprotein 19
Bile duct
  anastomosis, end-to-end 124
  injury 26, 114, 120, 121*t*
  mucosa 118
  sharp transection of 124
  stricture 122
Biliary anatomy, delineation of 25
Biliary anomalies 127

Biliary cirrhosis, secondary 126
Biliary enteric anastomosis 126
Biliary injury, management of 116
Biliary stricture
    benign 113, 113*t*, 118*t*, 126, 126*f*, 128, 129
    classification of 120
Biliary tract, surgery of 25
Biliary tree 26, 116
    anomalies 23
Bilioenteric anastomosis 113, 129
Biliopathy, portal 113
Biopsy 81*f*, 160
    forms of 253
    metastatic lesion 261
    pleural 195
Bipolar energy devices 67
Bisacodyl 179
Bismuth classification 121*t*
Bispectral index 7
Bleeding
    disorders 140
    duration of 139
    gastrointestinal 136, 143
    intestinal 136
    lesions 144
        types of 144, 144*t*
    occult 144
    overt 144
    pattern of 140
    rates 146
    source of 136
Bleomycin 269, 270
Blood
    circulation 35
    pressure 181
Blurred vision 90
Body
    mass index 198
    temperature 55
Botulinum injection 46
Bowel
    disease, inflammatory 137
    preparation 177, 181
        mechanical 173, 181
    severe hypoperfusion of 30
Branched-chain aminotransferase 232
Breast 153
    cancer 35, 216, 251
    carcinomas 214
    conservation surgery 253, 254
    Paget's disease of 249, 251*f*
    reconstruction 255*f*
    skin-saving mastectomy 255*f*
    surgery 30
    tumor 255

Buffalo hump 161
Burn wounds, grading of 35

C

Calcifications 128
Calcitonin gene-related peptide 238
Calcium
    channel blockers 156
    dobesilate 240
Calf muscle pump 224
    screening for 228
Calf perforator vein 227
Calot's triangle 26
Calprotectin, exclusion of 60
Cameron's erosions 141
Cancer 211
    cell 211
        invasive 255
    cervical 216
    colorectal 131, 214
    endometrial 216
    esophageal 195, 196, 216
    gallbladder 131
    head and neck 216
    immunotherapy 214
    increasing stage of 255
    prostate 219
    vaccines 218
Capecitabine 81*f*, 85
Capsule
    directed deep enteroscopy 145
    endoscopy 142-144, 144*t*, 148
Carbohydrates
    complex 176
    rich liquids 175
Carbon dioxide insufflator 42
Carboplatin 85, 273
    single cycle of 275
Carcinoid syndrome 77, 78, 95
    incidence of 77
    management of 83
    symptoms of 95
Carcinoid tumor 74, 137
Carcinoma 137
    adrenocortical 153-155
    colorectal 214
    embryonal 259, 268
    endometrial 217
    hepatocellular 6, 214
    invasive 249
    neuroendocrine 76, 76*f*, 86
    rectum 32*f*
    urothelial 216
Cardiac index 177

Cardiomyopathy, hypertrophic 140
Cardiopulmonary bypass oxygenator 34
Cardiothoracic surgery 33
    side hustle of 194
Cardiovascular disease, severe 138
Carinal resections 197
Catecholamines 153
    excessive 90
    hypersecretion 154
    production of 174
Central nervous system 218
    toxicity 272
Central venous catheter 21
Cerebral atrophy 272
Cerebrovascular surgery 32
Champagne glass sign 44f
Charge-coupled device 19
Chemoembolization, transarterial 96, 113
Chemokines 215
Chemotherapy 85, 273
    adjuvant 185, 254
    conventional dosage 273
    cycles of 275
    first cycle of 272
    high-dose 273
    hyperthermic intraperitoneal 8
Chest wall 194, 196
Chimeric antigen receptor T-cell
    therapy 217
Chlorhexidine-based solution 176
Cholangiocarcinoma 130, 131
Cholangiography 26
    intraoperative 24
Cholangiopancreatography 116
Cholangiopathy
    eosinophilic 113
    inflammatory 113
    single-operator 122
Cholecystectomy 26, 113
    laparoscopic 25
Cholecystitis, acute 26
Cholecystokinin 78
Choledochojejunostomy 129
Cholelithiasis, development of 83
Choriocarcinoma 259, 268
Chromogranin 75
Chronic venous disease 225
Ciltacabtagene autoleucel 218
Cirrhosis 138, 140
Cisplatin 85, 269, 270, 273
Clinical prediction rules 54, 55t, 57t
Clinical scoring system 54, 62f
Clot evacuation 196
Coagulation disorders 198

Coagulopathy 140
Coley's therapies 215
Colon adenocarcinomas 217
Colorectal anastomosis, vascularity of 27
Colorectal surgery, emergency 185
Common bile duct 26, 114, 121
    junction 27f
Complex oncological operations 195
Complex surgical procedure 11
Component separation techniques 108
Compression
    materials 237
    methods 237
    stockings 238
    therapy 236
Computed tomography 62, 80, 81f, 84f,
    92f, 118, 136, 145, 147, 148, 151,
    152, 158
    abdomen 61
    angiography 145
    contrast-enhanced 78, 87f, 261f,
        262f, 271f
    role of 230, 263
    three-dimensional 194, 202
Computer vision 2, 4f, 8
Concomitant vascular injury 120
Confocal laser endomicroscopy 118
Confusion 90, 218
Conn's adenoma 153, 161f, 165
Conn's syndrome 154
Continuous positive airway pressure 187
Cooper's ligaments 103
Corona phlebectatica 226
Coronary artery bypass surgery 33
Cortisol 78, 174
    hypersecretion 153
        diagnosis of 156
    levels 156
    secreting lesions 161
    simultaneous hypersecretion of 156
COVID-19 pandemic 186
Cowden disease 140
C-reactive protein 57
Crohn's disease 137, 143
Cronkhite-Canada syndrome 140
Cross-leg flaps 239
Crural vein 227
Cryptorchidism 260
Crystalloid administration,
    intraoperative 177
Cushing's adenoma 153, 161f
Cushing's syndrome 77, 162
    clinical features of 161
Cyanoacrylate embolization 244

Cystic duct 26
    clipping of 123
Cysts 153
Cytokine
    concentrations 234
    inflammatory 223
    release syndrome 218
Cytometry, advantage of 213
Cytotoxic T-lymphocyte antigen 215

D

da Vinci robotic surgical system 20, 21*f*
Deep enteroscopy 144, 147
    road map for 143
Deep learning 4*f*
Deep vein thrombosis 93, 224
Deficient mismatch repair 216, 217
Dehydration 239
Dehydroepiandrosterone sulfate 155
    testing serum levels of 156
Dense fibrous Glisson's sheath 23
Dense perihepatic fibrosis 25
Deoxyribonucleic acid 212
    damage, cisplatin-induced 274
Depression 93
Dermal backflow pattern 34
Dermatitis 93
Device-assisted deep enteroscopy 144, 145
Diabetes mellitus 46, 93, 176, 181
Diabetic autonomic neuropathy 47
Diaphragm 196
Diaphragmatic hernia repair 196
Diaphragmatic plication 196
Diarrhea 83, 85, 87*f*, 93, 94
Dieulafoy's lesion 137, 139
Diffuse neuroendocrine cell system 74
Digestive system tumors, WHO
    classification of 75
Digital subtraction angiography,
    intraoperative 32
Disseminated bilobar metastasis 96
Diverticula, multiple 139*f*
Dor's fundoplication 45
Double-balloon
    enteroscopy 144
    technique 144
Doxazosin 156
Drainage, percutaneous 69, 70
Ductal carcinoma in situ 251*f*
Ductal ectasia 252
Ductotomy 125
Duodenal nets 87
Duodenal neuroendocrine tumors 88*f*c

Duodenum 136
Dyspepsia 87*f*
Dysrhythmia, cardiac 163

E

Echocardiography, transthoracic 178
Eckardt score 45
Eczema 226
Edema 68, 226
Elastic bandages 237
Electroencephalogram 177
Electromagnetic therapy 238
Electronic health records 3
Electrosurgical unit 42
Embolization, transarterial 146
Emilos 105
Empyema thoracis 195
En bloc resection 49
Endoclips 49
Endocrine
    response 175
    symptoms 95
    system 174
Endoloops 42, 70
Endoscopes, high-definition 42
Endoscopic devices 42
Endoscopic fundoplication, role of 46
Endoscopic resection techniques 86
Endoscopic retrograde
    cholangiopancreaticography 116
    cholangiopancreatography 116, 118*t*
Endoscopic treatment 129, 130
Endoscopic ultrasound 79, 87*f*, 88, 118
    major advantage of 79
Endoscopy 146
    conventional 41
    gastrointestinal 5
Endothelial cell injury 223
Endotracheal tube 203
Endowrist instruments 199*f*
Energy metabolism 211
Enhanced recovery after surgery 148, 173,
        181, 182*f*
    elements 182*f*, 189*f*
Enteral nutrition, early 181
Enterochromaffin cells 74, 85
Enterography 146
Enteroscope, distal tip of 144
Enteroscopy 136, 143, 144*t*
    antegrade 144
    comparison of 144
    intraoperative 147
    retrograde 144

Epidermal growth factor receptor 216
Epidermal wound bed, gene expression of 232
Epidermotropic theory 250
Epirubicin 273
Epithelial membrane antigen 250
Epithelization, essential for 232
Esophageal lumen, dilatation of 43
Esophageal obstruction, complex 43
Esophageal spasm, diffuse 43
Esophageal sphincter pressure, lower 45
Esophagectomy 29, 183, 196
Esophagogastric junction 43
Esophagus 136, 194, 196
   abnormal contraction waves of 43
   restoration of 48
Estradiol 156
Estrogen receptor 251f, 255
Etoposide 85, 269, 270
European Association of Endoscopic Surgery 69
European Association of Urology guidelines 263
European Network for Study of Adrenal Tumors 166
European Neuroendocrine Tumor Society 76
European Organisation for Research and Treatment of Cancer 254
European Society for Medical Oncology 263
European Society of Endocrine Surgeons 166
European-African Hepato-Pancreato-Biliary Association 124
Everolimus 85
Ex vivo lung perfusion 202, 203, 204f
   systems 204f
Extracellular matrix 205
Extracorporeal sutures 102
Extrahepatic disease 97

F

Fat, subcutaneous 107
Femoral vein 227, 231
   common 227, 231
   deep 227
Fibrinous exudate 68
Fibroblast
   growth factor 234
   proliferation 234
Fibrogenesis 234
Fibrosis, pancreatic 128
Fibrous stroma 76f
Fine-needle aspiration 118

Flap reconstruction 239
Flatulence 83
Flu-like symptoms 218
Fluorescence 32f
   angiography 26, 28
   based flow cytometry 212
   cholangiography 26
   detector 20f
   emission wavelength spectrum of 18f
   guided brain tumor surgery 33
   guided surgery 17
      scores 17
   imaging system, basic configuration of 20f
   intravenous injection of 118
   microscopy 213
   properties 18
   visualization of 24
Fluorescent in situ hybridization 130
Fluorodeoxyglucose 81, 81f, 158, 166, 263, 269
   positron emission tomography 152
Fluorouracil 85
Four-D syndrome 93
Frank ischemia 30
Free tissue transfer 239
Frey's procedure 129
Functional adrenal lesion, removal of 164
Fungal infections 153

G

Gabapentin 177
Gallbladder 26, 131
   cancer 131
Gallium 80, 92f
Ganglioneuroma 153
Gangrenous appendix 68
Gardner syndrome 140
Gastrectomy, total 86
Gastric
   acid secretion 86
   adenocarcinoma 86
   antral vascular ectasia 137
   conduit formation 29
   decompression 173
   dysmotility 46
   emptying, delayed 176
   mucosa 85
   nets 85, 88fc
      classification of 86t
   peroral endoscopic myotomy 46, 47
   resection 114
Gastrin 78

Gastrinoma 91, 92
  symptoms of 93
  triangle 93
Gastrocnemius vein 227
Gastroduodenal
  neuroendocrine tumors 85
Gastroenteropancreatic nets, WHO
  classification for 76*t*
Gastroenteropancreatic neuroendocrine
  tumor 74, 75, 78
  principles of management of 82
  site-specific 85
Gastroenteropancreatic system,
  neuroendocrine tumors of 74
Gastroepiploic vessels 29
Gastroesophageal junction 43
Gastroesophageal reflux disease,
  post-treatment 43
Gastrointestinal stromal tumor 43,
  137, 138*f*
Gastrointestinal surgery 173
  elective upper 180
  emergency 184
  upper 46
Gastrointestinal system 74
Gastrointestinal tract 42*f*
  lower 136
  lumen of 41
Gastroparesis 43, 47
Gemcitabine 273
Gene
  expression 232
    profile 212
  minimal expression of 212
Genetic markers, nephrotoxicity-related 276
Germ cell
  neoplasia in situ 258, 267, 259
  tumors 259, 262
    management of 267
    nonseminomatous 259, 262, 266, 270*fc*
Glands, adrenal 151
Glucagon 78, 174
Glucagonoma 91, 93
Glucocorticoids 174
Glucose transporter, expression of 81
Glutathione S-transferase transporter
  protein 19
Goal-directed fluid therapy 177, 181, 187
Gome's grading 68
Gonadoblastoma 259
Gon-germ cell tumors 258
Graft
  dysfunction, primary 203
  failure, long-term 33

Granulocyte
  macrophage colony-stimulating factor,
    protein of 218
  monocyte colony-stimulating factor 238
Granulomatous diseases 153
Granulosa cell tumor 259
Great saphenous vein 227, 240
  high ligation of 240
  stripping 241
Gut
  enterochromaffin cells of 74
  gangrene 185
  neuroendocrine cells of 74

H

Handgrip dynamometry 176
Hannover classification 120
Harboring metastases 263
Health Insurance Portability and
  Accountability Act 13
Heart
  failure, congestive 154
  rate 181
Heartburn 93
Helicobacter pylori infection 93
Heller myotomy 45
Hemangioma 259
Hematemesis 140
Hematochezia 140
Hemicolectomy 95
Hemobilia 137
Hemorrhage 161*f*, 173
Hemostatic forceps 42
Hemosuccus pancreaticus 137
Heparin-binding epidermal growth
  factor 232
Hepatectomy 114, 125
  partial 113
Hepatic acute phase response
  mediators 174
Hepatic artery
  injuries 125
  thrombosis 113, 127
Hepatic duct 117*f*
  common 117*f*, 121
Hepatic extraction capacity 22
Hepatic metastatic lesions 24
Hepatic parenchyma, normal 25
Hepatic resection 10
  segmental 125
Hepatic surgery, major 22
Hepatic tumors, fluorescence imaging for 24
Hepaticojejunostomy 124-126
Hepaticotomy 125

Hepatobiliary iminodiacetic acid scan 116
Hepatoduodenal ligament 114
Hepatology intensive care unit 22
Hepp-Couinaud technique 26
Hernia
    defect 102*f*
    epigastric 107*f*
    infraumbilical incisional 109*f*
    minimally invasive repair of 108
    repair 104, 110
    sac 101
    ventral 101, 102*f*
Heyde syndrome 140
Hilum 23
Hirschsprung's disease 43, 48
Hodgkin's lymphoma 216
Holmium laser, use of 123
Hormonal hypersecretion, control of 168
Hormonal therapy 254
Hormone hypersecretion 151, 153
Horse chestnut extract 240
Hounsfield units 152, 157, 158, 159
Human amniotic membrane allografts 239
Hybrid
    intraperitoneal onlay mesh 102
    technique 107
    theory 250
Hybridization signal 212
Hydralazine 156
Hydroxyethylrutoside 240
Hyperaldosteronism, primary 164
Hyperbilirubinemia 115
Hypercatecholaminism, diagnosis of 157
Hyperchromatic nuclei 76*f*
Hypercortisolism 156
    causes of 156
Hyperemia 68
Hypergastrinemia, secondary 93
Hyperglycemia 85
Hyperplasia, intimal 33
Hypersecretion 153
    resolution of 165
Hypersecretory syndromes 168
Hypertension 161, 181
    gestational 163
    severe 154
    uncontrolled 176
    venous 223
Hypoglycemia 90
    intraoperative 176
Hypokalemia 77
    correction of 165
Hypoparathyroidism, long-term 31
Hypotension 113, 115, 203, 218

Hypothalamic-pituitary-adrenal axis 174
Hypoxemia 203
Hypoxia 218

I

Ifosfamide 269, 270
Ileocecal valve 142
Ileus
    earlier resolution of 185
    postoperative 179
Iliac fossa 56
Iliac vein
    common 227
    external 227
    internal 227
Immune
    cell profiling 211, 212*b*
        clinical applications of 214
        techniques 211
    checkpoint inhibitors 211, 216*t*
    effector cell-associated neurotoxicity
        syndrome 218
Immunoglobulin G4
    cholangiopathy 131
    sclerosing cholangitis 131
Immunohistochemistry 212
    conventional 213
    multiplexed 213
In situ carcinoma 249
In vivo lung perfusion 202, 205
Incidentally detected adrenal masses,
    management of 152*fc*
Incidentaloma 151, 160
    adrenal 151-153, 155*t*, 159*b*
Indocyanine green 17, 21, 27*f*, 29, 32*f*, 194
    drug kit 20*f*, 21*f*
    dye 18*f*
    elimination 23
    fluorescence
        angiography 27, 28*f*
        cholangiography 25
        imaging 233
    kinetics variables 23*t*
    molecule 17
    retention rate 24
    role of 22, 25
    use of 31
Indwelling urinary catheter 173
Inelastic bandages 237
Infections 85, 137
    genitourinary 59
    viral 219
Injection site subcutaneous nodules 83

Injury
  immunologically induced 127
  site of 114
Inotropes therapy 178
Insulin
  like growth factor-1 78
  regulated peripheral transport proteins,
    responsiveness of 174
  serum measurements of 78
Insulinoma 90, 92f
  diagnosis of 92f
Intelligent machines, concept of 1
Intensive care unit 184, 187, 195, 218
Intercostal nerve blocks 198
Intermittent pneumatic compression 179, 237
Internal-external biliary catheter
    placement 127
International Cancer Control, union for 75
International Germ Cell Cancer
    Collaborative Group 263, 266, 266t
Interstitial fluid 19
Interval appendectomy, role of 70
Intestinal obstruction
  acute 185
  lower incidence of adhesive 125
Intestine, small 137
Intracorporeal rectus aponeuroplasty,
    laparoscopic 103
Intraductal ultrasound 118
Intraepidermal clear cells 250
Intraepidermal theory 250
Intrahepatic biliary radicles 115
Intralesional injection 238
Intraperitoneal onlay mesh 100-102, 102f
Intratesticular mass 261
Intrinsic hepatic clearance 22
Invasive excision, laparoscopic 163
Invasive technique 146
Iodometomidate 167
Ionizing radiation 78
Ipilimumab 215, 216
Iron, deposition of 223
Ischemia
  gradual 122
  mesenteric 137
  warm 203

J

Jackhammer esophagus 43
Japan Esophageal Society 43
Jaundice 115
Jejunal diverticula 137, 138, 139f
Jejunum 139f, 142

K

Keratinocytes 239
Kidney failure 93
Krenning scale scoring system, modified 81
Kulchitsky cell tumors 74

L

Lactate dehydrogenase 262, 266
Lactiferous duct 253
Lanthanide metals 213
Laparoscopy 27f
Laparotomy, emergency 177, 186, 187b
Laser
  ablation, endovenous 240, 243
  speckle imaging 232
Leg
  surgery 224
  ulcer
    healing, venous 231
    nonhealing venous 232
  venous 223, 239
Leiomyoma 43
  esophageal 196
Lesions
  adrenal 153
  adrenocortical 167
  benign
    functional 161
    nonfunctional 168
  duodenal 87f
  multifocal 24
  submucosal 143
  ulcerative 143
Leucine-rich alpha-2-glycoprotein 60
Leukemia
  acute
    lymphoblastic 218
    myeloid 218
Leukocyte adhesion 240
Leukoencephalopathy, progressive
    multifocal 272
Levofloxacin 66
Leydig cell tumor 259
Ligation 123
Lipid-rich adrenal adenoma, diagnostic
    of 159
Lipodermatosclerosis 226
Liver
  blood flow 22
  disease
    chronic 23
    metastatic 96

extraction capacity 22
failure 126
function, dynamic assessment of 22
functional reserve 23
lesion 6, 9
metastasis 79*f*, 80*f*, 95
resection 22
segment 9
surgery 22
transplantation 22, 23, 82, 113, 126
Achilles heel of 127
Low-dose dexamethasone suppression test 155, 156
Low-molecular-weight heparin 179, 240
Lumbar hernias 103
Lung 153, 195
bioengineering 205
biopsy 195
cancer 195
staging thoracoscopy for 195
disease
emphysematous 195
end-stage 205, 206
injury, ventilator-associated 198
nodule biopsy 195
perfusion, isolated 202
resections, sublobar 201
transplantation 202, 203
tumors 202
Lymph node
biopsy 195
conglomerated mass of 261*f*
enlarged 255
interaortocaval 262*f*, 271*f*
mesenteric 95
para-aortic 95, 261
retroperitoneal 270
Lymphadenectomy 86, 114
locoregional 167
Lymphedema, treatment of 34
Lymphoma 137
Lymphovascular invasion 267
Lytic replication 219

M

Machine learning 2, 4*f*, 12
Macroscopic fat, large areas of 157
Magic bullet 11
Magnetic compression anastomosis 122
Magnetic resonance
cholangiopancreatography 23, 118
enterography 145
imaging 5, 78, 79, 80*f*, 152, 253*f*, 261

role of 262
scans 151
venography, role of 230
Makuuchi decisional algorithm 24*fc*
Malignancy 140, 157
clinical signs of 253
colorectal 30
extra-adrenal 153
features of 159*b*
primary operable 160
Maltodextrin 176
Mammogram 251*f*
Mammography 252
Mannheim peritonitis index 176
Mass, adrenal 157, 160
Mastectomy 253
Matrix
metallopeptidase 2 234
metalloproteinases 223
Maximum intensity projection 81*f*, 84*f*
May-Thurner syndrome 224
Mean arterial pressure 177
Mechanical obstruction, absence of 46
Meckel's diverticulum 137-139, 146
Mediastinum 195
Medico-legal litigation 9
Melanoma 153, 216
cutaneous 30
Melena 140
Mesenteric lymph node 95
metastasis 95
Mesh materials, types of 100
Mesh placement 101*f*, 106, 109*f*
rectrorectus space 107*f*
Mesoappendix dissection 67
Metal stents, self-expanding 122
Metastasectomy, pulmonary 205
Metastasis 153, 154, 160
colorectal 6
Metastatic disease 261
evaluation of 78
management of 89
staging of 78
Methylxanthine 240
Metoclopramide 46
Metronidazole 66
Microarrays technology 212
Microcalcifications 252
Micronized purified flavonoid fraction 240
Microwave 96
ablation, endovenous 240
Minimally invasive
adrenalectomy procedure 163
approach 90, 178

endoscopic procedure 42
excision 163
surgery 4f, 9, 25, 181, 195
techniques 175, 178, 194
thoracic surgery 194, 199
Mini-phlebectomy 241
Mirizzi syndrome 113
Mitotic rate 75
Mitral regurgitation, severe 140
Mobilization 235
Molecular mass 18
Molecular targeted therapy 85
Monoclonal antibody 218
Monopolar energy devices 67
Moon facies 161
Mucosa 47
   duodenal 47
Mucosal defect 42
Multicentric microcalcification 251f
Multilayer inelastic bandages 237
Multiorgan damage 218
Multiple endocrine neoplasia 75, 77, 86, 88, 154
Multiple intrahepatic strictures 130
Muscle wasting 175
Muscular vein 227
Myelolipoma 153, 161f
   adrenal 158f
   benign 157
Myotomy 42
   anterior 46
   endoscopic 44
   site of 46

N

Nasogastric tube 173
National Comprehensive Cancer Network 263
Natural killer 174
Natural orifice transluminal endoscopic surgery 4f, 41
Nausea 83, 177, 182f
Near-infrared spectroscopy 230
Necrolytic migratory erythema 93
Necrosis, transmural 30
Needle aspiration cytology 118
Negative predictive value 263
Negative pressure wound therapy 238
Nerve-sparing retro-peritoneal lymph node dissection 270
Neuroblastoma 153
Neuroendocrine liver metastases 96
   evaluation of 79
Neuroendocrine non-neuroendocrine neoplasm 76, 77
Neuroendocrine tumors 74-76, 81f, 84f, 86, 87f, 91, 92f, 152
   colorectal 95
Neurofibromatosis 75, 77, 154
Neuroglycopenia 90
Neurohormonal response 174
Neuromuscular blocking agents 198
Neuron-specific enolase 75
Neuropathy, autonomic 46
Neurosurgery 32
Neutropenia 85
Neutrophils, proportion of 59, 60
Nipple
   areola complex 249, 250, 252, 254
   reconstruction 254
   region 253
   complete destruction of 251
   Paget's disease of 249f
   reconstruction 255f
   removal of 253
Nociception level 11
Non-anastomotic biliary stricture 127
Noncardiac chest organs, surgical treatment of 194
Noninvasive ventilation 187
Nonlinear fluorescence quantum 36
Nonmetastatic disease 96
Nonoperative therapy 65
Nonsaphenous vein 227
Nonseminoma 268
Nonsmall cell lung cancer 215, 216
Nonsteroidal anti-inflammatory drugs 137, 139, 179
Nonthermal options involve sclerotherapy 240
Nontumescent options involve sclerotherapy 240
Normothermia 181
   intraoperative 178
North American Neuroendocrine Tumor Society guidelines 89
N-terminal pro-brain natriuretic peptide 78
Nuclear medicine-based functional imaging 79
Nutritional supplements 245

O

Obesity, central 161
Obstruction, venous 224
Off-pump coronary artery bypass grafting 34

Oncolytic viruses 219
Open appendectomy 67
Open surgery 100
    fluorescence imaging in 19
Opioid-free analgesics 184
Orchiectomy 266
Organ
    care system lung 203
    failure 30
    triangular-shaped 151
Outflow obstruction 43
Ovarian cyst 59
Ovarian epithelial-type tumors 259
Overnight dexamethasone suppression test 156
Oxaliplatin 273
Oxygen
    partial pressure, transcutaneous measurement of 233
    to-see method 233

P

Paclitaxel 269, 273
Paget's cells 249, 250
Pain 81*f*
    abdominal 1, 83, 115
    acute 261
    control 235
    flank 154
Palpitation 90
Pancreas, small neuroendocrine tumor of 9
Pancreatectomy 9
Pancreatic
    fistula, postoperative 11
    head lesion 92*f*
    islet tumors 74
    nets, functional 91*t*
    neuroendocrine tumor 74, 79*f*, 89
        functional 90
        nonfunctional 89
    resection 114
Pancreaticoduodenectomy 92*f*, 183
Pancreatitis
    acute 113
    autoimmune 131
    chronic 113, 128, 129, 129*f*
Paracrine mechanisms 239
Paraganglioma syndrome, familial 154
Parasitic infestation 113
Parathyroid
    glands 31
    surgery 31

Paravertebral blocks 198
Parkinson's disease 224
Partial hepatectomy 113
    indications for 125
Pediatric appendicitis score 54, 56, 57
Pelvic
    inflammatory disease 53, 59
    procedures 53
    vein 227
Pembrolizumab 216
    single agent 215
Pentoxifylline 240
Peptic ulcer disease 91
Peptide receptor radionuclide therapy 81*f*, 83, 84*f*
Percutaneous transhepatic
    approach 122
    balloon stricture dilatation 125
    biliary drainage 116
    cholangiography 116
    cholangioscopy 118
Periappendiceal adhesions increase 69
Periappendiceal phlegmon 68
Periareolar region 30
Peripheral opioid receptor blockers 181
Peripheral wide-bore cannula 21
Peritoneal tears, risk of 106
Peritoneum
    flaps 106
    incision 106
Peritonitis 30
    diffuse 68
Peroneal vein 227
Peroral cholangioscopy 118
Peroral endoscopic myotomy 41-43, 44*f*, 45
    steps of 44*b*
Per-rectal endoscopic myotomy 43, 48
Peutz-Jeghers syndrome 138, 140
Pharmacokinetics 19
Pheochromocytoma 153-155, 161*f*, 162, 163, 164*fc*
    contrast-enhanced computed tomography of 158*f*
    diagnosis of 157
    incidence of 163
    malignant 153
    recurrent 163
    small noninvasive 163
    subclinical 163
Phlegmon 61, 69
Photoplethysmography probes 229
Physical therapy 235
Placental site trophoblastic tumor 259

Plasma 165
  aldosterone concentration 164
  disappearance rate 23
  free metanephrines 157
  normetanephrine levels 157
  renin activity 156, 164
Plastic surgery 34
Platelet derived growth factor 238
Platinum
  based perioperative chemotherapy 90
  resistant disease 274
Plethora 161
Plethysmography 231
Pleural diseases 195
Pneumonia 7, 198
Pneumoperitoneum, creation of 101
Pneumothorax, recurrent 195
Polydioxanone 122
Polyglactic acid 122
Polymeric clips 70
Polymorphonuclear leukocytes,
     proportion of 57
Polyposis
  familial adenomatous 138
  syndromes 137, 140
    hereditary 138
Popliteal vein 227, 231
Portal venous system 97
Ports, placement of 101
Portsmouth physiological and operative
     severity score 176
Positive end-expiratory pressure 187
Positron emission tomography 80, 81f, 84f,
     92f, 158, 166, 263, 269
  machine 79
  role of 263
Postchemotherapy
  residual mass 276
  surgery 273
Postcholecystectomy
  bile duct injury 113
  bismuth 117f
Post-coronary artery bypass grafting 33
Posterior rectus sheath 100, 107f
Posterior sheath closure 109f
Post-liver transplantation benign biliary
     stricture 127
Postoperative peak expiratory flow rate 183
Post-thrombotic syndrome 223
Prazosin 156
Prednisone 131
Pregabalin 177
Pregnancy 163
Preterm labor 59

Primary tumor
  complete resection of 97
  locoregional spread of 78
  origin, regardless of 85
Progesterone 156
  receptor 251f, 255
Programmed cell death protein 1 215
Progression free survival 82, 219, 266
Progressive chronic venous disease 223
Prostate cancer, metastatic
     castrate-resistant 219
Prostatic acid phosphatase 218
Proteolysis 234
Proteomic-based technologies 213
Proton-pump inhibitor 46, 91, 152
Proximal strictures 121
Pseudoaneurysm 142f
Pulse
  dye densitometry 22
  pressure variation 177
Pyloric muscle ring 47
Pyloromyotomy
  laparoscopic 46
  peroral 46, 47
Pylorospasm 46
  endoscopic dilatation for 46

R

Radiation
  enteritis 137
  therapy 113
Radical mastectomy, modified 35
Radioembolization, transarterial 96
Radiofrequency 96
  ablation 240, 242
Radiology 5
Radionuclide
  scan 146
  therapy 83
Radiotherapy 269
Raja Isteri Pengiran Anak Saleha
     Appendicitis 54, 56-58
Randomized controlled trial 188
Rapamycin, mammalian target of 85
Rapid-sequence induction 187
Reactive oxygen 223
Recklinghausen disease 75
Rectal neuroendocrine tumor 80f
Red blood cell scan 142
Relook endoscopy 141
Renal cell
  cancers, metastatic 215
  carcinoma 216

Renal disease, chronic 138
Rendezvous techniques, use of 121
Residual mass after chemotherapy 269*fc*
Respiratory complications 177
Reticular veins 226, 227
Retrograde biliary interventions 119
Retroperitoneal lymph node 270
    dissection 274*f*
Retroperitoneum 32
    nonadrenal pathology of 153
Retrorectus space creation 109*f*
Retrorectus telescopic dissection 104*f*
Retzius space 103
Reverse totally extraperitoneal
    procedure 105
Rheumatologic disorders 138
Rib tumors, excision of 196
Ribonucleic acid 212
Rives-Stoppa technique 108
Robotic adrenalectomy 163
Robotic biliary-enteric reconstruction 125
Robotic surgery 4, 9, 10*f*, 106, 199*f*
    autonomous 13
Robotic-assisted thoracic surgery 194, 199
Rocuronium 181
Rouviere's sulcus 9
Roux-en-Y hepaticojejunostomy 118, 124

S

Salt supplementation 163
Salvage
    therapy 206
    treatment 273, 274
Samuel's pediatric appendicitis score 59
Saphenous vein
    anterior accessory 227
    small 227
Sarcoidosis 153
Sarcomas 153
Scintigraphy 147
Sclerosing cholangitis 130*f*
    primary 113, 129
    secondary 113
Sclerosis, tuberous 75, 77
Sclerotherapy 243
Scrotal swelling, differential
    diagnosis of 260
Scrotum 261
Segmentectomy 201
Seizures 90
    prophylaxis 218
Selective cyclooxygenase-2 inhibitors 139
Selective relaxant binding agent 181

Seminiferous tubules, germinal epithelium
    of 259
Seminoma 258, 259, 266, 268*fc*, 269,
    269*fc*, 272
Seminomatous components 259
Sentinel lymph node
    biopsy 254
    mapping, use for 30
Sepsis 7, 30, 115
    intra-abdominal 186
    screen for 187
Septum, sides of 47
Seroma, high incidence of 107
Sertoli cell tumor 259
Serum tumor marker
    characteristics of 262*t*
    levels 261
Sex cord-stromal tumors 258, 259
Shock lung 203
Short bowel syndrome 30, 95
Single photon emission computed
    tomography 80
Single-balloon enteroscopy 144
Single-cell
    assay 212
    droplets 213
    level 213
    RNA sequencing, advantage of 213
Single-incision laparoscopic
    appendectomy 67
Single-nucleotide polymorphisms 212
Skin
    decontamination of 176
    perfusion pressure 233
    saving mastectomy 254
Sleep apnea 198
Small benign adrenal masses 161
Small bowel
    gastrointestinal stromal tumors 143
    injury, drug-induced 137
    neoplasms 139
    varices 138
Small intestine
    erosions 139
    evaluation of 142
    neuroendocrine tumors 95
    tumor of 137
Small saphenous vein 227
    procedures, operative technique
        for 241
Society of American Gastrointestinal
    and Endoscopic Surgeons
    Guidelines 69
Soft-tissue tumors 153

Soleal vein 227
Somatostatin
  analog 82, 88, 91
  receptor 80, 83
    overexpression of 79
Somatostatinoma syndrome 94
Somnolence 218
Spermatocytic tumor 259
Spermatogenesis 259
Sphincterotomy 113
Spinal anatomy 198
Spironolactone 164
Static stiffness index 237
Steam ablation, endovenous 240, 243
Steep learning curve 104
Stenosis 127
  papillary 113
Stents
  migration 46
  number of 121
  types of 121
Stereotactic radiosurgery 272
Steroid precursors 153
Stewart-Way classification 120
Stomach 136
  adenocarcinomas 217
Strasberg classification 121*t*
Strasberg injuries 121
Streptococcus pyogenes 214
Streptozocin 85
Stroke volume
  measurements of 177
  variation 177
Subcutaneous onlay laparoscopic
    approach 106
Subfascial endoscopic perforator
    surgery 242
Submucosal tumors 43
  resection of 49
Submucosal tunneling endoscopic
  dissection 43
  resection 49
  septum division 47
Sugammadex 181
Sulodexide 240
Sunitinib 85
Superficial venous reflux 245
Suprafascial repairs 106
Suprainguinal venous obstruction
    evaluation 231
Surgery 1, 4, 123
  colorectal 177
  emergency 184
  endocrine 31

gastrointestinal 173
hepatopancreaticobiliary 183
laparoscopic 20, 160, 167
reconstructive 34
reoperative 25
role of 240
Surgical site infection 66, 100, 187
  rates of 183
  risk of 7
Surgical stress response 174, 174*fc*
Suture ligation 70
Sweating 90
  excessive 154
Swelling 260
  painless 261
  scrotal 260
Synaptophysin 75

T

Tachycardia 154
T-cell immune checkpoints 215
Telangiectasia 138, 226, 227
Temozolomide 81*f*, 85
Tenderness 115, 260
Teratoma 259, 268
  syndrome 272
Testes, primary lymphatic drainage
    pathway of 261
Testicle 261
Testicular cancer
  diagnosis of 261
  management of 261
Testicular germ cell tumors 265*t*
Testicular tumors 258, 262*t*
  classification of 259*b*
  clinical features 260
  diagnostic imaging 262
  epidemiology 258
  management of 258
  prognosis 264
  risk factors 260
  signs of 261*t*
  staging 264
  symptoms of 261*t*
Testosterone 156
Therapeutic blockade 215
Thermal ablation 96
Thick wall atherosclerotic
    vessels 33
Thigh perforator vein 227
Third-space endoscopy 41, 42, 49
  principle of 42*f*
  procedures 43*t*

Thoracic
    oncology 205
    surgery 194, 201
    surgical armamentarium 195
Thrombocytopenia 140
Thromboembolic events, risk of 175
Thromboembolism, venous 187
Thromboprophylaxis 179, 181
    mechanical 187
Thulium laser vaporization 123
Thyroid
    gland, dissection of 31
    surgery 31
Tidal volume 187
Tisagenlecleucel 218
Tissue 249
    perfusion, real-time assessment of 27
    scaffold, form of 205
Tocilizumab 218
Toe pressure 229
Toker cells 250
Total endoscopic-assisted linea alba reconstruction 107
Totally extraperitoneal technique 103
Tracheobronchial tree 194
Tracheo-broncho-esophageal fistula 196
Transabdominal preperitoneal repair 105
Transabdominal retromuscular repair 106, 107*f*
Transabdominal retrorectus space dissection 107*f*
Transforming growth factor-beta 1 232
Transillumination guided rendezvous technique 48
Trans-scrotal ultrasonography 260
Transverse colon, enhancement of 28*f*
Transversus abdominis
    plane 181
        blocks 179
    release 108, 109*f*
Trauma 113
    surgery 11
Treitz ligament 136
Tremelimumab 215
Tremor 90
Tricarbocyanine molecule 18
Tuberculosis 137, 143, 153
Tumor
    adrenal 151
    benign functional 152
    cells 76*f*
    excision 42
    functional 160
    grade 75
    hematolymphoid 259
    hypervascular 78
    infiltrating lymphocytes 275
    malignant 152
    mediastinal 195
    microenvironment 211
    mutational burden 217
    necrosis factor 174
    neuroendocrine 74-76, 81*f*, 84*f*, 86, 87*f*, 91, 92*f*, 152
    nonseminomatous 269, 272
    proportion score 216
    stromal 137
    subepithelial 49
    submucosal 43
    tissue 24
    transcriptome of 212
    types 259
Tyrosine kinase inhibitor 85

U

Ulcer 139
    chronic venous 237*f*
    clinical examination of 228
    duodenal 184
    healed 226
    healing 239
    lower leg 228
    prevent recurrence of 245
    recurrent venous 226
    venous 223, 232, 234, 240
Ulnar nerve stimulation 177
Ultrasound
    endoscopic 79, 87*f*, 88, 118
    examinations 151
    high-frequency 79
    high-intensity focused 240, 245
    intravascular 231
Unilateral aldosterone-producing adenomas 164
Unilateral cortisol-secreting adenomas 161
Uniportal surgery, advantages of 197
Ureter identification, use for 31
Ureteral stents, placement of 32
Urinary catheter, early removal of 181
Urinary fractionated metanephrines 157
Urinary tract infection, rates of 178
Urine aldosterone levels 165

V

Vagotomy 46
Valve incompetence 223

Valvular reflux 224
Varicose veins 223, 226
   endovenous technique for 242
Varicosities, local 241
Vascular ectasia 137
Vascular endothelial growth factor 234
Vascular injury 126
Vasculitis 137
Vasoactive intestinal
   peptide 78
   polypeptide 91, 238
Vater ampulla 89
Vein, anterior 227
Vena cava, inferior 34, 167, 227
VenaSeal sapheno closure system 244
Venoactive drug 240
Venography 231
Venous disease 223
Venous shear stress 223
Venous ulcer 223, 232, 234, 240
   treatment of 234
   typical location of 228f
Venous valve deterioration 240
Ventral hernia 102f
   left-sided 101
   repair 35, 100, 109t
   right-sided 101
Verapamil 156
Verner–Morrison syndrome 94
Vessels, mesenteric 95
Video capsule endoscopy 142, 147
Video-assisted thoracic surgery 194, 195, 196f
   indications of 195
   nonintubated 197
   types of 196
Video-capsule endoscopy, widespread use of 136
Video-laparoscopic cart 10
Vinblastine 269, 273
Vipoma 91, 94
Virtual-assisted lung mapping 201

Vomiting 177, 182f
von Hippel–Lindau
   disease 154
   syndrome 75
von Willebrand syndrome 140

W

Water jet 42
Weight
   loss 84f, 93, 94
   management 245
Werner syndrome 75
Whipple's operation 142f
Whipple's procedure 92f
Whipple's triad 92f
White blood cell 56, 57
   count 60
World Society of Emergency Surgery 68
   grading 68
Wound
   care 236
   healing 176, 232, 234
      venous 232
   infection 67, 238
   therapies 242

X

Xenobiotics 260
Xiphoid 105

Y

Yolk sac tumor 259, 268

Z

Zenker's diverticulum 43, 47
Zenker's peroral endoscopic myotomy 47
Zollinger–Ellison syndrome 77

EU GSPR Authorised Reprsentative
Logos Europe, 9 rue Nicolas Poussin
1700, La Rochelle, France
Phone: +33 (0) 6 67 93 73 78
E-mail: contact@logoseurope.eu

www.ingramcontent.com/pod-product-compliance
Ingram Content Group UK Ltd.
Pitfield, Milton Keynes, MK11 3LW, UK
UKHW050428150426
5217IPUK00019B/1286